# Recent Advances in Pediatric Medicine

## (Volume 1)

## (Synopsis of Current General Pediatrics Practice)

## Edited By

## Seckin Ulualp

*Division of Pediatric Otolaryngology Department of Otolaryngology-Head and Neck Surgery University of Texas Southwestern Medical Center Children's Health Dallas, Texas, USA*

# Recent Advances in Pediatric Medicine

*Volume # 1*

*Synopsis of General Pediatric Practice*

Editor: Seckin Ulualp

eISSN (Online): 2543-2249

ISSN (Print): 2543-2257

eISBN (Online): 978-1-68108-520-3

ISBN( Print): 978-1-68108-521-0

## General:

1. Any dispute or claim arising out of or in connection with this License Agreement or the Work (including non-contractual disputes or claims) will be governed by and construed in accordance with the laws of the U.A.E. as applied in the Emirate of Dubai. Each party agrees that the courts of the Emirate of Dubai shall have exclusive jurisdiction to settle any dispute or claim arising out of or in connection with this License Agreement or the Work (including non-contractual disputes or claims).
2. Your rights under this License Agreement will automatically terminate without notice and without the need for a court order if at any point you breach any terms of this License Agreement. In no event will any delay or failure by Bentham Science Publishers in enforcing your compliance with this License Agreement constitute a waiver of any of its rights.
3. You acknowledge that you have read this License Agreement, and agree to be bound by its terms and conditions. To the extent that any other terms and conditions presented on any website of Bentham Science Publishers conflict with, or are inconsistent with, the terms and conditions set out in this License Agreement, you acknowledge that the terms and conditions set out in this License Agreement shall prevail.

**Bentham Science Publishers Ltd.**
Executive Suite Y - 2
PO Box 7917, Saif Zone
Sharjah, U.A.E.
Email: subscriptions@benthamscience.org

**BENTHAM
SCIENCE**

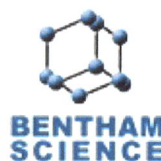

# CONTENTS

# PREFACE

The field of pediatric medicine encompasses a rapidly expanding volume of information. This book has been prepared by a diverse group of authors from a range of pediatric subspecialists to create a platform to review the recent advances quickly and efficiently. With authors from pediatric subspecialties, duplication of the information was reduced to a minimum by integrating the chapters effectively. The authors clearly explain etiology, pathophysiology, and management of commonly encountered pediatric disorders.

The book does not pretend to describe the all aspects of the management of the various problems discussed. Each contributor presented the scientific evidence and discussed the practice pathways to enhance effectiveness of readers in approaching commonly encountered medical problems in children. Concise information about the approach of pediatric subspecialists to common medical problems, that are frequently very complex, enhances the educational value of the book for everyone involved in the care of children.

It is my hope that, by presenting the breadth and depth of many of the typical problems encountered while caring for children in an evidence-based format, *Recent Advances in Pediatric Medicine; Synopsis of Current General Pediatrics Practice* will become a valuable asset for the pediatric practitioner, specialists, medical students, and others involved in the care of children.

A book like this is the result of the effort of many people. I am very grateful to my wife, Zerrin, for having gracefully accepted that many weekends were absorbed by the preparation of this book. Many thanks go to all authors trying the impossible and sparing time to write this book within their endless working schedule.

**Seckin Ulualp**
Division of Pediatric Otolaryngology
Department of otolaryngology-Head and Neck Surgery
University of Texas Southwestern Medical Center
Children's Health
Dallas, Texas
USA

# List of Contributors

| | |
|---|---|
| **Abha Choudhary** | Department of Otolaryngology, University of Texas Southwestern Medical Center, Dallas, TX, USA |
| **Amal Isaiah** | Department of Otolaryngology— Head and Neck Surgery, University of Texas Southwestern Medical Center, Dallas, TX, USA |
| **Amine Daher** | University of Texas Southwestern (UTSW) Medical Center, Dallas Children's Health, Dallas, TX, USA |
| **Anil Gungor** | Department of Otolaryngology – Head and Neck Surgery, Louisiana State University School of Medicine, Shreveport, LA, USA |
| **Anthony Sheyn** | Department of Otolaryngology, University of Tennessee Health Science Center, LeBonheur Children's Hospital, St. Jude Children's Research Hospital, TN 38105, USA |
| **Bailey LeConte** | Department of Otolaryngology, University of Texas Medical Branch, Galveston, TX, USA |
| **Bethany A. Auble** | Department of Pediatrics, Division of Endocrinology, Medical College of Wisconsin, Children's Hospital of Wisconsin, Milwaukee, WI, USA |
| **Carisse Orsi** | Department of Pediatrics, University of Texas San Antonio Health Science Center, San Antonio, TX, USA |
| **Catherine Blanchet** | Department of ENT and Head and Neck Surgery, University of Montpellier, Montpellier, France |
| **Dayton Young** | Department of Otolaryngology, University of Texas Medical Branch, Department of Otolaryngology, Galveston, TX, USA |
| **Derek L. Pepiak** | Department of Pediatrics, Ochsner for Children and The University of Queensland School of Medicine, Ochsner Clinical School, New Orleans, LA, USA |
| **Elia Escaname** | Department of Pediatrics, University of Texas San Antonio Health Science Center, San Antonio, TX, USA |
| **Emily Tignor** | Department of Otolaryngology, University of Texas Medical Branch, Department of Otolaryngology, Galveston, TX, USA |
| **Eric Velazquez** | Medical College of Wisconsin, Children's Hospital of Wisconsin, Milwaukee, WI, USA |
| **Harold Pine** | Department of Otolaryngology, University of Texas Medical Branch, Galveston, TX, USA |
| **Issam Saliba** | Division of Otorhinolaryngology Head & Neck Surgery, University of Montreal, Otology and Neurotology, Sainte-Justine University Hospital Center (CHUSJ) and University of Montreal Hospital Center (CHUM) Montreal, Quebec, Canada |
| **Jamie Flor** | Section of Pediatric Psychology, University of Arkansas for Medical Sciences, Little Rock, AR, USA |
| **Jayne Bellando** | Section of Pediatric Psychology, University of Arkansas for Medical Sciences, Little Rock, AR, USA |

| | |
|---|---|
| **Jesica F. Ramirez** | Centro Javeriano de Oncologia - Hospital Universitario San Ignacio, Bogota, Columbia Department of Pediatrics, University of Texas Health Science Center, San Antonio, TX, USA |
| **Jessica Hutchins** | Department of Pediatrics, University of Texas San Antonio Health Science Center, San Antonio, TX, USA |
| **Joshua L. Kennedy** | Department of Internal Medicine, Department of Pediatrics, Division of Allergy and Immunology, University of Arkansas for Medical Sciences, Little Rock, AR, USA |
| **Kathleen R. Billings** | Division of Pediatric Otolaryngology-Head and Neck Surgery, Ann & Robert H. Lurie Children's Hospital of Chicago, Chicago, IL, USA |
| **Kristine H. Schmitz** | Department of General and Community Pediatrics, Washington, DC, USA |
| **Leandra Godoy** | Department of Psychology, Children's National Health System, Washington, DC, USA |
| **Maria C. Veling** | Department of Otolaryngology – Head and Neck Surgery, Division of Pediatric Otolaryngology, University of Texas Southwestern Medical Center, Dallas, TX, USA |
| **Maria Rayas** | Department of Pediatrics, University of Texas San Antonio Health Science Center, San Antonio, TX, USA |
| **Maya Lopez** | Section of Pediatric Psychology, University of Arkansas for Medical Sciences, Little Rock, AR, USA |
| **Melissa Frei-Jones** | Department of Pediatrics, Division of hematology and Oncology, University of Texas Health Science Center, San Antonio, TX, USA |
| **Michel Mondain** | Department of ENT and Head and Neck Surgery, University of Montpellier, Montpellier, France |
| **Mi-Young Rhee** | Department of Psychology, Children's National Health System, Washington, DC, USA |
| **Mohamed Akkari** | Department of ENT and Head and Neck Surgery, University of Montpellier, Montpellier, France |
| **Musaed Alzahrani** | Department of Surgery, Division of Otolaryngology, King Fahad Specialist Hospital, Dammam, Saudi Arabia |
| **Neslihan Gungor** | Department of Pediatrics, Division of Endocrinology, Louisiana State University-Health Sciences Center/University Health, Shreveport, LA, Shreveport, LA, USA |
| **Olga Hardin** | Department of Internal Medicine, University of Arkansas for Medical Sciences, Little Rock, AR, USA |
| **Ricardo Medina-Centeno** | Department of Pediatrics, Division of Gastroenterology and Hepatology, University of Texas Southwestern Medical Center, Dallas, TX, USA |
| **Rinarani Sanghavi** | Department of Pediatrics, Division of Gastroenterology and Hepatology, University of Texas Southwestern Medical Center, Dallas, TX, USA |
| **S. Kamal Naqvi** | Division of Respiratory and Sleep Medicine, Department of Pediatrics, University of Texas Southwestern Medical Center, Dallas, TX, USA |

| | |
|---|---|
| **Seckin O. Ulualp** | Department of Otolaryngology- Head and Neck Surgery, Division of Pediatric Otolaryngology, University of Texas Southwestern Medical Center, Children's Health, Dallas, TX, USA |
| **Suparna N. Shah** | Department of Otolaryngology, University of Texas Medical Branch, Galveston, TX, USA |
| **Tanya M. Martinez-Fernandez** | University of Texas Southwestern (UTSW) Medical Center, Dallas Children's Health, Dallas, TX, USA |
| **Tomoko Makishima** | Department of Otolaryngology, University of Texas Medical Branch, Galveston, TX, USA |
| **Yadira M. Rivera-Sanchez** | University of Texas Southwestern (UTSW) Medical Center, Dallas Children's Health, Dallas, TX, USA |

# CHAPTER 1

# Update on the Management of Otitis Media

**Emily Tignor, Bailey LeConte, Dayton Young** and **Tomoko Makishima**[*]

*Department of Otolaryngology, University of Texas Medical Branch, Galveston, TX, USA*

**Abstract:** This chapter discusses the difference between acute otitis media, recurrent otitis media, and otitis media with effusion as well as the etiology, epidemiology, diagnosis and treatment of the distinct diseases. New 2016 guideline updates on Otitis Media with Effusion from the American Academy of Otolaryngology are incorporated.

**Keywords:** Antibiotics, Cholesteatoma, Ear, Effusion, Hearing, Infection, Myringosclerosis, Otitis media, Otorrhea, Tube, Tympanostomy.

## INTRODUCTION

Ear infections are one of the most common reasons for which children seek the care of a pediatrician before the age of three [1]. Parents know that ear infections are common and attribute a multitude of symptoms to the ears- fever, fussiness, pulling at ears, delayed speech, failure to respond when called. Therefore, it is vital for every clinician to have a strong knowledge of how and why ear infections occur, what distinguishes different types of infections and what is the standard of care management for these infections.

## Definition

Acute Otitis Media (AOM) is defined as inflammation of the middle ear associated with middle ear effusion [2]. It has a rapid onset and includes symptoms of pain and fever. The tympanic membrane (TM) may be erythematous and bulging outward from middle ear purulence or ruptured due to excessive middle ear positive pressure.

Otitis Media with effusion (OME) is defined as middle ear effusion without acute inflammatory signs or symptoms [3 - 5]. This has a longer duration with gradual onset and includes symptoms of conductive hearing loss and speech delay. Signs

[*] **Corresponding author Tomoko Makishima:** Department of Otolaryngology, University of Texas Medical Branch, Galveston, TX, USA; Tel: 409.772.9946; Fax: 409.772.1715; E-mail: tomakish@utmb.edu

**Seckin Ulualp (Ed.)**

include middle ear effusion with decreased tympanic membrane mobility and flat tympanogram.

Therefore, acute otitis media (AOM) is a separate entity from otitis media with effusion (OME) even though both are forms of middle ear effusion [2].

## PATHOPHYSIOLOGY

Middle ear disease stems from many interacting factors including anatomy, environment, infectious agents, and genetics.

### Anatomic Causes

The middle ear is an air-filled space medial to the tympanic membrane and lateral to the inner ear [6]. It has a mucosal lining of respiratory epithelium and contains three bones that form a lever mechanism (malleus, incus, and stapes). This lever mechanism is important for the conduction of sound. If the mechanism is damaged or function is decreased, a conductive hearing loss may follow.

The Eustachian tube (ET) plays an important role in middle ear pressure equalization and, therefore, middle ear disease [7]. The ET originates in the anterior middle ear space and courses anteriorly to empty into the lateral nasopharynx. The tensor veli palatini muscle controls opening and closing of the ET during swallow [6, 8, 9]. The Eustachian tube is essential to maintain a functional middle ear by providing ventilation, protection, and clearance. If any of these are impaired, otitis media may develop. Ventilation is the active process of regulating middle ear pressure which is accomplished by contraction of the tensor veli palatine during swallowing, jaw movements, and yawning [6]. This function is poor in children and improves with age [9]. Children who are prone to otitis media are more likely to have deficient active ET function *versus* children who are not [8]. Closure of the ET is a passive process which protects the middle ear from pharyngeal reflux [6].

The Eustachian tube is lined with ciliated respiratory epithelium. Mucociliary clearance contributes to ET function by propelling mucus and fluid from the middle ear into the nasopharynx. Known disorders of mucociliary clearance lead to an increase in middle ear disease [6].

The ET opens laterally in the nasopharynx and can be obstructed by midline adenoid growth or seeded by biofilm from chronic adenoiditis. Orientation of the ET affects reflux of fluid in the nasopharynx into the middle ear as well as drainage of fluid from the middle ear to the nasopharynx. In adults, the Eustachian tube empties into the nasopharynx at a 45 degree angle, while in children, this angle is closer to 90 degrees. In addition, any excess tissue in the nasopharynx can lead to ET obstruction (*e.g.* adenoid hypertrophy) and, in turn, middle ear disease.

However, despite the common acceptance and logical association of ET dysfunction to middle ear disease, much controversy still exists on causal relationship [9].

## Environmental Causes

### *Irritants*

Tobacco smoke is the leading preventable risk factor for the development of otitis media. Studies have consistently shown that tobacco smoke exposure, including second and third hand smoke, is associated with an increased incidence of otitis media and recurrent otitis media [10]. In addition, tympanic membrane perforation, cholesteatoma and other OME complications are increased in children exposed to smoke [11]. Suppression or modulation of the immune system, enhancement of the bacterial adherence factors, impairment of the mucociliary apparatus of the respiratory tract, or enhancement of toxins are suggested mechanisms related to tobacco smoke exposure [12].

### *Daycare*

Daycare is a well-studied risk factor for recurrent AOM: children enrolled in daycare are twice as likely to have AOM due to increased exposure to bacterial pathogens and viral infections [13].

### *Allergy*

Allergies are often blamed for middle ear effusion, and patients with skin test proven atopy and history of recurrent middle ear disease show resolution or significant improvement of middle ear disease after initiation of immunotherapy. This is explained by Th2 inflammatory response mediators (normally increased in the allergic response pathway) which have been found in the fluid of chronically diseased middle ears. No direct evidence exists linking ear disease and allergy at this time [14, 15].

### *Breast Feeding*

Breast feeding may be a protective factor; lower rates of otitis media have been seen in breastfed children for the first 11 months of life. In addition, these children have been noted to have increased serum IgG which may protect against AOM [13].

## Infectious Causes

Acute otitis media is the most common reason for an antibiotic prescription for pediatric patients in the United States; however, AOM is not always caused by bacteria.

### *Viruses*

Viral causes of AOM (Table **1**) account for only 10% of cases. However, 70% of AOM have viral isolates found in middle ear exudate. Recent evidence shows that viruses can lead to bacterial superinfection through inflammatory and anatomic pathways [16].

Table 1. Common causal pathogens for acute otitis media [16, 17].

| Viruses | Bacteria |
|---|---|
| • **Respiratory Syncytial Virus**<br>• Coronavirus<br>• Adenovirus<br>• Human bocavirus<br>• Rhinovirus | • *Streptococcus pneumoniae*<br>• *Non-typeable Haemophilus influenzae*<br>• *Moraxella catarrhalis* |

### *Bacteria*

Bacteria typically colonize the nasopharynx, but do not cause infection until a viral upper respiratory infection initiates it. See Table **1** for most common bacteria [17].

The pneumococcal conjugate vaccines have led to an overall decrease in AOM episodes in vaccinated children. However, an increase has been documented in non-vaccinated strains of *S. pneumoniae* [17].

In most cases of acute otitis media, bacteria can be cultured from the middle ear effusion. Because of difficulty isolating pathogens, OME was long thought to be a noninfectious or "sterile" process. Studies now show that bacteria are present in OME [18]. These bacteria are not in free planktonic form as in AOM, but in biofilm.

A biofilm is defined as "a community of interacting bacteria attached to a surface and encased in a protective glycocalyx or matrix of exopolylsaccharides" [18]. The majority of bacteria in the body exist in a biofilm and are able to survive in environments that free (planktonic) bacteria cannot [19]. The bacteria have decreased oxygen and nutrient requirements, an increase in resistance genes, the ability of cell to cell signaling, and poor antimicrobial penetration [19].

# Genetic Causes

## *Race, Ethnicities and Gender*

Studies have shown a difference in incidence/prevalence of OM based on race and ethnicities. Indigenous populations such as Australian Aborigines, Inuits, New Zealand Maoris, American Indians and Alaska natives are known to have high prevalence of otitis media [20 - 22]. Discrepancies in treatment have been shown also to be race related with children of minority less likely to receive broad spectrum antibiotics and more likely to have hospitalization from AOM complications [23].

## *Heritability*

Heritability estimates of recurrent acute otitis media are 0.49 [24] and accounted for by differences in anatomy, genetic syndromes/alterations, and susceptibility to viruses and bacteria [25]. Twin studies have shown that the concordance of otitis media is around 0.9 in monozygotic twins and increases with age, while in dizygotic twins the concordance was 0.65 [25].

## *Genetic Alterations*

Genetic susceptibility to otitis media is caused by alterations in genes coding for innate and adaptive immunity factors as well as random genetic alterations (Table **2**) [26 - 29]. Immune involvement in genetic risk for OM is supported by increased rates of otitis media in patients with combined variable immuno-deficiency compared to normal population [30].

**Table 2. Genes associated with otitis media.**

| Innate Immunity | Adaptive Immunity | Others |
|---|---|---|
| • TLR2<br>• CD14<br>• MBL2<br>• SP-α1 | • IL-1β<br>• IL-8<br>• IL-10<br>• TGF-β1<br>• TNFα | • MUSC5Ac<br>• CCR5<br>• PAI-1<br>• A2ML1 |

TLR2 = toll-like receptor 2, CD14 = cluster of differentiation 14, MBL2 = mannose-binding lectin 2, SP-α1 = surfactant protein A 1, IL-1β = Interleukin 1 beta, IL-8 = Interleukin 8, IL- 10 = Interleukin 10, TGF- β1 = transforming growth factor beta 1, TNFα = tumor necrosis factor alpha, MUSC3Ac = muscarinic receptor Ac, CCR5 = C-C chemokine receptor type 5, PAI-1 = plasmin activator inhibitor 1, A2ML1 = alpha-2-macroglobulin-like 1.

Mutations in genes related to innate immunity, adaptive immunity among others are associated with susceptibility to otitis media [26 - 28].

## *Cleft Palate*

Ninety percent of children with cleft palate (prevalence 6/10,000 live births) will have chronic OME. The cause of OME is the Eustachian tube dysfunction accompanying the cleft palate [31].

## *Down's Syndrome*

Eustachian tube dysfunction in patients with Down's Syndrome (prevalence 1/700 live births) is due to hypotrophy of the middle face and general musculature. Other associated features include narrow ear canal and hypertrophy of the nasopharyngeal lymphatic tissue [32]. The prevalence of OME in these patients is reported as 60-85% [33, 34].

## *Primary Ciliary Dyskinesia*

Primary Ciliary Dyskinesia (PCD) is a rare autosomal recessive disorder with unknown prevalence which affects the motility of cilia. Because the middle ear mucosa is lined with ciliated epithelium, in those with PCD there is decreased mucous motility, increased stasis, increased infection, increased biofilm, and decreased hearing due to fluid collection. The use of tubes for treatment of OME is controversial in patients with PCD due to the persistence of tube otorrhea [35].

## ACUTE OTITIS MEDIA

### Definition

Acute otitis media (AOM) is an infection of the middle ear space characterized by a neutrophil rich middle-ear effusion in conjunction with signs and symptoms of middle-ear inflammation [2]. Recurrent acute otitis media (RAOM) is defined as 3 or more episodes of AOM in 6 months, or 4 or more in 12 months [2].

### Epidemiology

The average child will have had 1.7 episodes of AOM by the age of three. The incidence of AOM before three years is 50% [1, 13] and prevalence decreasing from 34% to 24% from 1997 to 2007. Rates of AOM remain highest in children younger than 3 years normally being found between ages 6-12 months [13]. Decrease in prevalence may be due to implementation of pneumococcal vaccine, decrease in smoke exposure, increase in breast feeding, or increase in stringent diagnostic criteria [2, 13].

## Clinical

### History and Physical

The typical presentation of a child with AOM includes rapid onset of irritability, fever and ear pain [6]. In infants with symptoms of an upper respiratory infection, the probability of AOM is increased if the child attends daycare and parents are able to identify ear pain and cough. Ear pulling is not predictive of AOM [1].

On physical exam the tympanic membrane is erythematous, bulging with fluid pressing the ear drum laterally. In some instances, thin yellow or green otorrhea may be present in the external auditory canal, which is associated with tympanic membrane perforation.

### Diagnosis

Diagnosis of acute otitis media is made clinically with otoscopic examination and pneumatic otoscopy or tympanometry to verify middle ear effusion [33, 34].

### Complications

Complications of ear infections are uncommon, but, due to the high prevalence of the disease, still seen by primary care providers. Complications can be divided into subgroups based on anatomy.

Intratemporal complications (complications which remain confined to the ear) include common complications such as tympanic membrane perforation which occurs in 7% of acute infections, and rarer complications which include mastoiditis, labyrinthitis, vertigo, conductive or sensorineural hearing loss, cholesteatoma, facial nerve paralysis, ossicular discontinuity [6, 36, 37].

Intracranial complications typically arise after mastoiditis and are more serious in nature [6]. These may include meningitis (most common), epidural or brain abscess, and dural sinus thrombosis.

Long term complications of acute otitis media are few unless one of the above complications occurred [6]. A high number of AOM episodes has been associated with adult onset hearing loss [38].

## Treatment

### Acute Otitis Media, Single Episode

Treatment options include symptomatic treatment alone, delayed antibiotic treatment and immediate antibiotic therapy. AOM is the most common reason that a child receives antibiotic therapy in the United States [39].

Because 60% of AOM usually resolves in 24 hours without treatment, symptomatic treatment with acetaminophen or NSAIDs for mild pain and fever is an appropriate option for AOM with reevaluation in 48-72 hours [2, 39, 40]. A 48-72 hour observation prior to antibiotic dispensation in patients with non-severe AOM can be considered, which will in turn decrease medication side effects such as nausea, vomiting, and diarrhea [39]. In children without symptom resolution within 72 hours or worsening symptoms, antibiotics should be started [2, 40]. Antibiotics should be started at diagnosis for children with systemic symptoms, serious illnesses, or selectively in children less than 2 years of age with bilateral AOM or with otorrhea [2, 40]. Recommendations for antibiotic therapy is listed in Table **3** [40]. Five days of antibiotics will usually suffice for children 2 years or older, but it may be necessary to give up to 10 days if less than 2 years of age or with a tympanic membrane perforation [2]. Patients should be followed in 4-8 weeks to assess response to treatment.

Table 3. Recommended antibiotics for treatment of acute otitis media [40].

|  | **First-line Treatment** | **Alternative** |
|---|---|---|
| **Initial Treatment** | Amoxicillin or Amoxicillin-clavulanate | • Cefdinir<br>• Cefuroxime<br>• Cefpodoxime<br>• Ceftriaxone |
| **After Treatment Failure** | Amoxicillin-clavulanate or Ceftriaxone | • Ceftriaxone<br>• Clindamycin<br>• Clindamycin + 2$^{nd}$ or 3$^{rd}$ generation cephalosporins |

## *Recurrent Acute Otitis Media*

Treatment options for recurrent otitis media include antibiotics, vaccination, and tympanostomy tubes. Vaccines administered during infancy can reduce the incidence of AOM. Tympanostomy tubes have been shown to be an effective treatment for recurrent otitis media [2, 3, 5, 41]. Recent 2016 guideline updates by the American Academy of Otolaryngology recommend ventilation tubes if bilateral or unilateral middle ear effusion is present at the time of assessment. If no middle ear effusion at the time of examination in either ear, observation for a 3-6 months period is recommended unless the patient is deemed high risk (history of autism, syndromic and craniofacial disorders, cleft palate, prior hearing loss, vision impairment, speech delay) [5].

# OTITIS MEDIA WITH EFFUSION

## Definition

Otitis media with effusion (OME) is characterized by the presence of fluid in the middle ear without signs or symptoms of acute otitis media, such as fever and earache. Other names for OME include glue ear, serous otitis media, and ear fluid [33, 34].

Chronic OME is middle ear effusion persisting for more than 3 months from date of onset or date of diagnosis [33, 34].

## Epidemiology

OME is the most common cause of hearing impairment in children in developed countries with a prevalence of 80% before the age of 4 years. Half of these cases will resolve within 3 months and 95% within 1 year. Recurrence of OME present in 30-40% of children, yet only 10% will still have fluid 3 months after AOM [5, 42]. The incidence of OME per year is 2.2 million in the United States [33, 34]. Most cases of OME occur during the ages of 6 months to 4 years, with no predilection for race or gender.

## Clinical

### *History and Physical*

Children with OME may present with conductive hearing loss, difficulties at school, behavioral issues, ear discomfort, recurrent AOM, or reduced quality of life [33, 34]. Children with OME lack the signs of acute inflammation found in AOM, such as fever, otalgia, otorrhea, and tympanic membrane erythema. However, these children may have decreased gross motor proficiency and behavioral problems such as distractibility, withdrawal, frustration, and aggressiveness.

### *Diagnosis*

OME may present asymptomatically and serous middle ear fluid is difficult to distinguish with otoscopy alone as the appearance of the TM is affected by many factors. Adding pneumatic otoscopy to the exam can clarify the diagnosis by demonstrating decreased TM movement [33, 34]. If pneumatic otoscopy is inconclusive, tympanometry should be used.

Formal audiometry should be performed in children with OME persisting for 3 months or longer or if high risk features present (TM retraction pockets, ossicular erosion, accumulation of keratin) [5, 33, 34].

## Complications

In most cases, OME resolves spontaneously with no adverse outcomes. Potential short-term complications include hearing loss, speech delay, and problems in school. Long term sequelae include adult hearing loss, which is more common and more profound in those with a history of OME and cholesteatoma [38, 43].

## Treatment

### Acute Treatment

#### Watchful Waiting

After the diagnosis of OME has been established, the clinician should monitor the patient for 3 months. Parents should be informed that reduced hearing may be experienced while waiting for the effusion to resolve and techniques to optimize learning should be utilized [33, 34].

If the effusion is still present after 3 months, watchful waiting may be continued if no symptoms of hearing loss are experienced. Surveillance should occur every 3 to 6 months [5].

Unless other indications are present, nasal steroids, antibiotics, and antihistamines/decongestants are not recommended for the treatment of OME [33, 34].

#### Autoinflation

Autoinflation is a technique to reopen the Eustachian tube by forced exhalation against a closed mouth and nose or using a Politzer device. This could provide benefit if performed during the watchful waiting period due to low cost and no potential risks [44].

### Recommendations for Tympanostomy Tubes

If fluid is present for 3 or more months, tympanostomy tubes may be recommended especially if hearing loss is present. Tympanostomy tubes may be considered before 3 months of watchful waiting for children at risk for developmental delays as additional hearing loss may have detrimental consequences [5, 33, 34].

# TYMPANOSTOMY TUBES

## Effectiveness

Tympanostomy tube placement is the most common surgery performed in children [3]. For children with OME, tympanostomy tubes are more effective at decreasing hearing loss than other treatments in the first 6 months after placement [45]. No studies have been done to evaluate effects on speech, language, and development [46]. Tympanostomy tubes do not decrease overall prevalence of otitis media, but do decrease frequency of recurrent episodes, duration of the recurrent episodes, and increase the ease of treatment [47].

## Indications (Table 4)

Recurrent acute otitis media [5, 40]:

- Middle ear effusion (unilateral or bilateral) at time of assessment.
- 3 episodes in 6 months, or 4 episodes in 1 year with 1 episode in the preceding 6 months.

Otitis media with effusion [5, 33, 34]:

- Middle ear effusion for at least 3 months with complications (hearing loss, balance problems, poor school performance, ear discomfort, reduced quality of life)
- High risk children (history of autism, craniofacial anomaly, cleft palate, syndrome, prior hearing loss, vision impairment, speech delay)

Table 4. Current guidelines for tympanostomy tube placement [5, 33, 34].

| Indications for Tympanostomy Tubes | |
| --- | --- |
| **Recurrent Acute Otitis Media** | **Otitis Media with Effusion** |
| • Middle ear effusion at time of otolaryngologic assessment<br>• 3 infections in 6 months<br>• 4 infections in 1 year with 1 in last 6 months | • Middle ear effusion for ≥ 3 months with complications (hearing loss, balance problems, poor school performance, ear discomfort, reduced quality of life)<br>• high risk children |

## Complex Cases

With all complex cases, a multi-disciplinary team should be utilized. For children with Down's syndrome, important considerations include: severity of hearing loss, age, difficulty of insertion, risks, and likelihood of extrusion [48]. Cleft palate patients often have tympanostomy tubes placed at the same time as the palatal repair. However, individual circumstances may warrant insertion at initial lip repair surgery or suggest hearing aids as a better option [48]. Hearing aids play an important role in complex cases and may be a good alternative to surgical intervention.

## Complications

### *Otorrhea*

Otorrhea, or drainage from the ear, is the most common complication after tube insertion. One fourth of patients will have drainage for more than two weeks after surgery and one third of patients will have recurrent episodes of otorrhea [49, 50].

Otorrhea is caused by viruses in 20% and polymicrobial bacteria (including *H. influenzae*, *S. aureus*, *P. aeruginosa*) in 80% of cases [51].

The most common treatments are oral or topical antibiotics, with other options including oral or topical steroids, aural toilet, and antiseptics. Pediatricians are more likely to give oral antibiotics, while otolaryngologists are more likely to give topical antibiotics [49, 52, 53]. Previously, it was believed there was no difference in resolution rates between oral and topical antibiotics. However, recent evidence suggests topical therapy is superior to oral [54].

Half of children who have had tympanostomy tube placement will require the same procedure again [55]. The general approach is to perform adenoidectomy at the same time as second myringotomy. In children less than 4 years of age, new recommendations are to only perform adenoidectomy at this time if a distinct indication such as chronic adenoiditis or nasal obstruction exists. If the child is 4 years old or greater, a separate indication for adenoidectomy is not required [33, 34, 49].

### *Myringosclerosis*

Myringosclerosis is a localized reaction of the tympanic membrane characterized by sclerosis, hyaline degeneration in the lamina propria, calcium and phosphate deposition, and is histologically similar to atherosclerosis [56]. It originates from inflammation in the middle ear- either from recurrent infections or tympanostomy tubes themselves, and is the most common long term sequela from tympanostomy tube placement [56 - 59]. Myringosclerosis rarely leads to hearing loss except in severe cases involving the entire tympanic membrane as well as the ossicles (known as tympanosclerosis). Tympanosclerosis may require surgical intervention.

## Tympanic Membrane Perforation

Tympanic membrane perforation is found in 1% of children after tube extrusion. The percentage increases if the tubes have to be manually removed or if multiple sets of tubes have been placed [50, 60]. Perforations may require surgical repair by otolaryngologist with either myringoplasty or tympanoplasty depending on severity.

## Follow-up

### Appointments

No agreement has been reached on timing of follow-up appointments, or whether the child needs to be seen at all. Most otolaryngologists do follow these children with an audiogram [61].

### Water Exposure

In a 2016 Cochrane review, recommendations were made against otic water precautions for children with ear tubes [62]. Tube extrusion and hearing loss rates are unaffected by water precautions, but tube otorrhea may be slightly increased if no water precautions are followed [62, 63].

## CONCLUSION

In conclusion, otitis media is a common process that all clinicians who see children will encounter. The disease is complex in origin with many contributing risk factors and causes. It is vital for clinicians to distinguish between recurrent acute episodes and chronic middle ear effusion as treatments are different. Work up should always include pneumatic otoscopy. Initial treatment of AOM may include watchful waiting for 48-72 hours. New recommendations indicate that placement of tympanostomy tubes should only be recommended if middle ear fluid is present in examination of children with ROM or if middle ear fluid is present for more than 3 months in OME.

## CONFLICT OF INTEREST

The authors declares no conflict of interest, financial or otherwise.

## ACKNOWLEDGEMENTS

We thank Dr. Tasnee Chonmaitree and Ms. Rebecca Cook for careful reading of the manuscript and for their valuable feedback.

# REFERENCES

[1]     McCormick DP, Jennings K, Ede LC, Chonmaitree T. Use of symptoms and risk factors to predict acute otitis media in infants. Int J Pediatr Otorhinolaryngol 2016; 81: 55-9.
[http://dx.doi.org/10.1016/j.ijporl.2015.12.002]

[2]     Wasson JD, Yung MW. Evidence-based management of otitis media: a 5S model approach. J Laryngol Otol 2015; 129(2): 112-9.
[http://dx.doi.org/10.1017/S0022215114003363]

[3]     Principi N, Marchisio P, Esposito S. Otitis media with effusion: benefits and harms of strategies in use for treatment and prevention. Expert Rev Anti Infect Ther 2016; 14(4): 415-23.
[http://dx.doi.org/10.1586/14787210.2016.1150781]

[4]     Rosenfeld RM, Culpepper L, Yawn B, Mahoney MC. Otitis media with effusion clinical practice guideline. Am Fam Physician 2004; 69(12): 2776-2778-2779.

[5]     Rosenfeld RM, Schwartz SR, Pynnonen MA, *et al.* Clinical practice guideline: Tympanostomy tubes in children. Otolaryngol Head Neck Surg 2013; 149(1) (Suppl.): S1-S35.
[http://dx.doi.org/10.1177/0194599813490141]

[6]     Mm L, Pw F, Eds. Casselbrant, M.L. and M. EM, Acute Otitis Media and Otitis Media with Effusion. Cummings Pediatric Otolaryngology. Philadelphia: Elsevier Saunders 2015; pp. 209-27.

[7]     Daly KA, Hunter LL, Levine SC, Lindgren BR, Giebink GS. Relationships between otitis media sequelae and age. Laryngoscope 1998; 108(9): 1306-10.
[http://dx.doi.org/10.1097/00005537-199809000-00008]

[8]     Stenstrom C, Bylander-Groth A, Ingvarsson L. Eustachian tube function in otitis-prone and healthy children. Int J Pediatr Otorhinolaryngol 1991; 21(2): 127-38.
[http://dx.doi.org/10.1016/0165-5876(91)90143-Y]

[9]     Straetemans M, van Heerbeek N, Schilder Anne GM, *et al.* Eustachian tube function before recurrence of otitis media with effusion. Arch Otolaryngol Head Neck Surg 2005; 131(2): 118-23.
[http://dx.doi.org/10.1001/archotol.131.2.118]

[10]    Yilmaz G, Hizli S, Karacan C, Yurdakök K, Coşkun T, Dilmen U. Effect of passive smoking on growth and infection rates of breast-fed and non-breast-fed infants. Pediatr Int 2009; 51(3): 352-8.
[http://dx.doi.org/10.1111/j.1442-200X.2008.02757.x]

[11]    Zhou S, Rosenthal DG, Sherman S, Weitzman M. Physical, behavioral, and cognitive effects of prenatal tobacco and postnatal secondhand smoke exposure. Curr Probl Pediatr Adolesc Health Care 2014; 44(8): 219-41.
[http://dx.doi.org/10.1016/j.cppeds.2014.03.007]

[12]    Kum-Nji P, Meloy L, Herrod HG. Environmental tobacco smoke exposure: prevalence and mechanisms of causation of infections in children. Pediatrics 2006; 117(5): 1745-54.
[http://dx.doi.org/10.1542/peds.2005-1886]

[13]    Hoffman HJ, Daly KA, Bainbridge KE, *et al.* Panel 1: Epidemiology, natural history, and risk factors. Otolaryngol Head Neck Surg 2013; 148(4) (Suppl.): E1-E25.
[http://dx.doi.org/10.1177/0194599812460984]

[14]    Hurst DS. Efficacy of allergy immunotherapy as a treatment for patients with chronic otitis media with effusion. Int J Pediatr Otorhinolaryngol 2008; 72(8): 1215-23.
[http://dx.doi.org/10.1016/j.ijporl.2008.04.013]

[15]    Kvaerner KJ, Kristiansen HA, Russell MB. Otitis media history, surgery and allergy in 60-year perspective: a population-based study. Int J Pediatr Otorhinolaryngol 2010; 74(12): 1356-60.
[http://dx.doi.org/10.1016/j.ijporl.2010.09.002]

[16]　Nokso-Koivisto J, Marom T, Chonmaitree T. Importance of viruses in acute otitis media. Curr Opin Pediatr 2015; 27(1): 110-5.
[http://dx.doi.org/10.1097/MOP.0000000000000184]

[17]　Casey JR, Adlowitz DG, Pichichero ME. New patterns in the otopathogens causing acute otitis media six to eight years after introduction of pneumococcal conjugate vaccine. Pediatr Infect Dis J 2010; 29(4): 304-9.

[18]　Post JC. Direct evidence of bacterial biofilms in otitis media. 2001. Laryngoscope 2015; 125(9): 2003-14.
[http://dx.doi.org/10.1002/lary.25291]

[19]　Coticchia JM, Chen M, Sachdeva L, Mutchnick S. New paradigms in the pathogenesis of otitis media in children. Front Pediatr 2013; 1: 52.
[http://dx.doi.org/10.3389/fped.2013.00052]

[20]　McCallum J, Craig L, Whittaker I, Baxter J. Ethnic differences in acute hospitalisations for otitis media and elective hospitalisations for ventilation tubes in New Zealand children aged 0-14 years. N Z Med J 2015; 128(1416): 10-20.

[21]　Daly KA, Hoffman HJ, Kvaerner KJ, *et al.* Epidemiology, natural history, and risk factors: panel report from the Ninth International Research Conference on Otitis Media. Int J Pediatr Otorhinolaryngol 2010; 74(3): 231-40.
[http://dx.doi.org/10.1016/j.ijporl.2009.09.006]

[22]　Singleton RJ, Holman RC, Plant R, *et al.* Trends in otitis media and myringotomy with tube placement among American Indian/Alaska native children and the US general population of children. Pediatr Infect Dis J 2009; 28(2): 102-7.
[http://dx.doi.org/10.1097/INF.0b013e318188d079]

[23]　Fleming-Dutra KE, Shapiro DJ, Hicks LA, Gerber JS, Hersh AL. Race, otitis media, and antibiotic selection. Pediatrics 2014; 134(6): 1059-66.
[http://dx.doi.org/10.1542/peds.2014-1781]

[24]　Bhutta MF. Epidemiology and pathogenesis of otitis media: construction of a phenotype landscape. Audiol Neurootol 2014; 19(3): 210-23.
[http://dx.doi.org/10.1159/000358549]

[25]　Rovers M, Haggard M, Gannon M, Koeppen-Schomerus G, Plomin R. Heritability of symptom domains in otitis media: a longitudinal study of 1,373 twin pairs. Am J Epidemiol 2002; 155(10): 958-64.
[http://dx.doi.org/10.1093/aje/155.10.958]

[26]　Miljanovic O, Cikota-Aleksić B, Likić D, *et al.* Association of cytokine gene polymorphisms and risk factors with otitis media proneness in children. Eur J Pediatr 2016; 175(6): 809-15.
[http://dx.doi.org/10.1007/s00431-016-2711-0]

[27]　Mittal R, Robalino G, Gerring R, *et al.* Immunity genes and susceptibility to otitis media: a comprehensive review. J Genet Genomics 2014; 41(11): 567-81.
[http://dx.doi.org/10.1016/j.jgg.2014.10.003]

[28]　Santos-Cortez RL, Chiong CM, Reyes-Quintos Ma Rina T, *et al.* Rare A2ML1 variants confer susceptibility to otitis media. Nat Genet 2015; 47(8): 917-20.
[http://dx.doi.org/10.1038/ng.3347]

[29]　Esposito S, Marchisio P, Orenti A, *et al.* Genetic Polymorphisms of Functional Candidate Genes and Recurrent Acute Otitis Media With or Without Tympanic Membrane Perforation. Medicine (Baltimore) 2015; 94(42): e1860.
[http://dx.doi.org/10.1097/MD.0000000000001860]

[30]    Magliulo G, Iannella G, Granata G, *et al.* Otologic evaluation of patients with primary antibody deficiency. Eur Arch Otorhinolaryngol 2016.
[http://dx.doi.org/10.1007/s00405-016-3956-y]

[31]    Tierney S, O'Brien K, Harman NL, *et al.* Risks and benefits of ventilation tubes and hearing aids from the perspective of parents of children with cleft palate. Int J Pediatr Otorhinolaryngol 2013; 77(10): 1742-8.
[http://dx.doi.org/10.1016/j.ijporl.2013.08.006]

[32]    Austeng ME, Akre H, Øverland B, *et al.* Otitis media with effusion in children with in Down syndrome. Int J Pediatr Otorhinolaryngol 2013; 77(8): 1329-32.
[http://dx.doi.org/10.1016/j.ijporl.2013.05.027]

[33]    Rosenfeld RM, Shin JJ, Schwartz SR, *et al.* Clinical Practice Guideline: Otitis Media with Effusion (Update). Otolaryngol Head Neck Surg 2016; 154(1) (Suppl.): S1-S41.
[http://dx.doi.org/10.1177/0194599815623467]

[34]    Rosenfeld RM, Rosenfeld RM, Rosenfeld RM, *et al.* Clinical Practice Guideline: Otitis Media with Effusion Executive Summary (Update). Otolaryngol Head Neck Surg 2016; 154(2): 201-14.
[http://dx.doi.org/10.1177/0194599815624407]

[35]    Morgan LC, Birman CS. The impact of Primary Ciliary Dyskinesia on the upper respiratory tract. Paediatr Respir Rev 2016; 18: 33-8.
[http://dx.doi.org/10.1016/j.prrv.2015.09.006]

[36]    Licse JG, Silfverdal SA, Giaquinto C, *et al.* Incidence and clinical presentation of acute otitis media in children aged <6 years in European medical practices. Epidemiol Infect 2014; 142(8): 1778-88.
[http://dx.doi.org/10.1017/S0950268813002744]

[37]    Nankivell PC, Pothier DD. Surgery for tympanic membrane retraction pockets. Cochrane Database Syst Rev 2010; (7): CD007943.

[38]    Aarhus L, Tambs K, Kvestad E, Engdahl B. Childhood Otitis Media: A Cohort Study With 30-Year Follow-Up of Hearing (The HUNT Study). Ear Hear 2015; 36(3): 302-8.
[http://dx.doi.org/10.1097/AUD.0000000000000118]

[39]    Venekamp RP, Sanders S, Glasziou PP, Del Mar CB, Rovers MM. Antibiotics for acute otitis media in children. Cochrane Database Syst Rev 2015; (6): CD000219.

[40]    Lieberthal AS, Carroll AE, Chonmaitree T, *et al.* The diagnosis and management of acute otitis media. Pediatrics 2013; 131(3): e964-99.
[http://dx.doi.org/10.1542/peds.2012-3488]

[41]    McDonald S, Langton Hewer CD, Nunez DA. Grommets (ventilation tubes) for recurrent acute otitis media in children. Cochrane Database Syst Rev 2008; (4): CD004741.

[42]    Tos M. Epidemiology and natural history of secretory otitis. Am J Otol 1984; 5(6): 459-62.

[43]    Kuo CL. Etiopathogenesis of acquired cholesteatoma: prominent theories and recent advances in biomolecular research. Laryngoscope 2015; 125(1): 234-40.
[http://dx.doi.org/10.1002/lary.24890]

[44]    Perera R, Glasziou PP, Heneghan CJ, McLellan J, Williamson I. Autoinflation for hearing loss associated with otitis media with effusion. Cochrane Database Syst Rev 2013; (5): CD006285.

[45]    Berkman ND, Wallace IF, Steiner MJ, *et al.* Otitis Media With Effusion: Comparative Effectiveness of Treatments. Rockville MD: Agency for Healthcare Research and Quality (US) 2013.

[46]    Browning GG, Rovers MM, Williamson I, *et al.* Grommets (ventilation tubes) for hearing loss associated with otitis media with effusion in children. Cochrane Database Syst Rev 2010; (10): CD001801.
[http://dx.doi.org/10.1002/14651858.CD001801]

[47]    Cheong KH, Hussain SS. Management of recurrent acute otitis media in children: systematic review of the effect of different interventions on otitis media recurrence, recurrence frequency and total recurrence time. J Laryngol Otol 2012; 126(9): 874-85.
[http://dx.doi.org/10.1017/S0022215112001338]

[48]    Khanna R, Lakhanpaul M, Bull PD. Surgical management of otitis media with effusion in children: summary of NICE guidance. Clin Otolaryngol 2008; 33(6): 600-5.
[http://dx.doi.org/10.1111/j.1749-4486.2008.01844.x]

[49]    Williamson I. Otitis media with effusion in children. BMJ Clin Evid 2011; 2011

[50]    Van Heerbeek N, De Saar GM, Mulder JJ. Long-term ventilation tubes: results of 726 insertions. Clin Otolaryngol Allied Sci 2002; 27(5): 378-83.
[http://dx.doi.org/10.1046/j.1365-2273.2002.00599.x]

[51]    van Dongen TM, Venekamp RP, Wensing AM, *et al.* Acute otorrhea in children with tympanostomy tubes: prevalence of bacteria and viruses in the post-pneumococcal conjugate vaccine era. Pediatr Infect Dis J 2015; 34(4): 355-60.
[http://dx.doi.org/10.1097/INF.0000000000000595]

[52]    Strachan D, Clarke SE, England RJ. The effectiveness of topical treatment in discharging ears with in-dwelling ventilation tubes. Rev Laryngol Otol Rhinol (Bord) 2000; 121(1): 27-9.

[53]    Vaile L, Williamson T, Waddell A, Taylor G. Interventions for ear discharge associated with grommets (ventilation tubes). Cochrane Database Syst Rev 2006; (2): CD001933.

[54]    Dohar J, Giles W, Roland P, *et al.* Topical ciprofloxacin/dexamethasone superior to oral amoxicillin/clavulanic acid in acute otitis media with otorrhea through tympanostomy tubes. Pediatrics 2006; 118(3): e561-9.
[http://dx.doi.org/10.1542/peds.2005-2033]

[55]    Hong HR, Kim TS, Chung JW. Long-term follow-up of otitis media with effusion in children: comparisons between a ventilation tube group and a non-ventilation tube group. Int J Pediatr Otorhinolaryngol 2014; 78(6): 938-43.
[http://dx.doi.org/10.1016/j.ijporl.2014.03.019]

[56]    Koc A, Uneri C. Sex distribution in children with tympanosclerosis after insertion of a tympanostomy tube. Eur Arch Otorhinolaryngol 2001; 258(1): 16-9.
[http://dx.doi.org/10.1007/PL00007517]

[57]    De Beer BA, Schilder AG, Zielhuis GA, Graamans K. Natural course of tympanic membrane pathology related to otitis media and ventilation tubes between ages 8 and 18 years. Otol Neurotol 2005; 26(5): 1016-21.
[http://dx.doi.org/10.1097/01.mao.0000185058.89586.ed]

[58]    Caye-Thomasen P, Stangerup SE, Jørgensen G, *et al.* Myringotomy *versus* ventilation tubes in secretory otitis media: eardrum pathology, hearing, and eustachian tube function 25 years after treatment. Otol Neurotol 2008; 29(5): 649-57.
[http://dx.doi.org/10.1097/MAO.0b013e318173035b]

[59]    Mohammed H, Martinez-Devesa P. Complications of long-term ventilation tubes. J Laryngol Otol 2013; 127(5): 509-10.
[http://dx.doi.org/10.1017/S0022215113000388]

[60]    O'Niel MB, Cassidy LD, Link TR, Kerschner JE. Tracking tympanostomy tube outcomes in pediatric patients with otitis media using an electronic database. Int J Pediatr Otorhinolaryngol 2015; 79(8): 1275-8.
[http://dx.doi.org/10.1016/j.ijporl.2015.05.029]

[61]   Spielmann PM, McKee H, Adamson RM, *et al.* Follow up after middle-ear ventilation tube insertion: what is needed and when? J Laryngol Otol 2008; 122(6): 580-3.
[http://dx.doi.org/10.1017/S0022215107001168]

[62]   Moualed D, Masterson L, Kumar S, Donnelly N. Water precautions for prevention of infection in children with ventilation tubes (grommets). Cochrane Database Syst Rev 2016; (1): CD010375.

[63]   Hebert RL II, King GE, Bent JP III. Tympanostomy tubes and water exposure: a practical model. Arch Otolaryngol Head Neck Surg 1998; 124(10): 1118-21.
[http://dx.doi.org/10.1001/archotol.124.10.1118]

# CHAPTER 2

# Contemporary Management of Children with Hearing Loss

**Musaed Alzahrani**[1] and **Issam Saliba**[2,*]

[1] *Department of Surgery, Division of Otolaryngology, King Fahad Specialist Hospital, Dammam, Saudi Arabia*

[2] *Division of Otorhinolaryngology Head & Neck surgery, University of Montreal, Otology and Neurotology, Sainte-Justine University Hospital Center (CHUSJ) and University of Montreal Hospital Center (CHUM), Montreal, Quebec, Canada*

**Abstract:** Hearing loss has a significant impact on children's ability to develop adequate language and communication skills and often interferes with educational performance as well as limits long-term employment opportunities. Hearing loss is categorized into three broad categories: Conductive, Sensorineural, and Mixed. Audiology workup aims to identify the category and the level of hearing loss; evaluation is divided into subjective and objective tests. Rehabilitation is available to almost all kinds and degrees of hearing loss if diagnosed and managed in a timely manner. For that, we need to increase the awareness of the families and health care providers as well about the screening programs and advocate its implementation in all maternity and child care centers. In this chapter, we discuss acquired and congenital causes of hearing loss. We will also address the diagnostic workup, and finally will discuss in detail the recent developments in pediatric hearing rehabilitation.

**Keywords:** Cochlear implant, Congenital, Genetics, Hearing aids, Hearing loss, Pediatrics, Syndrome.

## INTRODUCTION

Pediatric hearing loss is the most common sensory deficit with an estimated incidence of 1-4 per 1000 newborns [1, 2]. Clinically, 20 dB HL in both ears is considered the normal hearing threshold for children, adolescents, and adults [1]. Any increase in the threshold level is regarded as hearing loss and is classified according to specified degrees of increase (*i.e.,* mild (20 to 40 dB HL), moderate (41 to 55 dB HL), moderately severe (56 to 70 dB HL), severe (71 to 90dB HL) and profound (91 to dB HL) as shown in Fig. (**1**). In a recent fact sheet, the WHO

* **Corresponding author Issam Saliba**: Department of Otolaryngology, Sainte-Justine University Hospital Center (CHU SJ), 3175, Côte Sainte-Catherine, Montreal (QC) H3T 1C5, Canada; Tel: (514) 507-7722; Fax: (514) 507-9014; E-mail: issam.saliba@umontreal.ca

Seckin Ulualp (Ed.)

has estimated that about "360 million people worldwide have disabling hearing loss, 32 million (9%) of these are children" [3].

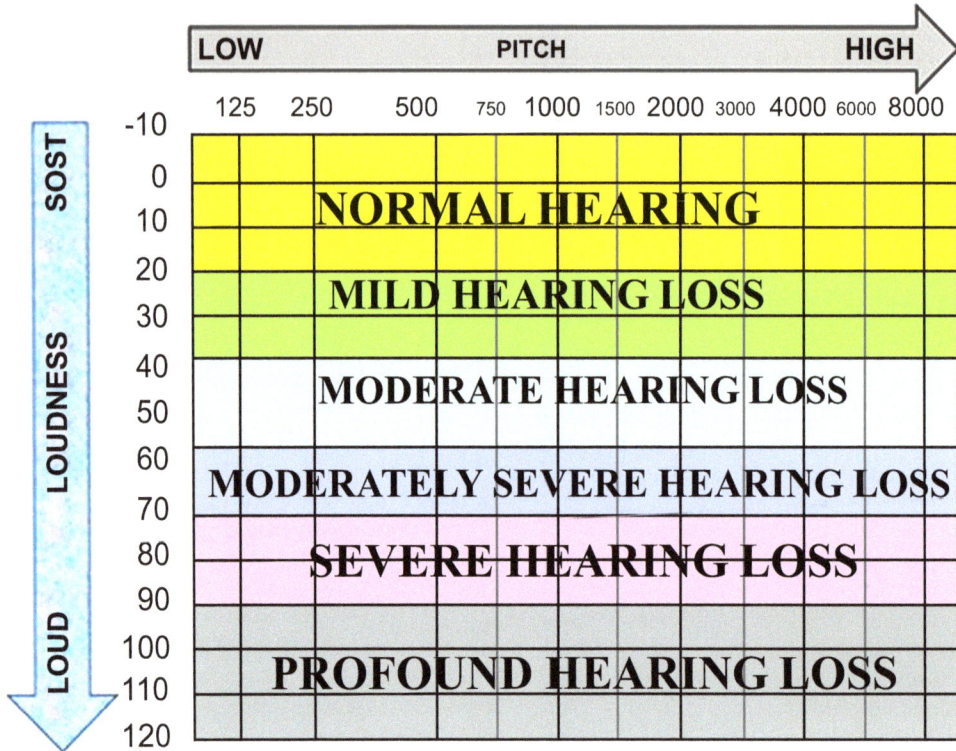

**Fig. (1).** An illustration showing the levels of hearing loss.

Hearing loss has a significant impact on children's ability to develop adequate language and communication skills [4, 5]; and often interferes with educational performance as well as limits long-term employment opportunities [2]. This impact can be reduced by early diagnosis through neonatal hearing screening programs and childcare clinics, as well as providing adequate educational and social services to affected children and their families [6].

Children diagnosed as clinically deaf have no or very little hearing, do not develop normal speech, and have no other recourse but to use sign language for communication. They may however, benefit from cochlear implants and develop variably normal speech if implanted during the speech development period, which is roughly before the age of five years [7]. However, "hard of hearing" children who suffer from mild to severe bilateral hearing loss develop spoken language and may benefit from hearing aids that amplify incoming sound signals [5, 7].

In this chapter, we discuss acquired and congenital causes of hearing loss. We will also address the diagnostic workup, and finally will discuss in detail the recent developments in pediatric hearing rehabilitation.

## DEFINITIONS

Hearing loss is caused by different etiologies affecting the external, the middle or the inner ear thus obstructing or damaging a part of the auditory system. The different types of hearing loss are categorized into three broad categories: Conductive, Sensorineural, and Mixed.

Conductive hearing loss refers to an impairment of the conductive part (*i.e.,* external and middle ears) of the auditory system in which the inner ear is usually normal, but air conducted sound is inadequately delivered or prevented from reaching the sensorineural apparatus of the inner ear in a normal way. Although sensitivity to sound is diminished, it may be perceptible if produced at a sufficient tone.

In this form of hearing loss, the bone conduction threshold is normal (less than 20 dB HL) while the air conduction threshold is increased resulting in what is called an air/bone gap (ABG). By definition, an ABG of more than 15 dB HL averaged over 500, 1000 and 2000 Hz is considered a conductive hearing loss [8].

Sensorineural hearing loss is associated with a pathological change, damage, or dysfunction in the structures within the inner ear or in the cochlear nerve. When the neural elements involved in the conduction or interpretation of nerve impulses originating in the cochlea are damaged or are dysfunctional, then either the perception or the interpretation of sound is impaired. The pure tone audiometry shows an increase of air and bone conductions thresholds (more than 20 dB HL), however, the ABG is less than 15 dB HL [8]. Sensorineural hearing loss may further divided into the following subcategories:

a. Sensory hearing loss occurs from an impairment confined to cochlea.
b. Neural hearing loss is related to the impairment of the cochlear nerve.
c. Central hearing loss (a rare occurrence of sensorineural) is a result of a deformity of the central nerve system rostral to the cochlear nerve.

Mixed hearing loss refers to hearing loss of a mixed nature, conductive and sensorineural. On pure tone audiometry, air and bone conduction thresholds are greater than 20 dB with an ABG of 15 dB HL or more.

Some forms of hearing loss may follow certain pattern according to the involved frequencies, such as low frequencies hearing loss (affecting selectively frequencies less than 500 Hz), mid frequencies or U-shaped hearing loss (from 500 to 2000 Hz) and High frequencies or sloping hearing loss (frequencies 2000-8000 Hz).

Furthermore, hearing loss can be defined as temporary or permanent. Temporary hearing loss is most commonly of the conductive type (although not always), for example, otitis media with effusion and otosclerosis, which can be reversed spontaneously, medically or by surgical management. Permanent hearing loss on the other hand is not reversible and cannot be restored medically or surgically.

Various forms of hearing loss can be bilateral or unilateral (asymmetrical hearing loss) affecting only one ear. Studies regarding Audiometric Asymmetric hearing loss define it as a difference of 15 dB HL or more in at least two frequencies with a pure tone average less than 20 dB HL of the better ear [8].

Finally, hearing loss can be described as progressive if the hearing threshold deteriorates by greater than 15 dB HL within a 10-year period [8].

## AUDIOLOGY WORKUP

### Objective Tests

### *1. Auditory Brainstem Responses (ABR)*

ABR test the auditory response to an external auditory stimulus. Results are plotted as waveforms representing the action potentials generated by the cochlear nerve up to the higher brain auditory centers (Fig. **2**) [9, 10]. Five waveforms are described as early responses representing the auditory pathway and it correlates with the hearing sensitivity in the 1500-4000 Hz range:

- Wave I originates from the cochlea and distal CN VIII.
- Wave II originates from the proximal CN VIII.
- Wave III is believed to correspond to cochlear nucleus in the brainstem.
- Wave IV from the superior olivary complex.
- Wave V originates from the inferior colliculus.

### *2. Otoacoustic Emissions (OAE)*

OAE are produced by the contractile outer hair cells of the inner ear. Positive OAE test indicates a hearing level better than 30 dB HL [10 - 12]. OAE are most commonly used nowadays, among other indications, as a neonatal hearing-screening test for newborns [13].

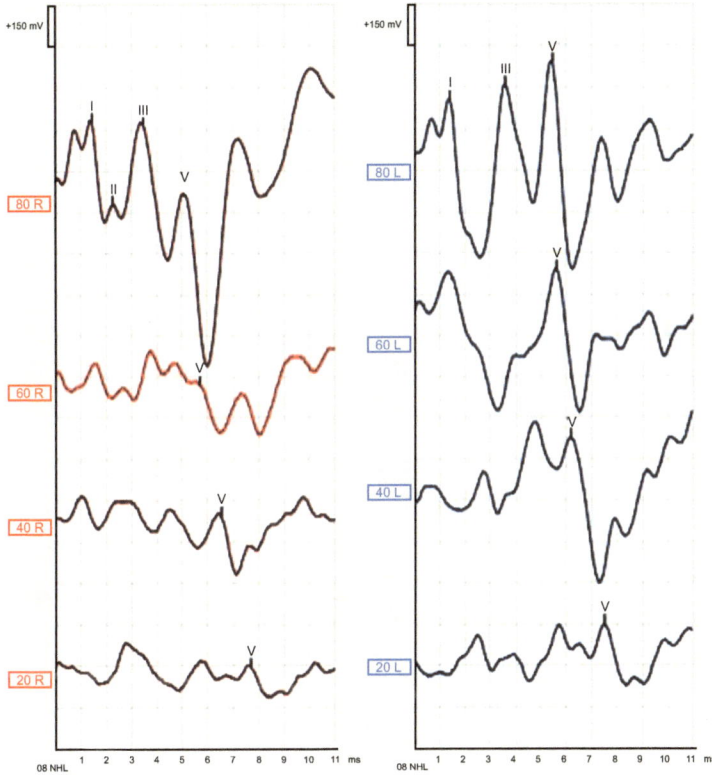

**Fig. (2).** Normal looking auditory brainstem Response, Left ear in blue, Right ear in red.

## 3. Immitancemetry

a. Tympanometry continuously records the middle ear impedance by modulating the air pressure in the sealed external auditory canal [10, 14]. Three finding can be described:

   i. Type A: normal pressure.
   ii. Type B: middle ear effusion.
   iii. Type C: negative pressure.

b. Acoustic reflexes: measurement of the contractions of the stapedius muscle in response to high intensity volume, more than 80 dB HL. It is useful in locating site of pathology along the auditory pathway from the middle ear to the auditory brainstem.

## Subjective Tests

*Pure Tone Audiometry* measures the hearing sensitivity at octave frequencies from 250 Hz to 8000 Hz. It is the most commonly used test to evaluate hearing threshold. An example of blotted audiogram result is shown in Fig. (**3**). This test requires cooperation of the child, which is difficult in young children. So, according to the age of the child, modified forms are used to evaluate his hearing level [8, 14].

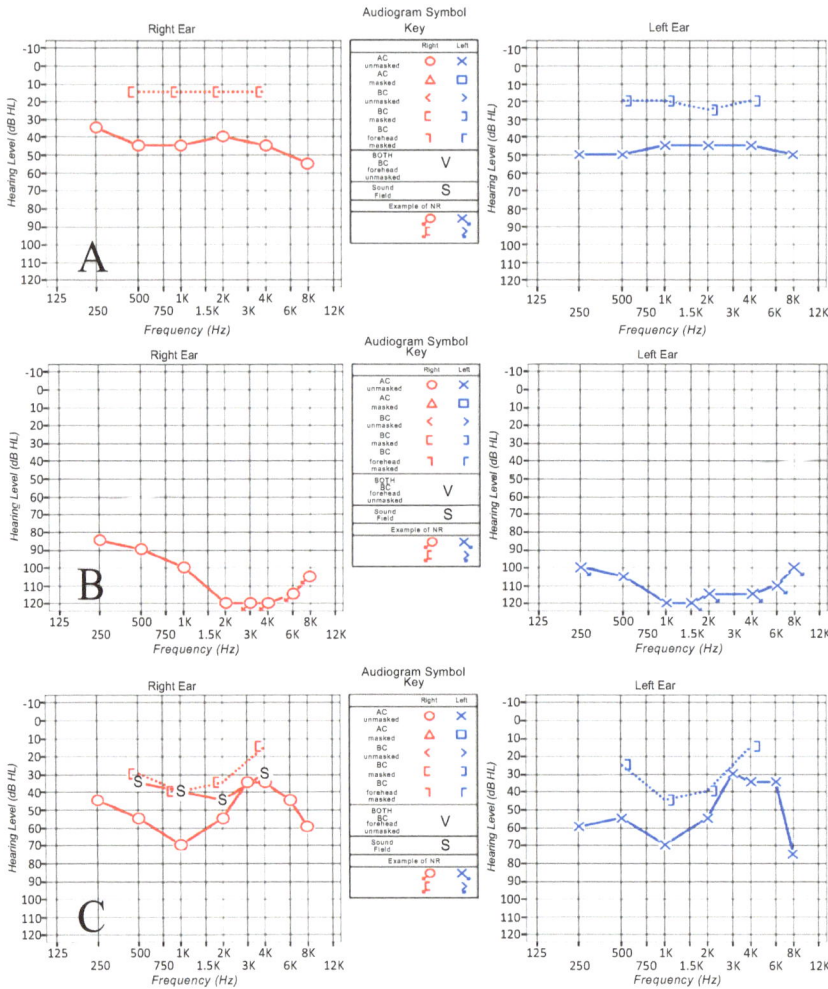

**Fig. (3).** Examples of hearing loss blotted on audiogram, A: conductive hearing loss, B: Sensorineural hearing loss and C: Mixed hearing loss.

A. Behavioral Audiometry: for children less than 3 years of age.
   i. Behavioral observational audiometry: for children less than 6 months of age. A skillful audiologist can detect the hearing impaired child.
   ii. Visual reinforcement audiometry: from 6 months to 3 years of age. In cooperative children, an audiogram can be obtained to determine the hearing level.

B. Conventional Audiometry:
  i. Conditional play audiometry: for children between 3 and 5 years of age.
  ii. Pure tone audiometry and speech audiometry: for children more than 5 years of age.

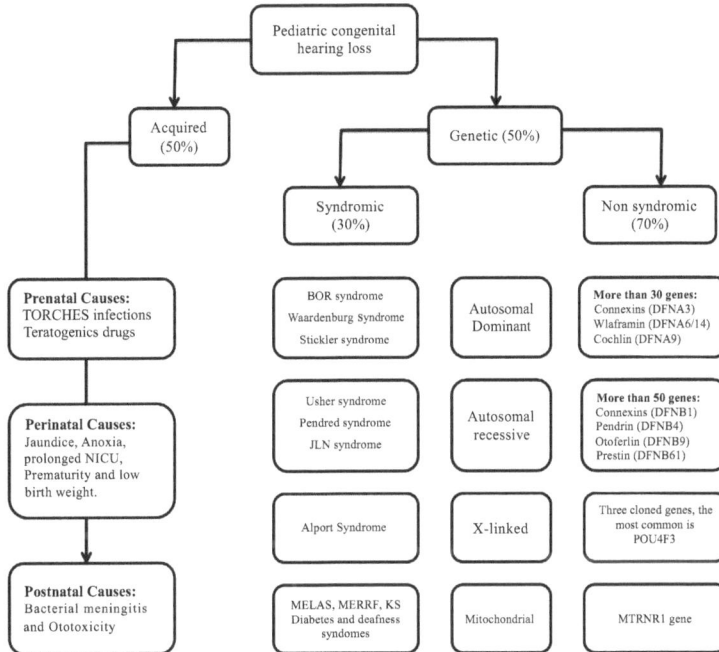

**Fig. (4).** A diagram showing the pediatric causes of hearing loss.
BOR: branchio-oto-renales JLN: Jervell and Lange-Nielsen MELAS: Mitochondrial myopathy, encephalopathy, lactic acidosis MERRF: Myoclonic epilepsy with ragged-red fibers KS: Klinefelter

## HEARING LOSS ETIOLOGIES

Causes of pediatric congenital hearing loss fall into two main categories: genetic and acquired (Fig. **4**) [15 - 25]. Identifying the cause can be achieved in more than 50% of the cases. Proper diagnosis can provide the caregiver and the child's family great support in planning appropriate rehabilitation, and anticipating the hearing sense prognosis. It is important to differentiate between acquired causes that occur during the prenatal period (*i.e.,* as TORCHES infections), and perinatal period (*i.e.,* Jaundice, prolonged NICU, *etc.,*) from truly occurring acquired postnatal causes (such as otitis media with effusion, trauma and meningitis) [26]. Almost half of the congenital hearing loss occurrences in children are acquired and may present with late onset with varying degrees, either pre or post lingual hearing loss [26].

This classification is helpful to reach the proper diagnosis. However for management purposes, it is not as much helpful because many of those causes can present with different forms of hearing loss and consequently different treatment [15]. For example, Pendred syndrome (an autosomal recessive syndromic disease which accounts for 7.5% of all congenital hearing loss) may present with variable degrees of hearing loss from mild to profound, pre or post lingually [27]. Another example is Cytomegalovirus infection, which is the most common cause of non-genetic sensorineural hearing loss [28]. Only 10% are symptomatic at birth while the majority of infected children present with late onset mild to profound, unilateral or bilateral and pre- or postlingual hearing loss [29]. Consequently, when treating a hearing-impaired child, it is wise to consider the type and degree of hearing loss rather than the cause. However, the etiological workup provides as substantial role in preventive management such as in children with enlarged vestibular aqueduct (EVA). Once the diagnosis is made by high resolution CT scan (midpoint diameter more than 1.5 mm), parents are advised to keep the child away from contact sports because any head trauma might exacerbate the degree of hearing loss [30, 31].

## IIEARING LOSS REHABILITATION

Hearing rehabilitation is dependent on the severity and type of hearing loss rather than the etiology. The most common scenario in profoundly deaf children is when parents seek medical advice at approximately 3 to 6 months of age because the child is not responding to sounds stimuli. In milder forms or progressive forms of hearing loss, diagnosis might be delayed beyond that. Moreover, it is not uncommon to diagnose unilateral forms of hearing loss at toddler's age because the child has normal contralateral hearing and acquire normal speech.

For the child to develop normal speech it is important to have a normal or near normal auditory stimulation during the first 5 years of age, which is the speech acquisition period. Moreover, Children with profound sensorineural hearing loss have the maximum benefit if they were rehabilitated during the first 24 months of age [32, 33].

### Medical/Surgical Rehabilitation

Conductive hearing loss due to otitis media with effusion, for example, can be corrected either medically (Antibiotics +/- corticotherapy) or surgically (transtympanic ventilation tubes +/- adenoidectomy) [34]. Other causes, such as juvenile otosclerosis are correctable surgically by stapedectomy [35]. External auditory canal (EAC) atresia traditionally is managed surgically by re-permeating the EAC. However, recently the rehabilitation may also be achieved surgically by bone conduction prosthesis such as bone-anchored hearing aids [36 - 38].

## Prosthetic Rehabilitation

In cases where medical of surgical rehabilitation is not possible, hearing restoration can be achieved through three mechanisms:

1. Acoustical stimulation
2. Mechanical stimulation
3. Electrical / Electro acoustic stimulation

Acoustical stimulation: Hearing aids, a medical device that delivers amplified acoustic signal to the ear, represent this mode of stimulation. It is the most common mode of hearing rehabilitation [39]. It works by amplifying acoustic signals through air conduction pathway. Recent model of hearing aids are powerful enough to fit for wide range of hearing loss up to severe degree. However it has some limitations such as: anatomical abnormality (EAC atresia), infections (chronic otorrhea), skin disorders (EAC eczema) and profound sensorineural hearing loss.

Many styles of hearing aids are available and the choice of one style over another may depend on its functionality or for cosmetic reasons:

1. Behind the ear (BTE) aids.
2. In the ear (ITE) aids.
3. In the canal (ITC) aids.
4. Completely in the canal (CIC) aids.
5. For patients with special needs:

 i. Body aids.
ii. Eyeglass aids.

Children who present with unilateral hearing loss (single sided deafness) may be aided through contralateral routing of signal (CROS) amplification. In this style, the child wears two hearing aids; the sound signal is received through the hearing aid of the deaf ear and rerouted through Bluetooth signal to the normal ear [40].

### *Components and Function*

Basic components of most hearing aids include: a microphone, an amplifier, a receiver, battery, volume control and on-off switch (Fig. **5**). The role of each structure is reported in Fig. (**6**).

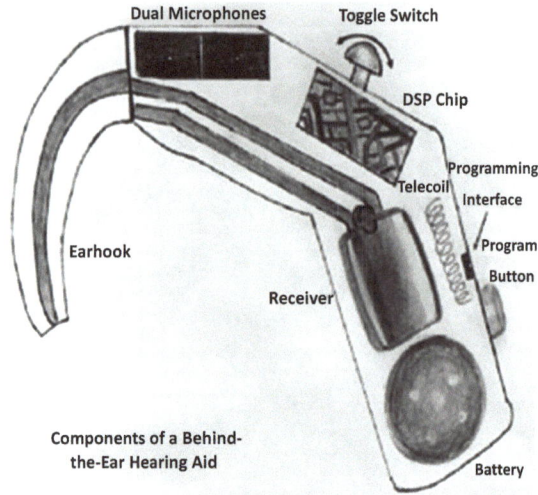

**Fig. (5).** Schematic drawing showing the components of the classical form of the hearing aid.

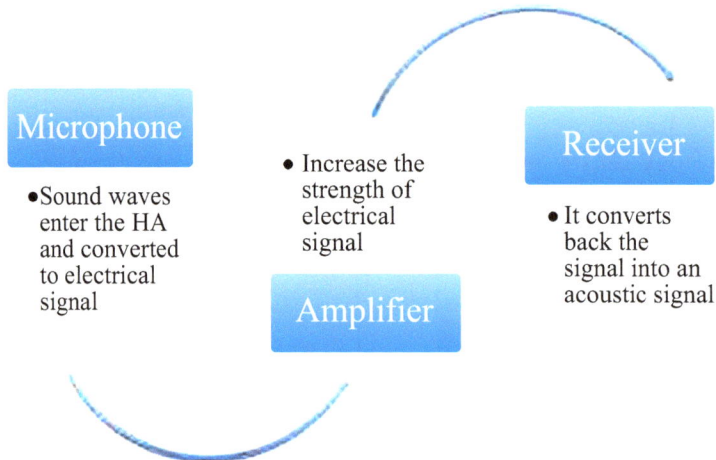

**Fig. (6).** This diagram shows the function of the different part of the hearing aid.

## Mechanical Stimulation

This mode of rehabilitation uses the bone conduction pathway for hearing restoration. In cases where acoustic stimulation (hearing aids) is not appropriate, mechanical stimulation through bone conduction is indicated [41 - 43].

The Bone-Anchored Hearing Aids are prostheses implanted surgically in the temporal bone that allow for the transmission of sound waves to the ipsilateral cochlea through direct bone conduction. Another mechanism of hearing restoration in patients with single sided deafness is through sound transfer to a normal contralateral cochlea across the skull [42]. However, in young children, where the temporal bone thickness is less than 3 mm, it is surgically contraindicated due to technical difficulties. Alternatively, it can be attached over a headband until the age of 4 to 5 years. Indication for mechanical stimulation includes single sided deafness, mild to severe conductive or mixed hearing loss, external ear pathologies such as atresia or eczema and chronic otorrhea [36].

## Electrical Stimulation

### *Cochlear Implants*

Also referred to as Bionic ear (Bionic being defined as application of technology and engineering to biological system). Cochlear implant is an electronic device that transmits sound to the central auditory system (cochlear nerve) by passing the external/middle and inner ears (Fig. 7) [44]. This makes it different from hearing aids, which simply amplifies the sound signal reaching the inner ear through external auditory canal and middle ears. Additionally, cochlear implant is composed of two parts, one is surgically implanted under the skin and the other is worn externally, whereas hearing aids are only worn externally.

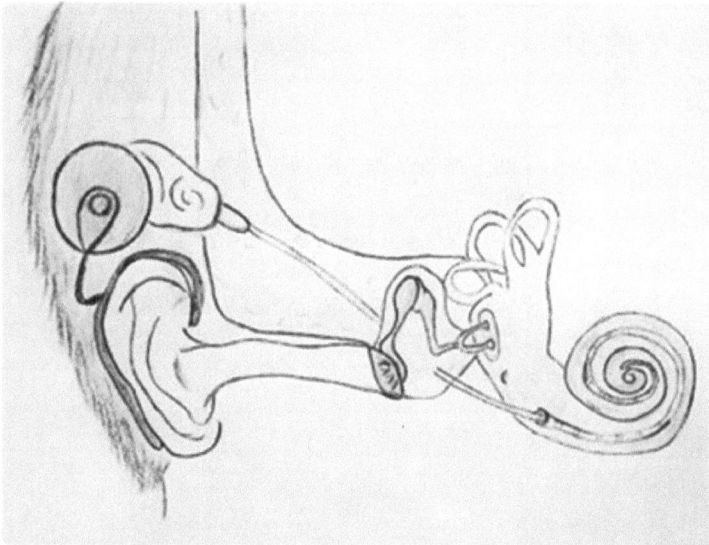

**Fig. (7).** Components of the cochlear implant:

In recent years, the number of children receiving cochlear implant for profound sensorineural hearing loss has significantly increased. The implementation of neonatal hearing screening programs has led to a very early diagnosis of hearing loss and consequently earlier age of implantation. The encouraging results, continuous technology improvement and increased awareness of its safety have resulted in global increase in cochlear implant recipients [32, 45]. There has been a lot of research on the advantages of early implantation suggesting that children receiving cochlear implant before the age of two may catch up with their normal peers [46].

### *Auditory Brain Stem Implant (ABI)*

It was developed in the 1970s, initially for patient with neurofibromatosis type 2. The indications of ABI are expanded to children who are not candidates of cochlear implants due cochlear agenesis, labyrinthitis ossificans or cochlear nerve agenesis. Although the results are less spectacular compared to cochlear implants, it may provide some degree of speech perception [47].

## CONCLUSION

Hearing loss has a significant impact on the child and his family. It limits the normal acquisition of speech and interferes with the child educational performance. Rehabilitation is available to almost all kinds and degrees of hearing loss if diagnosed and managed in a timely manner. For that, we need to increase the awareness of the families and health care providers as well about the screening programs and advocate its implementation in all maternity and child care centers.

## CONFLICT OF INTEREST

The authors declares no conflict of interest, financial or otherwise.

## ACKNOWLEDGEMENTS

We acknowledge Dr Tagrid Alrashidi for her contribution to this chapter by providing the drawings

## REFERENCES

[1]    Smith RJ, Bale JF, White KR. Sensorineural hearing loss in children. Lancet Lond Engl 2005; 365(9462): 879-90.
       [http://dx.doi.org/10.1016/S0140-6736(05)71047-3]

[2]    Davis AC. The prevalence of hearing impairment and reported hearing disability among adults in Britain. Int J Epidemiol 1989; 18(4): 911-7.
       [http://dx.doi.org/10.1093/ije/18.4.911]

[3]    WHO | Deafness and hearing loss [Internet]. WHO. Available from: http://www.who.int/ mediacentre/factsheets/fs300/en/ , [cited 2016 Apr 18];

[4]    Lescanne E, Al Zahrani M, Bakhos D, Robier A, Morinière S. Revision surgeries and medical interventions in young cochlear implant recipients. Int J Pediatr Otorhinolaryngol 2011; 75(10): 1221-4.

[http://dx.doi.org/10.1016/j.ijporl.2011.07.003]

[5]     Tharpe AM, Gustafson S. Management of Children with Mild, Moderate, and Moderately Severe Sensorineural Hearing Loss. Otolaryngol Clin North Am 2015; 48(6): 983-94.
[http://dx.doi.org/10.1016/j.otc.2015.07.005]

[6]     Katbamna B, Crumpton T, Patel DR. Hearing impairment in children. Pediatr Clin North Am 2008; 55(5): 1175-88. [ix.].
[http://dx.doi.org/10.1016/j.pcl.2008.07.008]

[7]     Iseli C, Buchman CA. Management of Children with Severe, Severe-profound, and Profound Sensorineural Hearing Loss. Otolaryngol Clin North Am 2015; 48(6): 995-1010.
[http://dx.doi.org/10.1016/j.otc.2015.06.004]

[8]     Katz J. Handbook of Clinical Audiology. 7th ed., Philadelphia: Wolters Kluwer Health 2015.

[9]     Auditory Brainstem Response Audiometry , 2013 Nov 7; [cited 2014 Sep 10]; Available from: http://emedicine.medscape.com/article/836277-overview#aw2aab6b3

[10]    Hall JW, Mueller HG. Audiologists' Desk Reference A Singular Audiology Text. San Diego: Singular Pub.Group 1997; Vol. I.

[11]    Kemp DT. Otoacoustic emissions, their origin in cochlear function, and use. Br Med Bull 2002; 63: 223-41.
[http://dx.doi.org/10.1093/bmb/63.1.223]

[12]    Otoacoustic Emissions , 2012 Jun 17; [cited 2014 Sep 10]; Available from: http://emedicine.medscape.com/article/835943-overview

[13]    Colella-Santos MF, Hein TAD, de Souza GL, do Amaral MIR, Casali RL. Newborn hearing screening and early diagnostic in the NICU. BioMed Res Int 2014; 2014: 845308.
[http://dx.doi.org/10.1155/2014/845308]

[14]    Jr JB, Wackym PA. Ballenger's Otorhinolaryngology Head and Neck Surgery. 17th edition., Shelton, Conn.; Hamilton, Ont.; London: Pmph USA 2008.

[15]    Alzahrani M, Tabet P, Saliba I. Pediatric hearing loss: common causes, diagnosis and therapeutic approach. Minerva Pediatr 2015; 67(1): 75-90.

[16]    Cummings Otolaryngology - Head and Neck Surgery. 3-Volume Set: Expert Consult: Online and Print, 5e 5 edition. Philadelphia: Mosby 2010.

[17]    Lammens F, Verhaert N, Devriendt K, Debruyne F, Desloovere C. Aetiology of congenital hearing loss: a cohort review of 569 subjects. Int J Pediatr Otorhinolaryngol 2013; 77(9): 1385-91.
[http://dx.doi.org/10.1016/j.ijporl.2013.06.002]

[18]    Morton NE. Genetic epidemiology of hearing impairment. Ann N Y Acad Sci 1991; 630: 16-31.
[http://dx.doi.org/10.1111/j.1749-6632.1991.tb19572.x]

[19]    Reardon W. Genetic deafness. J Med Genet 1992; 29(8): 521-6.
[http://dx.doi.org/10.1136/jmg.29.8.521]

[20]    Rehm HL. A genetic approach to the child with sensorineural hearing loss. Semin Perinatol 2005; 29(3): 173-81.
[http://dx.doi.org/10.1053/j.semperi.2004.12.002]

[21]    Schrijver I. Hereditary non-syndromic sensorineural hearing loss: transforming silence to sound. J Mol Diagn JMD 2004; 6(4): 275-84.
[http://dx.doi.org/10.1016/S1525-1578(10)60522-3]

[22]    Smith RJ, Shearer AE, Hildebrand MS, Van Camp G. Deafness and Hereditary Hearing Loss Overview. In: Pagon RA, Adam MP, Ardinger HH, Bird TD, Dolan CR, Fong C-T, Eds. GeneReviews(®). Seattle, WA: University of Washington, Seattle 1993. [Internet][cited 2014 Aug 17]

[23]   De Leenheer EM, Janssens S, Padalko E, Loose D, Leroy BP, Dhooge IJ. Etiological diagnosis in the hearing impaired newborn: proposal of a flow chart. Int J Pediatr Otorhinolaryngol 2011; 75(1): 27-32.
[http://dx.doi.org/10.1016/j.ijporl.2010.05.040]

[24]   Huang BY, Zdanski C, Castillo M. Pediatric sensorineural hearing loss, part 1: Practical aspects for neuroradiologists. AJNR Am J Neuroradiol 2012; 33(2): 211-7.
[http://dx.doi.org/10.3174/ajnr.A2498]

[25]   Huang BY, Zdanski C, Castillo M. Pediatric sensorineural hearing loss, part 2: syndromic and acquired causes. AJNR Am J Neuroradiol 2012; 33(3): 399-406.
[http://dx.doi.org/10.3174/ajnr.A2499]

[26]   Kenna MA. Acquired Hearing Loss in Children. Otolaryngol Clin North Am 2015; 48(6): 933-53.
[http://dx.doi.org/10.1016/j.otc.2015.07.011]

[27]   Shaukat S, Fatima Z, Zehra U, Waqar AB. Syndromic and non-syndromic deafness, molecular aspects of Pendred syndrome and its reported mutations. J Ayub Med Coll Abbottabad JAMC 2003; 15(3): 59-64.

[28]   Pediatric Cytomegalovirus Infection , 2013 Feb 19; [cited 2014 Aug 18]; Available from: http://emedicine.medscape.com/article/963090-overview#a0199

[29]   Kenneson A, Cannon MJ. Review and meta-analysis of the epidemiology of congenital cytomegalovirus (CMV) infection. Rev Med Virol 2007; 17(4): 253-76.
[http://dx.doi.org/10.1002/rmv.535]

[30]   Saliba I, Gingras-Charland M-E, St-Cyr K, Décarie J-C. Coronal CT scan measurements and hearing evolution in enlarged vestibular aqueduct syndrome. Int J Pediatr Otorhinolaryngol 2012; 76(4): 492-9.
[http://dx.doi.org/10.1016/j.ijporl.2012.01.004]

[31]   Gopen Q, Zhou G, Whittemore K, Kenna M. Enlarged vestibular aqueduct: review of controversial aspects. Laryngoscope 2011; 121(9): 1971-8.

[32]   May-Mederake B, Kuehn H, Vogel A, Keilmann A, Bohnert A, Mueller S, *et al.* Evaluation of auditory development in infants and toddlers who received cochlear implants under the age of 24 months with the LittlEARS) Auditory Questionnaire. Int J Pediatr Otorhinolaryngol 2010; 74(10): 1149-55.
[http://dx.doi.org/10.1016/j.ijporl.2010.07.003]

[33]   Kosaner J, Sonuguler S, Olgun L, Amann E. Young cochlear implant users' auditory development as measured and monitored by the LittlEARS® Auditory Questionnaire: a Turkish experience. Int J Pediatr Otorhinolaryngol 2013; 77(8): 1359-63.
[http://dx.doi.org/10.1016/j.ijporl.2013.05.036]

[34]   Rosenfeld RM, Shin JJ, Schwartz SR, Coggins R, Gagnon L, Hackell JM, *et al.* Clinical Practice Guideline: Otitis Media with Effusion Executive Summary (Update). Otolaryngol--Head Neck Surg Off J Am Acad Otolaryngol-. Head Neck Surg 2016; 154(2): 201-14.
[http://dx.doi.org/10.1177/0194599815624407]

[35]   Vincent R, Wegner I, Vonck BM, Bittermann AJ, Kamalski DM, Grolman W. Primary stapedotomy in children with otosclerosis: A prospective study of 41 consecutive cases. Laryngoscope 2016; 126(2): 442-6.
[http://dx.doi.org/10.1002/lary.25403]

[36]   Saliba I, Froehlich P, Bouhabel S. One-stage *vs.* two-stage BAHA implantation in a pediatric population. Int J Pediatr Otorhinolaryngol 2012; 76(12): 1814-8.
[http://dx.doi.org/10.1016/j.ijporl.2012.09.007]

[37]   Saliba I, Woods O, Caron C. BAHA results in children at one year follow-up: a prospective longitudinal study. Int J Pediatr Otorhinolaryngol 2010; 74(9): 1058-62.
[http://dx.doi.org/10.1016/j.ijporl.2010.06.004]

[38]   Bouhabel S, Arcand P, Saliba I. Congenital aural atresia: bone-anchored hearing aid *vs.* external auditory canal reconstruction. Int J Pediatr Otorhinolaryngol 2012; 76(2): 272-7.
[http://dx.doi.org/10.1016/j.ijporl.2011.11.020]

[39]   Johnson CE, Danhauer JL, Ellis BB, Jilla AM. Hearing Aid Benefit in Patients with Mild Sensorineural Hearing Loss: A Systematic Review. J Am Acad Audiol 2016; 27(4): 293-310.
[http://dx.doi.org/10.3766/jaaa.14076]

[40]   Hol MK, Kunst SJ, Snik AF, Cremers CW. Pilot study on the effectiveness of the conventional CROS, the transcranial CROS and the BAHA transcranial CROS in adults with unilateral inner ear deafness. Eur Arch Oto-Rhino-Laryngol Off J Eur Fed Oto-Rhino-Laryngol Soc EUFOS Affil Ger Soc Oto-Rhino-Laryngol -. Head Neck Surg 2010; 267(6): 889-96.

[41]   Hol MK, Nelissen RC, Agterberg MJ, Cremers CW, Snik AF. Comparison between a new implantable transcutaneous bone conductor and percutaneous bone-conduction hearing implant. Otol Neurotol Off Publ Am Otol Soc Am Neurotol Soc Eur Acad Otol Neurotol 2013; 34(6): 1071-5.
[http://dx.doi.org/10.1097/MAO.0b013e3182868608]

[42]   Colquitt JL, Loveman E, Baguley DM, Mitchell TE, Sheehan PZ, Harris P, *et al.* Bone-anchored hearing aids for people with bilateral hearing impairment: a systematic review. Clin Otolaryngol Off J ENT-UK Off J Neth Soc Oto-Rhino-Laryngol Cervico-Facial Surg 2011; 36(5): 419-41.

[43]   Shin J-W, Kim SH, Choi JY, Park H-J, Lee S-C, Choi J-S, *et al.* Surgical and Audiologic Comparison Between Sophono and Bone-Anchored Hearing Aids Implantation. Clin Exp Otorhinolaryngol 2016; 9(1): 21-6.
[http://dx.doi.org/10.21053/ceo.2016.9.1.21]

[44]   Forli F, Arslan E, Bellelli S, Burdo S, Mancini P, Martini A, *et al.* Systematic review of the literature on the clinical effectiveness of the cochlear implant procedure in paediatric patients. Acta Otorhinolaryngol Ital 2011; 31(5): 281-98.

[45]   Vlastarakos PV, Proikas K, Papacharalampous G, Exadaktylou I, Mochloulis G, Nikolopoulos TP. Cochlear implantation under the first year of age--the outcomes. A critical systematic review and meta-analysis. Int J Pediatr Otorhinolaryngol 2010; 74(2): 119-26.
[http://dx.doi.org/10.1016/j.ijporl.2009.10.004]

[46]   Tomblin JD, Barker BA, Spencer LJ, Zhang X, Gantz BJ. The effect of age at cochlear implant initial stimulation on expressive language growth in infants and toddlers. J Speech Lang Hear Res 2005; 48(4): 853-67.
[http://dx.doi.org/10.1044/1092-4388(2005/059)]

[47]   Shah PV, Kozin ED, Kaplan AB, Lee DJ. Pediatric Auditory Brainstem Implant Surgery: A New Option for Auditory Habilitation in Congenital Deafness? J Am Board Fam Med JABFM 2016; 29(2): 286-8.
[http://dx.doi.org/10.3122/jabfm.2016.02.150258]

CHAPTER 3

# Overview of Management of Recurrent Tonsillitis

**Suparna N. Shah** and **Harold Pine**[*]

*Department of Otolaryngology, University of Texas Medical Branch, Galveston, TX, USA*

**Abstract:** An understanding of the anatomy and physiology of Waldeyer's tonsillar ring is important to learning as how to diagnose and treat diseases in the upper aerodigestive tract. The physician should have an understanding of the many disease processes that can affect this region and how to treat them. The clinician should be aware of the possible complications of diseases in Waldeyer's ring and the common presentations so these can be recognized and immediate treatment can be initiated. The physician should be knowledgeable of the current indications for tonsillectomy and adenoidectomy and be aware of the potential complications during the postoperative course.

**Keywords:** Adenoidectomy, Adenoids, Clinical guidelines, Nonsuppurative complications, Palatine tonsils, Pharyngitis, Post-tonsillectomy hemorrhage, Suppurative complications, Tonsillectomy, Tonsillitis, Waldeyer's tonsillar ring.

## INTRODUCTION

Infectious and inflammatory diseases of the pharynx, tonsils, and adenoids make up a large portion of childhood illnesses and health care expenditures resulting in two of the most common pediatric surgical procedures today in the United States, tonsillectomy and adenoidectomy. The most common indications for adenotonsillectomy or tonsillectomy currently are obstructive sleep apnea followed by recurrent tonsillitis. In this chapter, we will review pharyngitis and adenotonsillar disease processes. We will review current guidelines to help ensure appropriate referral to specialists. Finally, we will review some pitfalls in taking care of children with tonsillar disease as well as some pearls for those who need help with post-operative management.

### Anatomy

The palatine tonsils laterally, the lingual tonsils anteriorly, and the pharyngeal tonsils also known more commonly as the adenoids posterosuperiorly making up

[*] **Corresponding author Harold Pine**: Department of Otolaryngology, University of Texas Medical Branch, Galveston, TX, USA; Tel: 409-772-2701; Fax: 406-772-1715; E-mail: hspine@UTMB.EDU

Seckin Ulualp (Ed.)

a ring of lymphoid tissue around the upper part of the pharynx known as Waldeyer's tonsillar ring which is illustrated in Fig. (**1**). All three of the aforementioned structures in Waldeyer's tonsillar ring have similar histology, which leads to the probability of similar function [1].

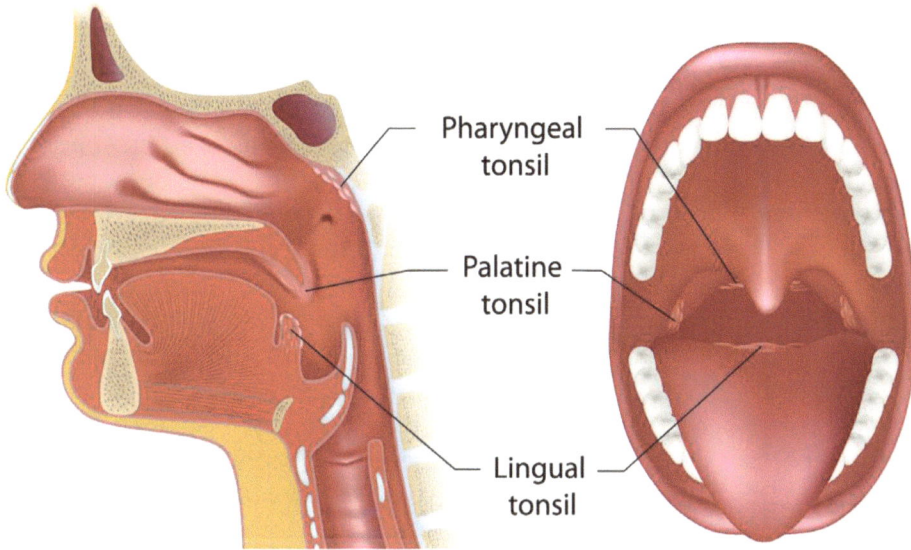

**Fig. (1).** Anatomy of Waldeyer's tonsillar ring, lateral and anterior views [4].

The palatine tonsils are the largest accumulations of tissue and the only structure in this ring with a capsule. The palatine tonsil is more compact than the other structures and consists of tonsillar crypts, which are blind tubules lined with stratified squamous epithelium that extend deep into its core [2]. The crypts are designed to maximize exposure to surface antigen, but they can also hold debris and bacteria causing recurrent infections [3]. The fibrous capsule, which is a specialized portion of the pharyngobasilar fascia, covers the tonsil and forms septa extending deep into the tonsil to conduct the nerves and vessels [1]. Therefore, when surgically excising the tonsils from the tonsillar fossa in which they are housed, the dissection should occur along the loose connective tissue plane between the capsule and the tonsillar bed since the capsule is not easily separated from the tonsillar tissue.

The tonsillar fossa consists of 3 muscles predominantly. The anterior pillar is made up of the palatoglossus muscle, the posterior pillar is the palatopharyngeal muscle, and the base of the fossa is made up of the pharyngeal constrictors, mainly the superior constrictor muscle [3]. The muscular wall of the tonsillar bed is thin and immediately under is the glossopharyngeal nerve and deeper the neurovascular structures of the carotid sheath. Great care needs to be taken to avoid violating the

muscular wall and damaging the nerve during a tonsillectomy [1]. Even without actual damage to the nerve, patients can still experience transient loss of taste over the posterior third of the tongue and referred otalgia caused by edema after a tonsillectomy [3].

The arterial blood supply of the palatine tonsils is primarily based at the inferior pole and consists of several branches from the external carotid artery. The inferior pole is supplied by the tonsillar and ascending palatine branches of the facial artery and the tonsillar branch of the dorsal lingual artery. The superior pole gets its blood supply from the ascending pharyngeal artery and the palatine branches of the maxillary artery. The main blood supply however is the tonsillar branch of the facial artery [5]. Venous blood drains through a peritonsillar plexus into the lingual and pharyngeal veins, which subsequently drain into the internal jugular vein [3]. Lymphatic drainage is to the superior deep cervical and jugular digastric lymph nodes. The nerve supply of the tonsillar region is primarily through the tonsillar branches of the glossopharyngeal nerve and there is lesser contribution from the descending branches of the lesser palatine nerve [1].

The adenoids or pharyngeal tonsils are located on the posterior wall of the nasopharynx and the lingual tonsils are located at the base of the tongue, still within the ring of lymphoid tissue that surrounds the oropharyngeal opening. The adenoids and lingual tonsils are covered by a specialized, pseudostratified, ciliated columnar epithelium that forms plicated surface folds similar to the tonsillar crypts to maximize the surface area of the tissue [3].

The blood supply of the adenoids includes the ascending pharyngeal artery, the ascending palatine artery, the pharyngeal branch of the maxillary artery, the artery of the pterygoid canal, and contributing braches from the tonsillar branch of the facial artery. Venous drainage is to the pharyngeal plexus communicating with the pterygoid plexus and all draining into the internal jugular and facial veins. Lymphatic drainage is to the retropharyngeal and pharyngomaxillary lymph nodes and nerve supply is from the pharyngeal plexus [1].

## Physiology

The lymphoid tissue of Waldeyer's tonsillar ring consists predominantly of B-cell lymphocytes with some T-cell lymphocytes and mature plasma cells. These cells are found in four distinct zones of the adenoids and tonsils, the reticular cell epithelium, the extrafollicular area, the mantle zone of the lymphoid follicle, and the germinal center of the lymphoid follicle [3].

The primary functions of these tissues are inducing secretory immunity and regulating immunoglobulin production [1]. This tissue has specialized endothelium-covered channels that facilitate antigen uptake directly into the tissue, similar to Peyer patches in the colon. The independence of this system from the lymphatics offers an advantage to directly uptake airborne antigens. The location and exposure at the entrance of upper aerodigestive tract allows direct access to foreign antigens maximizing the development of immunologic memory. These tissues hypertrophy during its most active stage from the ages of 4-10 and then regress after puberty. Along with decreasing in size, the tissue still has the same function but not as the same level as in childhood [3].

**Normal Flora**

Establishment of normal flora in the upper respiratory tract begins at birth. Around 6–8 months of age, *Actinomyces, Fusobacterium, and Nocardia* are acquired. Subsequently, *Bacteriodes, Leptotrichia, Propionibacterium,* and *Candida* take hold as a part of the normal oral flora [6]. Anaerobic and aerobic bacteria both exist as part of the oral flora and in saliva. Depending on oxygen concentration throughout the upper respiratory tract, the ratio of anaerobic to aerobic is approximately 10:1.

Healthy children can carry known aerobic pathogens, *Streptococcus pneumoniae* was found in 19%, *Haemophilus influenzae* in 13%, group A *Streptococcus* in 5%, and *Moraxella catarrhalis* in 36% of healthy children. The amount of bacteria is known to decrease as children age possibly due to increased immunity. During periods of viral upper respiratory tract infection compared to healthy periods, the oral pharyngeal colonization for gram negative enteric organisms and *S. Aureus* was found to be significantly increased. Gram negative enteric bacteria and *S. Aureus* colonization during healthy periods varies from 12-18% and 5-15% respectively whereas during periods of illness, the percentages increase to 60% and 43%. A similar increase is seen in healthy *versus* diseased adenoids. Bacterial cultures showed no growth of normal flora in most healthy children *versus* only 45% showed no growth in the infected children. The bacteria found in the diseased state were likely β-lactamase producers [1].

Since healthy children are known to carry aerobic pathogens, bacterial cultures along with clinical presentation are necessary to diagnose any type of upper respiratory infection.

**Infections**

Many organisms can infect the structures of Waldeyer's ring. These include aerobic and anaerobic bacteria, viruses and fungi. Because of the normal flora, most infections in this area are polymicrobial [3]. Most common cause of pharyngitis is viral and the second most common cause is bacterial infection of which the predominant is Group A β-hemolytic streptococcus (GABHS), which causes strep throat [1].

The added complication when addressing polymicrobial infections is that many antimicrobial resistant organisms can aid sensitive organisms by secreting a compound to degrade the antibiotic. In addition, because some patients are carriers of pathogenic bacteria, diagnosis of an infection can be difficult even with a bacterial culture [3].

## *Fungal Pharyngitis*

Oropharyngeal candidiasis, also referred to as thrush, usually presents in immunocompromised patients or patients treated with a prolonged course of antibiotics. Patients usually present with white cottage-cheese appearing plaques on an erythematous base that are adherent to the pharyngeal mucosa and cause bleeding if forcibly removed. Treatment is usually topical nystatin, clotrimazole lozenges, or systemic antifungals for refractory cases along with addressing any underlying disease processes [3].

## *Viral Pharyngitis*

Viral pharyngitis is usually mild in presentation compared to its bacterial counterpart. Patients usually present with a sore throat and dysphagia. Some may have a fever. On physical exam erythema of the pharyngeal mucosa and enlarged tonsils with no exudate are the common findings [1]. The organisms implicated in this disease process include adenovirus, rhinovirus, influenza virus, parainfluenza virus, coxsackievirus, echovirus, reovirus, and respiratory syncytial virus [6].

## *Epstein Barr Virus*

Epstein Barr Virus (EBV) causes the mononucleosis syndrome, which manifests as high fevers, general malaise, lymphadenopathy, hepatosplenomegaly, sore throat, odynophagia, and large edematous tonsils that are covered with a grayish-white exudate and can compromise the airway. Petechiae at the junction of the soft and hard palates is another classic sign of EBV infection but not pathognomonic [1]. EBV is contracted through oral contact [3].

Diagnosis of EBV involves a complete blood count characteristically showing 50% lymphocytosis with 10% atypical lymphocytes [5]. A Monospot test is more sensitive and specific than a heterophil antibody test, which can be falsely negative in the first few weeks of illness [3]. Only 60% of patients with EBV have a positive result within the first 2 weeks and that percentage goes to 90% after 1 month. Some practitioners order EBV Viral Capsid Antigen (VCA)-IgG and VCA-IgM titers. These tests for EBV antibodies are used to help diagnose infectious mononucleosis if a person is symptomatic but has a negative mono test [7]. Treatment of EBV is mostly supportive with intravenous fluids and rest. Care should be taken to avoid any excessive trauma to the abdomen while hepatosplenomegaly may be present [3]. Antibiotics would only needed if a secondary bacterial infection is suspected. Amoxicillin should be avoided because a rash could develop even if no prior issues when taking this antibiotic [1]. Finally, an evaluation of the airway should be undertaken to make sure no significant upper airway obstruction is present. If enlarged tonsils cause airway obstruction, then initial management includes a course of systemic steroids. Rarely, a nasopharyngeal airway, nasotracheal intubation, or tracheotomy may be needed to secure the airway [3].

### *Bacterial Pharyngitis*

Group A β-hemolytic *Streptococcus* (GAS) is the most common pathogen causing acute bacterial tonsillitis. This infection manifests with dry sore throat, malaise, fever, cervical lymphadenopathy, odynophagia, dysphagia, otalgia, headache, and chills [5]. On physical exam, erythematous enlarged tonsils with yellowish spots are usually noted but severe cases can have a purulent exudate. Acute streptococcal tonsillitis is primarily a disease of childhood, mostly around the ages of 5-6 but has been shown to occur in children under 3 years old and in the elderly as well [1].

However, how common is bacterial pharyngitis in the many different causes of sore throat? Most patients who seek medical attention for sore throat are concerned about streptococcal tonsillopharyngitis, but fewer than 10% of adults and 30% of children actually have a streptococcal infection. Group A beta-hemolytic streptococci (GAS) are most often responsible for bacterial tonsillopharyngitis, although Neisseria gonorrhea, Arcanobacterium haemolyticum (formerly Corynebacterium haemolyticum), Chlamydia pneumoniae (TWAR agent), and Mycoplasma pneumoniae have also been suggested as possible, infrequent, sporadic pathogens. Viruses or idiopathic causes account for the remainder of sore throat complaints [8].

The clinical importance of this infection is not only the frequency of the infection which is the basis of the Paradise criteria which guides clinicians to proceed with surgical management but also as the precursor of two serious sequelae, acute rheumatic fever and poststreptococcal glomerulonephritis [3].

Diagnosis of acute streptococcal tonsillitis is usually made after a clinical exam.

However, distinguishing between streptococcal and nonstreptococcal pharyngitis is difficult with just clinical parameters. Therefore, the gold standard for diagnostic confirmation of streptococcal pharyngitis is a throat culture. However the downside of a throat culture is the length of time to get results which can be anywhere from 18-48 hours delaying treatment and increasing the time children have to be kept out of school or other activities and can spread the infection to others [1]. For this reason, many rapid tests based on ELISA (enzyme-linked immunosorbent assay) or latex agglutination have been developed to detect the streptococcal antigen. These tests can be conducted in the office or hospital setting with results available in minutes allowing treatment to be started immediately. The rapid strep test, though highly specific, is not as sensitive as a throat culture. The accepted clinical standard when a child with high suspicion for acute streptococcal tonsillitis presents is to employ the rapid strep test and if found negative but suspicion is still high, then to proceed with a throat culture [9]. Data from numerous published studies in which a high-sensitivity antigen test (rapid strep test) were evaluated against a variety of gold standards, the sensitivity and specificity of the high-sensitivity antigen test were 95% and 89.1%, respectively which leads to the possibility of a false negative test. Therefore, in these cases, a throat culture is done. The sensitivity and specificity of blood agar plate throat culture were 83.4% and 99%, respectively [10].

Treatment is usually with penicillin; however if no response is evident in 48 hours, then β-lactamase-producing organisms should be suspected and therapy changed to amoxicillin with clavulanic acid, a β-lactamase inhibitor. Another alternative could be clindamycin. For penicillin allergic patients, a suitable alternative is erythromycin. The use of antibiotics shortens the course of the illness but also more importantly minimizes the chance of suppurative complications and developing acute rheumatic fever [5]. Schwartz and colleagues demonstrated that a full 10 days of therapy as opposed to 7 days have lower recurrence rates [11].

**Tonsiliths**

Normally, the contents of the tonsillar crypts drain into the oral cavity, but in deep or stenotic crypts, retained material and bacterial growth can stagnate developing into concretions even if the patient does not have a history of infections in the adenoids or tonsils. Patients with tonsilloliths can present with halitosis or sore throat with whitish, expressible, foul tasting and smelling concretions. Management of this condition initially begins with oral hygiene and attempts to clean the tonsils with jets of water and progression to silver nitrate to chemically cauterize and obliterate the crypts. However, if the condition persists, then tonsillectomy as definitive therapy is needed [3].

## Complications of Tonsillitis

Tonsillar complications can be broken down into 2 categories, nonsuppurative and suppurative. The main nonsuppurative complications include scarlet fever, acute rheumatic fever, and poststreptococcal glomerulonephritis. Fortunately, the use of antibiotics has decreased the incidence of nonsuppurative complications. However, the suppurative complications, which are the result of abscess formation, are still common [1].

### Nonsuppurative Complications

Scarlet fever follows streptococcal infection and is a manifestation due to the endotoxin produced by the bacteria [1]. Symptoms of scarlet fever may include sore throat, fever, lymphadenopathy, a yellowish exudate covering the tonsils, pharynx and nasopharynx, a diffuse erythematous rash, facial flush, petechiae in body folds, and a red tongue with desquamation of the papillae, referred to as strawberry tongue [3]. Diagnosis is made by culture and the Dick test, which is an intradermal injection of the streptococcal toxin [1]. Although scarlet fever is not a severe complication, identification and treatment are necessary to prevent other complications. Treatment is with penicillin [3].

Acute rheumatic fever incidence has decreased in the United States due to rapid treatment with antibiotics of streptococcal pharyngitis, down to 0.3%. This illness usually occurs 18 days after being infected with group A β-hemolytic *Streptococcus*. The basis of this illness involves streptococcal antibodies cross reacting with heart tissue leading to irreversible damage of all 3 layers, pericardium, myocardium, and endocardium. The current accepted management is to place patients on penicillin prophylaxis and undergo tonsillectomy to completely eliminate the reservoir for further infections [1].

Poststreptococcal glomerulonephritis usually occurs 10 days after an acute streptococcal tonsillitis or a skin infection. An acute nephritic syndrome develops at first due to a common antigen between the glomerulus and the streptococcus bacteria. The pathogenic mechanism involves injury to the glomerulus by deposition of the immune complexes and circulating autoantibodies of the streptococcal antigen. Therapy does not decrease the attack rate on the kidney or affect the natural progression. Tonsillectomy may be needed to eliminate the source of infection completely [3].

Finally, a disease has been identified called PANDAS (pediatric autoimmune neuropsychiatric disorders associated with streptococcal infections), which is a set of obsessive-compulsive disorders (OCDs) and tics associated with an acute streptococcal pharyngitis infection. Symptoms include obsessive thoughts and fears, ritualistic compulsions, tics, and anxiety disorders. PANDAS usually occurs within a few weeks of the pharyngotonsillar infection. The working mechanism is a cross reactivity antistreptococcal antibodies neurons in the basal ganglia. Management includes antibiotics and tonsillectomy, which has shown a decrease in symptoms [12].

## Suppurative Complications

Peritonsillar abscesses mostly occur in patients with recurrent tonsillitis or chronic tonsillitis that has not been adequately treated. The bacterial infection of the tonsils extends beyond the tonsillar capsule and into surrounding tissues developing into a peritonsillar abscess [1]. The abscess is usually unilateral and develops in the space between the tonsillar capsule and the pharyngeal muscle bed causing tonsillar displacement to the midline or beyond and reflection of the uvula toward the opposite side [13]. The manifestation of a peritonsillar abscess includes sore throat, severe trismus, dysphagia, odynophagia, and lymphadenopathy [3]. The odynophagia can subsequently cause dehydration and drooling. Treatment is incision and drainage of the abscess. This can be done on an awake patient with local anesthesia. Patients usually find immediate relief and reduction in symptoms after the procedure. A tonsillectomy or Quinsy tonsillectomy, tonsillectomy performed when the patient is acutely infected, may be indicated if the abscess tends to recur [1].

Deep neck infections are another complication associated with acute or chronic tonsillitis. However, with the widespread use of antibiotics, these complications have significantly decreased. Clinical presentations of severe odynophagia, trismus, and shortness of breath should alert the clinician to a possible deep neck infection. On examination, there may be asymmetric pharyngeal swelling extending more inferiorly than the tonsillar region into the hypopharynx. Definitive diagnosis is made by computed tomography (CT) scan of the neck with contrast. Management includes control of the airway if needed, intravenous antibiotics, and surgical drainage of the abscess [3].

## Clinical Guidelines [14]

The American Academy of Otolaryngology-Head and Neck Surgery (AAO-HNS) have released evidence-based recommendations on the preoperative, intraoperative, and postoperative care and management of children 1 to 18 years old under consideration for tonsillectomy. The primary purpose of the guidelines is to provide clinicians with evidence-based guidance in identifying children who are the best candidates for tonsillectomy. Secondary objectives are to optimize the perioperative management of children undergoing tonsillectomy, emphasize the need for evaluation and intervention in special populations, improve counseling and education of families of children who are considering tonsillectomy for their child, highlight the management options for patients with modifying factors, and reduce inappropriate or unnecessary variations in care.

The following statements were made by the panel followed by their recommendation.

Statement 1 – Watchful waiting for recurrent throat infection: Clinicians should recommend watchful waiting for recurrent throat infection if there have been fewer than 7 episodes in the past year or fewer than 5 episodes per year in the past 2 years or fewer than 3 episodes per year in the past 3 years. – RECOMMENDATION.

Statement 2 – Recurrent throat infection with documentation: Clinicians may recommend tonsillectomy for recurrent throat infection with a frequency of at least 7 episodes in the past year or at least 5 episodes per year for 2 years or at least 3 episodes per year for 3 years with documentation in the medical record for each episode of sore throat and one of more of the following: temperature >38.3°C, cervical adenopathy, tonsillar exudate, or positive test for GABHS. – OPTIONAL

The paradise criteria for tonsillectomy as the above statements refer to are detailed in Table **1**.

**Table 1. Paradise Criteria for Tonsillectomy.**

| Criterion | Definition |
|---|---|
| Minimum frequency of score throat episodes | 7 or more episodes in the preceding year, OR |
| | 5 or more episodes in each of the preceding 2y, OR |
| | 3 or more episodes in each of the preceding 3 y |
| Clinical features (sore throat plus the presence of one or more qualifies as a counting episode) | Temperature > 38.3 °C, OR |
| | Cervical lymphadenopathy (tender lymph nodes or >2 cm), OR |
| | Tonsillar exudate, OR |
| | Positive culture for group A β-hemolytic streptococcus |
| Treatment | Antibiotics had been administered in conventional dosage for proved or suspected streptococcal episodes |
| Documentation | Each episode and its qualifying features had been substantiated by contemporaneous notation in a clinical record, OR |
| | If not fully documented, subsequent observance by the clinician of 2 episodes of throat infection with patterns of frequency and clinical features consistent with the initial history[a] |

[a]This last statement allows children who meet all other criteria for fonsillectomy except documentation to nonetheless qualify for surgery if the same pattern of reported illness is observed and documented by the clinician in 2 subsequent episodes. Because of this tendency to improve with time, a 12-month period of observation is usually recommended prior to consideration of tonsillectomy as an intervention.

Statement 3 – Tonsillectomy for recurrent infection with modifying factors: Clinicians should assess the child with recurrent throat infection who does not meet criteria in Statement 2 for modifying factors that may nonetheless favor tonsillectomy, which may include but are not limited to multiple antibiotic allergy/intolerance, PFAPA (periodic fever, aphthous stomatitis, pharyngitis, and adenitis), or history of peritonsillar abscess. – RECOMMENDATION

Statements 4, 5, and 6 are guidelines associated with sleep-disordered breathing and as such out of scope for this chapter.

Statement 7 – Intraoperative Steroids: Clinicians should administer a single, intraoperative dose of intravenous dexamethasone to children undergoing tonsillectomy. – STRONG RECOMMENDATION

Statement 8 – Perioperative antibiotics: Clinicians should not routinely administer or prescribe perioperative antibiotics to children undergoing tonsillectomy. – STRONG RECOMMENDATION

Statement 9 – Postoperative pain control: The clinician should advocate for pain management after tonsillectomy and educate caregivers about the importance of managing and reassessing pain. – RECOMMENDATION

Most practitioners are avoiding Tylenol with codeine and only using narcotics in children with caution and when absolutely necessary. A good regimen to employ for postoperative pain control could be alternating Tylenol and ibuprofen around the clock for the first week in essence to stay ahead of the pain so the patient does not avoid eating/drinking due to pain. In our practice, we have seen a greater number of post-tonsillectomy hemorrhages in children who avoid oral intake probably due to pain and become dehydrated.

Statement 10 – Posttonsillectomy hemorrhage: Clinicians who perform tonsillectomy should determine their rate of primary and secondary posttonsillectomy hemorrhage at least annually. – RECOMMENDATION

Based on the Paradise Criteria for tonsillectomy, we, at the University of Texas Medical Branch, have created the tonsil card featured in Figs. (**2**) and (**3**). The tonsil card is meant to aid pediatricians and parents in keeping track of the number of recurrent tonsil infections and when a referral to an otolaryngologist is warranted. We have provided instructions on the back of the card which can be read in Fig. (**3**) about how to use the card and exactly when a referral to an otolaryngologist should be considered. We hope the tonsil card makes the compliance with the Paradise criteria easier and more accurate as well as takes the guessing out of when surgery may be indicated.

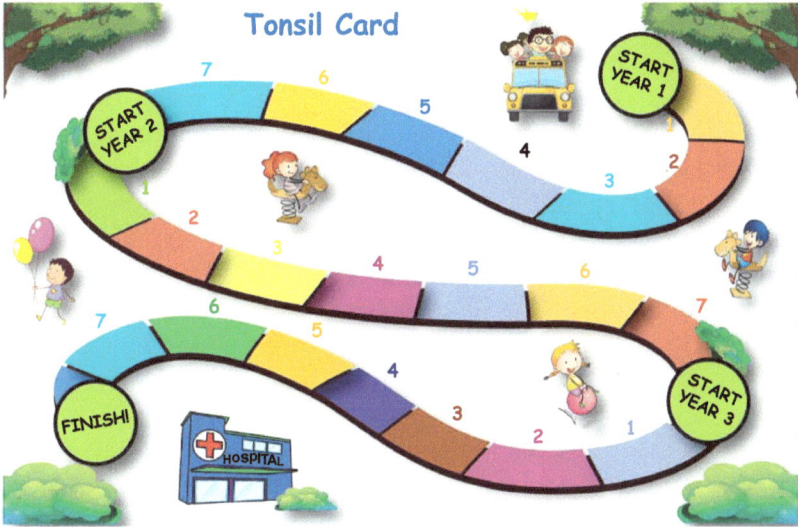

**Fig. (2).** Tonsil card front.

**Fig. (3).** Tonsil card back.

## Management

Tonsillectomy is one of the most common pediatric surgical procedures, more than 530,000 performed annually in the United States [1]. The management algorithm for patients with recurrent sore throat is outlined in Fig. (**4**). The current indications for tonsillectomy and adenoidectomy after significant clinical research due to widespread performance of tonsillectomy based on fear instead of thorough clinical management of complications are listed in Table **2** (indications for obstructive disease is included for completeness even though this topic is not being covered in this chapter). With rapid diagnosis and antibiotic use, the complication rate of tonsillitis has decreased and no longer is immediate tonsillectomy indicated [3]. In all cases, the potential benefits of tonsillectomy should be weighed against the significant morbidity of the procedure and the potential postoperative complications. When discussing a tonsillectomy, the adenoids having the same function and location should also be evaluated. An adenoidectomy does not add significant morbidity on top of a tonsillectomy and should be performed simultaneously if indicated [3]. The indications for an adenoidectomy alone are listed in Table **3**.

**Table 2. Surgical indications for tonsillectomy and adenoidectomy [3].**

- Infectious Disease
  - o Recurrent, acute tonsillitis, with 7 or more episodes in one year, 5 episodes per year for 2 years, or 3 episodes per year for 3 years
  - o Recurrent, acute tonsillitis with recurrent febrile seizures, or cardiac valvular disease
  - o Chronic tonsillitis, unresponsive to medical therapy or local measures
  - o Peritonsillar abscess with history of tonsillar infections
- Obstructive Disease
  - o Heroic snoring with chronic mouth breathing
  - o Obstructive sleep apnea or sleep disturbances
  - o Adenotonsillar hypertrophy with dysphagia or speech abnormalities
  - o Adenotonsillar hypertrophy with craniofacial growth or occlusive abnormalities
  - o Mononucleosis with obstructive tonsillar hypertrophy, unresponsive to steroids
- Other
  - o Asymmetric growth or tonsillar lesion suspicious for neoplasm (with adenoidectomy)

**Table 3. Surgical indications for adenoidectomy [3].**

- Infectious Disease
  - o Adenoid hypertrophy with eustachian tube dysfunction and persistent ear infection or middle ear effusion
  - o Adenoid hypertrophy associated with chronic sinusitis, unresponsive to medical therapy
  - o Obstructive adenoid hypertrophy
  - o Heroic snoring with chronic mouth breathing
  - o Obstructive sleep apnea or sleep disturbances
  - o Craniofacial growth or occlusive abnormalities
- Other
  - o Adenoid mass or lesion or asymmetric enlargement
  - o Patients requiring second or multiple sets of ear tubes

Referral to Evaluate for Recurrent Sore Throat

>7 episodes of tonsillitis or streptococcal pharyngitis in the preceding year OR >5 episodes in the preceding 2 yrs OR >3 episodes in the preceding 3 yrs

Recurrent viral pharyngitis OR Bacterial tonsillitis/Streptococcal pharyngitis that does not meet the Paradise criteria*

Continue observation +/- antibiotics as needed for bacterial pharyngitis

Frequency of tonsillitis or pharyngitis worsens

Eventual compliance with Paradise criteria* or presentation of modifying factors**

Eventual resolution as adenoids/tonsils regress as child ages

Tonsillectomy +/- Adenoidectomy

*Paradise criteria - As defined in Table 1
**Modifying factors - Include but are not limited to multiple antibiotic allergy/intolerance, PFAPA (periodic fever, aphathous stomatitis, pharyngitis, and adenitis), or history of peritonsillar abscess

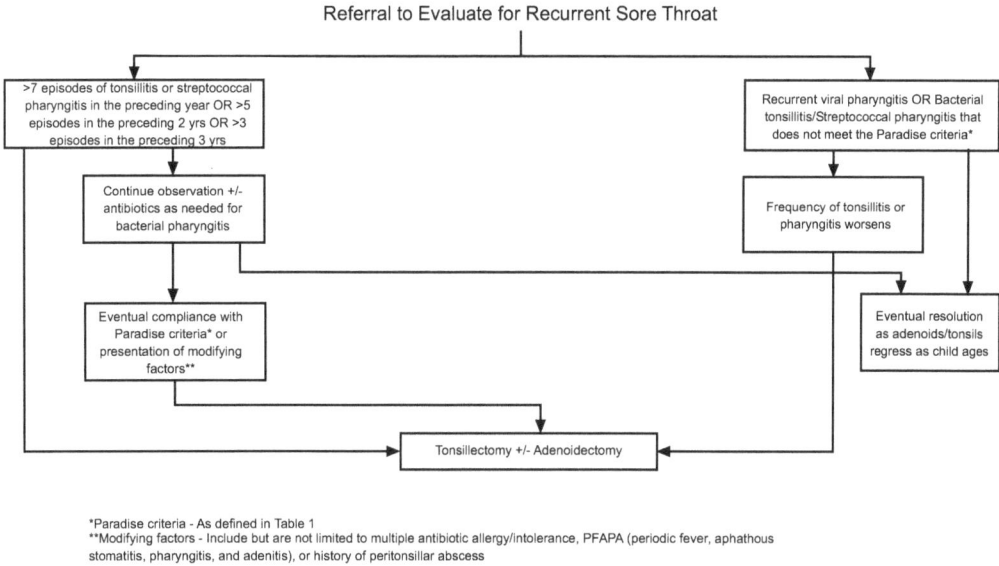

**Fig. (4).** Management algorithm for pediatric pharyngitis.

The tonsillar fossa after a tonsillectomy to the untrained eye could lead some practitioners to believe pathology may be present; however, the tonsillar fossa for a couple of weeks after surgery will have a whitish eschar from the cauterization tool used to excise the tonsil. This could last up to 2 weeks and is normal. The tonsillar fossa on day 8 is depicted in Fig. (5). However, the postoperative course of a tonsillectomy can have significant morbidity and potential complications. Patients experience considerable pain, odynophagia, and general malaise. Recovery can take anywhere from 4 days to 2 weeks. Patients can become dehydrated from the odynophagia and refusal to drink due to pain requiring hospital admission for intravenous fluids. One of the major complications of tonsillectomy, which can be life-threatening due to airway compromise is post-tonsillectomy hemorrhage [15]. A traditional adenoidectomy involves removal of the adenoid tissue under general anesthesia. The morbidity and complication rate of this procedure is low and there is minimal pain [3].

In our practice, we have found the immunological sequelae of a tonsillectomy in children has been a source of concern for many parents. Through our research and clinical practice, we have found that a tonsillectomy or adenotonsillectomy does not have any clinically significant negative effects on the immune system. Furthermore, Bitar and colleagues reviewed 35 separate articles in the literature which included in total 1997 patients and found only 4 studies that suggested a tonsillectomy could have negative effects on the immune system. Even with these few studies, there is enough evidence to reasonably conclude that a tonsillectomy does not have long term negative clinical sequelae on the immune system [16].

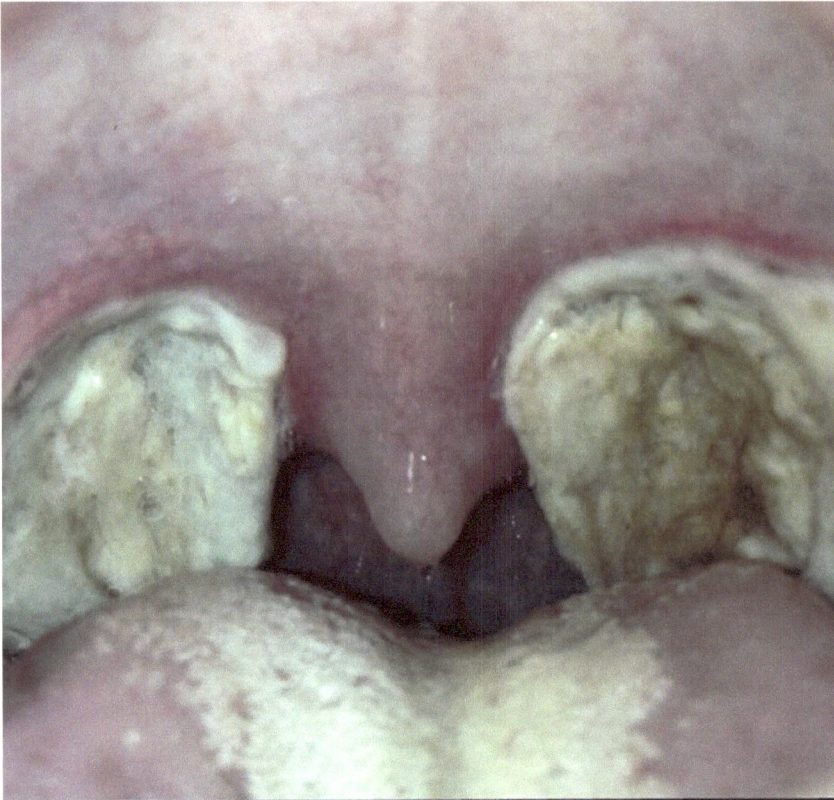

**Fig. (5).** Normal presentation on Day 8 after tonsillectomy [17].

## CONCLUSION

Recurrent tonsillitis turns out to be more of a pediatric condition than adult, possibly due to multiple factors. First the tonsils are more active at a young age when the immune system is developing making them larger in size and more susceptible due to an increase in surface area to a variety of airborne organisms [1]. Second, the location at the entrance of the oropharyngeal airway makes the palatine tonsils the first line of defense for airborne organisms entering the airway potentially on each breath [3]. Also, the anatomy of the palatine tonsil includes tonsillar crypts, which may be necessary for immunological function but also lend to more organisms seeding in the core of the tonsil causing repeated infections [6]. Finally, the normal flora of the oral cavity does include pathogenic bacteria, which are kept under control by other bacteria in the oral cavity, however with antibiotic use, pathogenic bacteria can outgrow their normal concentrations and cause disease [5]. Pediatricians should keep tonsillitis in their differential diagnosis when children are presented with sore throat, fever, chills, dysphagia, general malaise, cough or lymphadenopathy. When tonsillitis is suspected and treatment decisions are being considered, a rapid strep test is a useful tool to get an immediate diagnosis of streptococcal pharyngitis, however, there is a small chance for a false negative. In the case of a negative rapid strep but with high suspicion, a throat culture would be the next step in management. Rapid strep tests help guide treatment decisions and assist clinicians in using antibiotics appropriately without overuse. Many times, children could be present with the above symptoms and have a viral infection which would not require antibiotics. However, because of the possibility of a false negative rapid strep and the inherent nature of throat cultures which take 48-72 hours to provide diagnostic results, some clinicians may choose to treat with antibiotics based on the highly suspicious nature of the child's symptoms [18]. Pediatricians should also keep good medical records of acute streptococcal episodes as these numbers help guide surgical decisions. The paradise criteria explained above has strict guidelines about when a tonsillectomy should be performed for recurrent tonsillitis. When a child meets these guidelines, a referral to an otolaryngologist is necessary for surgical evaluation.

The tonsillectomy continues to be one of the most common pediatric surgical procedures today; subsequently clinical guidelines based on extensive research have been developed to assist clinicians with when the procedure is indicated and its management needs to be carried out [1].

## CONFLICT OF INTEREST

The authors declares no conflict of interest, financial or otherwise.

## ACKNOWLEDGEMENTS

Declared none.

## REFERENCES

[1]    Shirley W. "Pharyngitis and Adenotonsillar Disease". In: Flint Paul W, Ed. Cummings Otolaryngology. 5th ed., 2010.

[2]    Pasha R. Otolaryngology-Head and Neck Surgery. 4th ed., San Diego: Plural Publishing Inc 2014.

[3]    Yelizaveta S, Lee KC, Bernstein JM. Management of Adenotonsillar Disease. Current Diagnosis and Treatment in Otolaryngology - Head and Neck Surgery Anil K Lalwani. 2nd ed. New York: McGraw-Hill Companies, Inc. 2008; pp. 340-7.

[4]    What Are Tonsils? (With Pictures) wiseGEEK Np 2016. Web. 11 Nov. 2016.

[5]    Thompson LD. "Pharyngitis" Head & Neck Surgery - Otolaryngology Byron J Bailey, Jonas T Johnson and Shawn D Newlands. 4th ed. Lippincott Williams & Wilkins 2006; pp. 600-20.

[6]    Regauer S. Nasopharynx and Waldeyer's Ring. Pathology of the Head and Neck Antonio Cardesa and Pieter J Slootweg. 1st ed. Heidelberg: Springer 2006; pp. 184-7.
       [http://dx.doi.org/10.1007/3-540-30629-3_6]

[7]    Carey Roberta B. EBV Antibodies: The Test | EBV Antibodies Test: Epstein-Barr Virus Antibodies | Lab Tests Online Labtestsonlineorg NP 2016. Web. 8 Mar. 2016.

[8]    Pichichero ME. Antibiotic Therapy for Acute Otitis, Rhinosinusitis, and Pharyngotonsillitis. Pediatric Otolaryngology for the Clinician Ron B Mitchell and Kevin D Pereira. 1st ed. London: Humana Press 2009; pp. 9-12.
       [http://dx.doi.org/10.1007/978-1-60327-127-1_1]

[9]    Bisno AL, Gerber MA, Gwaltney JM, Kaplan EL, Schwartz RH. Practice Guidelines For The Diagnosis And Management Of Group A Streptococcal Pharyngitis. Clin Infect Dis 2002; 35(2): 113-25. [Web].
       [http://dx.doi.org/10.1086/340949]

[10]   Mersch John. Rapid Strep Test: Get The Facts On Accuracy Of This Test MedicineNet Np 2016. Web. 17 Mar. 2016.

[11]   Schwartz RH. Penicillin V For Group A Streptococcal Pharyngotonsillitis. A Randomized Trial Of Seven *Vs* Ten Days' Therapy. JAMA 1981; 246(16): 1790-5. [Web].
       [http://dx.doi.org/10.1001/jama.1981.03320160022023]

[12]   Orvidas LJ, Slattery MJ. Pediatric Autoimmune Neuropsychiatric Disorders And Streptococcal Infections: Role Of Otolaryngologist. Laryngoscope 2001; 111(9): 1515-9. [Web].
       [http://dx.doi.org/10.1097/00005537-200109000-00005]

[13]   Bull PD. The Tonsils and Oropharynx. Lecture Notes on Diseases of the Ear, Nose, and Throat PD Bull. 9th ed. Oxford: Blackwell Science 2002; pp. 111-5.

[14]   Baugh RF, Archer SM, Mitchel RB, *et al.* Clinical Practice Guideline: Tonsillectomy in Children. Otolaryngol Head Neck Surg 2010; 144(1) (Suppl.): S1-S30.

[15]   Bull PD. Tonsillectomy. Lecture Notes on Diseases of the Ear, Nose, and Throat PD Bull. 9th ed. Oxford: Blackwell Science 2002; pp. 111-5.

[16]   Bitar MA, Dowli A, Mourad M. The Effect Of Tonsillectomy On The Immune System: A Systematic Review And Meta-Analysis. Int J Pediatr Otorhinolaryngol 2015; 79(8): 1184-91.
       [http://dx.doi.org/10.1016/j.ijporl.2015.05.016]

[17]   Tooke Greg. Tonsillectomy Recovery Tips Tonsillectomy Recovery Tips Np 2016. Web. 17 Mar. 2016.

[18]   Webb KH. Does Culture Confirmation Of High-Sensitivity Rapid Streptococcal Tests Make Sense? A Medical Decision Analysis. Pediatrics 1998; 101(2): e2-2.
       [http://dx.doi.org/10.1542/peds.101.2.e2]

# CHAPTER 4

# Therapies for Pediatric Chronic Rhinosinusitis

## Anthony Sheyn[*]

*University of Tennessee Health Science Center, Department of Otolaryngology, LeBonheur Children's Hospital, St. Jude Children's Research Hospital, TN 38105, USA*

**Abstract:** Pediatric Chronic Rhinosinusitis (PCRS) is a common condition in otolaryngological practice. PCRS remains ill-defined as a condition as it remains difficult to establish as a diagnosis. PCRS may co-exist with other widespread conditions such as allergic rhinosinusitis and adenoiditis. Recent efforts have been targeted at defining this condition and to develop stepwise treatment. A consensus of statement was recently put out defining PCRS as at least 90 continuous days of nasal symptoms with corresponding endoscopic and/or image findings in a patient who is 18 years old or younger. With a working definition, research has focused on developing stepwise treatments ranging from medical management to endoscopic sinus surgery. This chapter focuses on discussing the developed treatments for PCRS.

**Keywords:** Adenoiditis, Balloon sinuplasty, Chronic rhinosinusitis, Endoscopic Sinus surgery.

## INTRODUCTION

Pediatric chronic rhinosinusitis (PCRS) is a difficult, but common problem in the otolaryngologic practice arising mainly from poor understanding of the disease. The differential diagnosis for PCRS includes viral upper respiratory infections, acute bacterial sinusitis, allergic rhinitis, nasal foreign body, and congenital abnormalities such as choanal atresia and pyriform aperture stenosis. Arriving at a diagnosis is often difficult, but a recent clinical consensus statement from the American Academy of Otolaryngology has developed a working definition of PCRS with the intent of helping with diagnosis and guiding treatment strategies. PCRS is defined as at least 90 continuous days of symptoms of purulent rhinorrhea, nasal obstruction, facial pressure/pain, or cough with corresponding endoscopic and/or CT findings in a patient who is 18 years of age or younger [1].

PCRS may also co-exist with other widespread conditions such as allergic rhinitis

---

[*] **Corresponding author Anthony Sheyn**: University of Tennessee Health Science Center, Department of Otolaryngology, LeBonheur Children's Hospital, St. Jude Children's Research Hospital, TN 38105, USA; Tel: (513) 225-2288; Email: tsheyn@gmail.com

**Seckin Ulualp (Ed.)**

and adenoid disease [2] and has the potential to exacerbate asthma, which affects approximately 2-20% of children [3]. Improvements in asthma have been observed in children following surgery for PCRS.

The pathogenesis of PCRS in poorly understood and is likely multifactorial. Mucociliary clearance defects, allergic rhinitis, chronic bacterial infection, environmental factors and social factors all contribute to the development of disease. Over the past 10-15 years, bacterial biofilms have been identified as an additional factor in disease progression [4]. A recent study indicated that a hereditary contribution exists as well. Siblings of patients with PCRS had a 57.5 fold increased risk, first cousins had a 9.0 increased risk and second cousins had a 2.7 increased risk [5].

Anatomic variants may also contribute to the disease process, although controversy still exists. The most frequent anatomic variants noted in CRS are pneumatized middle turbinate, uncinate hyperplasia, deviation of the uncinate, large ethmoid bulla, large agger nasi cells, and Haller cells. Nasal polyps in children are rare, except in cases of CF. Antrochoanal polyps are more likely but still quite rare and may cause obstructive symptoms and rhinorrhea.

In addition to health related problems, the treatment of PCRS is a prominent public health issue and incurs a high financial cost. PCRS visits are second to well child visits for pediatricians. The actual cost of treating chronic sinusitis is difficult to estimate, but over $2 billion is spent annually on over-the-counter medications alone [6].

As our understanding of PCRS grows, treatment options are improved and now occur in a step wise fashion. Currently, long term antibiotic therapy is the first line therapy. Alternatives to oral antibiotic therapy and treatment of refractory disease include a variety of surgical therapies. Adenoidectomy is generally considered the primary surgical therapy. Additional procedures include endoscopic sinus surgery and balloon catheter dilation.

## DIAGNOSIS

The diagnosis of PCRS is based on the presence of specific symptoms present for 3 months or more with associated image or endoscopic findings. The major and minor criteria used for diagnosis are the same as those used for diagnosing acute bacterial rhinosinusitis (Table **1**). The usual symptom complex for children includes cough, nasal congestion, and rhinorrhea [7].

Physical examination should always include an anterior rhinoscopy and a nasal endoscopy. Anterior rhinoscopy is quite often unreliable and very non-specific.

Nasal endoscopy is more sensitive procedure for examining a patient in the office. It allows for evaluation of septal, turbinate, meatal, and nasopharyngeal abnormalities. These areas should be carefully inspected for presence and quality of secretions, presence of inflammation, patency of choanae, nasopharyngeal masses, and adenoid hypertrophy.

**Table 1. Major and Minor Criteria for Bacterial Sinusitis.**

| Major Criteria | Minor Criteria |
|---|---|
| Facial pain or pressure | Headache |
| Facial congestion or fullness | Fever (for chronic) |
| Nasal congestion or obstruction | Halitosis |
| Nasal discharge, purulence, or discolored nasal discharge | Fatigue |
| Hyposmia or anosmia | Dental pain |
| Fever (for acute) | Cough |
| Purulence on intranasal examination | Ear pain, pressure, fullness. |

Radiologic studies are not routinely indicated in the initial management of suspected PCRS. If necessary, imaging should be CT Maxillofacial scan without contrast to examine the paranasal sinuses. While plain radiographs have been described as having a sensitivity of 84.2% and a specificity of 76.6% when compared to nasal endoscopy, it is a challenge to differentiate between a mass, polyp, infection, or mucosal disease in opacified sinuses [8, 9]. With CT, the Lund-McKay scoring system can be used to increase the predictive value of imaging. It is important to consider that in children, a score of 5 is the cutoff for being consistent with the presence of sinus disease [10]. While MRI is better at examining soft tissues, it has worse bony resolution when compared to CT, and is inadequate for surgical planning or intraoperative guidance if sinus surgery is necessary. Finally, it is important to remember that abnormal imaging findings may persist for some time after symptom resolution [11]. In cases of complicated PCRS, especially with suspicion of cystic fibrosis or primary ciliary dyskinesia, additional lab work may be necessary and will be discussed in a later section.

## MEDICAL MANAGEMENT OF PCRS

PCRS is a very difficult disease to treat due to difficulties with diagnosis and the many contributing factors to the pathophysiology of the disease. There is agreement that a step wise approach should be adopted to the treatment of children with this disease, beginning with medical management. Treatment generally begins with antibiotics and adjuvant medical management, progressing to surgical treatment in recalcitrant cases. A recent consensus has also been reached that management of children 12 years and younger is distinctly different than managing those 13 to 18 years of age [1].

## Antibiotics

Long term antibiotics should be the first step in treatment of PCRS. The Clinical Consensus statement came to the conclusion that 20 consecutive days of antibiotics may produce a better clinical response when compared to the clinical response in patients who receive shorter courses [1]. Other authors recommend treatments for as long as 6 weeks.

Empiric antibiotics should be directed at the most common bacteria causing PCRS; gram-positive cocci such as coagulase-negative staphylococci and *S. aureus,* as well as gram negative bacilli such as *H. influenza* and *M. catarrhalis* [12]. First line therapy is usually Amoxicillin or Amoxicillin-Clavulanate. Penicillin resistance is common and is more common in children attending daycare, younger than 2, and those who were recently treated with antibiotics and had a rapid recurrence of symptoms [11]. In penicillin allergic or resistant patients, first line therapy may be a second or third generation cephalosporin or a macrolide. In children older than 6 months, cefdinir has been shown to be just as effective as Amoxicillin-Clavulanate [13]. In penicillin resistant patients, clindamycin and Bactrim may also be effective, especially if *S. aureus* is the suspected pathogen.

Culture directed antibiotic therapy may improve outcomes in those patients who have not responded to long term empiric therapy [1]. Maxillary sinus irrigation and aspiration and middle meatus culture and biopsies are two ways of obtaining specimen for culture. In one study maxillary sinus irrigation had a culture sensitivity of 80% and middle meatus culture had a sensitivity of 73% for pathogenic bacteria [4]. The patients in this study had previously been treated unsuccessfully. Based on cultures they were started on double antibiotic therapy based on cultures and had complete resolution of symptoms between 4.9 and 8.8 weeks.

Intravenous antibiotics have also been described as an additional medical therapy in patients who fail oral antibiotics in hopes of avoiding surgical treatments. Majority of data on IV antibiotics in PCRS is from uncontrolled retrospective reviews. Short term results range from 29-89%, but with a high relapse rate and complications [14, 15]. Complications may include superficial thrombophlebitis, serum sickness, pseudomembranous colitis, and drug fevers.

## Steroids

Adjuvant therapies which have been described for PCRS include topical and oral steroids, antihistamines, nasal saline irrigation and anti-reflux medication with varying degrees of success. Topical nasal steroid spray and topical nasal irrigation have been found to be the most beneficial in treating PCRS [1].

Topical nasal steroids suppress local inflammation and come in a wide variety of formulations with similar efficacies. These medications are typically used in combination with antibiotic therapy. Steroids tend to shorten symptoms but do not appear to hasten resolution of PCRS [16]. Given their long list of potential complications, systemic steroids are not typically indicated in uncomplicated PCRS. The use of systemic steroids has shown utility in the treatment of PCRS with nasal polyps, allergic fungal rhinosinusitis, and PCRS due to cystic fibrosis.

## Nasal Irrigation

Intranasal irrigations with saline are also a useful adjunct to the treatment of PCRS. Children can use irrigations with varying degrees of assistance from adults depending on age. Saline irrigation has been shown to cause subjective and objective improvement in compliant patients between 65.9% and 73.5% [17, 18]. Objective measures were obtained by utilizing CT scans and the Lund-McKay score. Children in the middle age range, between 6 and 8 years of age, appear to have a better compliance rate with this therapy when compared to younger and older children [18]. Reasons for stopping use may include difficulty of administration, aural fullness, otalgia, and little perceived effectiveness.

## Antihistamines

Systemic antihistamines have no proven benefit in the treatment of PCRS [7]. They may provide some relief of symptoms such as nasal congestion and nasal drainage but do decrease the overall duration of the diseases process. It has also been shown that the effects of antihistamines on the nasal mucosa may adversely affect the ability of the nose and paranasal sinuses to manage inflammation and infection [19].

## Gastroesophageal Reflux

There have been multiple studies that have made mention of the relationship between gastroesophageal reflux (GER) and PCRS. In one study, GER was found to be present in 40% of patients presenting with symptoms of rhinorrhea, nasal congestion, and chronic cough based on esophageal biopsies [20]. A smaller study of 11 patients with PCRS and 11 controls with normal CT findings, identified that reflux was much more likely in patients with PCRS than those without [21].

Some small scale studies have found improvements in treatment of GER in the resolution of PCRS symptoms, but these were retrospective and had a small number of patients between them [22, 23].

## Biofilms

The presence of biofilms on adenoid tissue has been implicated in the persistence of chronic rhinosinusitis despite adequate medical management. Biofilms are aggregates present on a surface within a matrix of polysaccharides, nucleic acids, and proteins [24]. Antibiotics may suppress symptoms of infection by killing free floating bacteria that are released from the bacterial biofilm; due to the protective nature of the polysaccharide matrix, antibiotics fail to eradicate the bacteria completely. When the active course of antibiotics is completed, the remaining bacteria may act as a source of recurrent infections [24, 25]. In a study comparing presence of biofilms in children with CRS (who failed at least 4 weeks of antibiotics) and those of children who underwent adenoidectomy as part of sleep apnea procedures, 94.9% of adenoid surface was found to be covered with biofilms compared to 1.9% of surface area coverage in children with sleep apnea and no CRS symptoms [26]. The presence of biofilms may help explain why surgical therapy is the best therapy for patients who fail adequate medical management as discussed before in this chapter.

## Surgical Therapy

### *Adenoidectomy*

Adenoid tissue has been implicated in chronic sinus disease for a very long time. With the identification of bacterial biofilms on adenoid surfaces, removing the tissue has become a mainstay of treatment of medically refractory PCRS. The size of adenoid tissue does not appear to play a role in the presence and/or severity of symptoms [27]. Lack of a size relationship with severity of symptoms of PCRS makes sense because of the growing amount of evidence that shows that adenoid biofilms play a major role in the disease process.

It is agree that adenoidectomy should be the first line surgical therapy for PCRS. It is a quick and easy procedure, which is able to be performed on an outpatient basis and has very few side effects. The effectiveness of adenoidectomy appears to vary with age. Adenoidectomy appears to be the most effective in children up to age 6, with less improvement in those aged 6-12. It is unclear whether adenoidectomy alone offers any benefit in pediatric patients 13 years and older [1]. This may be due to the fact that as children become older the adenoid tissue tends to recede, thereby making it less likely to be a contributor to PCRS symptoms. Tonsillectomy offers no benefit in the treatment of PCRS.

A meta-analysis of nine studies on adenoidectomy revealed that symptomatic improvement was found in 69.3% of patients [28]. In a prior study, 75% of patients who failed medical therapy benefited from an adenoidectomy [29]. Most studies report a success rate of at least 50% or greater, and none report success greater than 75% [29, 30].

There is no clear consensus on why adenoidectomy fails in a large proportion of the population. Ramadan attempted to elucidate reasons for failure in another study. The study found that the mean time to failure was 23.7 months. The best predictors of failure, especially early failure, were age and the presence of asthma. Children younger than age 7 appeared to have a higher and earlier failure rate when compared to older patients. Gender, CT findings, and presence of allergic rhinitis did not appear to be associated with failure [31].

Given the presence of persistent disease despite adenoidectomy, a significant amount of research has been on done on identifying adjunctive treatment which can be done in addition to adenoidectomy. Deckard *et al* investigated two groups of patients. One group underwent maxillary sinus irrigation with aspiration and adenoidectomy and second underwent middle meatus culture and biopsies with adenoidectomy. Both groups were then started on culture directed antibiotics with resolution rates of 94.6% and 92.6%, respectively [4]. Additionally, Ramadan compared children who underwent adenoidectomy with maxillary sinus wash versus those who underwent adenoidectomy alone. Those who underwent a sinus wash had a symptom resolution rate of 87.5% when compared to the adenoidectomy alone group of 60.7% [32]. Other studies have come to a similar conclusion, although the patient number remains low in each study [33].

### Balloon Catheter Dilation

No additional adjunctive treatments have been described and there continues to be a relatively higher failure rate following adenoidectomy, especially in older children. The usual next step was endoscopic sinus surgery (ESS). However, in the past several years balloon catheter dilation (BCD) or balloon sinuplasty has been emerging as an alternative to ESS.

The rise in popularity of BCD is due in part to it being a technique of tissue preservation with less post-operative bleeding and tissue disruption. In one study, patients with persistent symptoms following an adenoidectomy were treated with BCD. Based on pre- and post-operative SN-5 (Sino-Nasal 5 quality of life questionnaire for children) scores, 81% of patients were treated successfully [34].

An earlier study by the same author in children between age 2 and 11 showed no adverse effects but a lower rate of symptom improvement [35].

BCD when performed with adenoidectomy seems to have a beneficial effect when compared to adenoidectomy alone. One study had an improvement in symptoms in 80% of patients who underwent BCD with adenoidectomy when compared to those who had adenoidectomy alone (52.6%) [36].

BCD with ethmoidectomy has also been compared to ESS. Both treatment groups noted improvement in symptoms, with the BCD group noting a higher improvement in symptoms (80%) compared to ESS (64.3%). The authors hypothesize that this may be due to decreased debris following BCD, but the follow-up is short and a small sample size and they state that the results are not statistically significant [37]. Additionally, the improvement in symptoms following BCD and ethmoidectomy may be due to the ethmoidectomy alone and the resultant openness of the osteomeatal complex.

Children with asthma, allergic rhinitis, and GERD were more likely to have BCD when compared to children without those co-morbidities [38]. Additionally, operating room time does not appear to be decreased when comparing BCD with standard maxillary antrostomy and charges to the patient were increased with BCD.

The available literature shows that BCD is safe for treating children with PCRS, but not enough data is available to determine if it is just as or more effective than ESS.

### *Endoscopic Sinus Surgery*

The extent of endoscopic sinus surgery in the pediatric population depends on the extent of the disease as well as the patient's age due to the progressive development of the paranasal sinuses. In the younger population, ESS is generally limited to a partial (anterior) ethmoidectomy and maxillary antrostomy. With increasing age, ESS may include all the paranasal sinuses depending on the extent of the disease.

Prior to ESS, it has been shown that a CT scan of the sinuses is indicated to assess for presence of anatomical abnormalities and extent of disease [1]. Obtaining a CT is also useful if surgical guidance is necessary, which it typically is in extensive disease and revision surgery.

In the past there has been concern that ESS in the pediatric population may effect facial growth. This comes primarily from studies involving animal data. Carpenter showed an impact on piglet facial growth following ESS [39]. Studies of human children have not shown any change in facial growth after pediatric ESS [40 - 42]. Based on these studies the clinical consensus is that there is a lack of convincing evidence that ESS causes clinically significant impairment in facial growth [1].

In an early study by Rosenfeld, 100% of patients who underwent ESS following failed medical management and adenoidectomy reported improvement in symptoms [29]. Most studies report success rate between 82% - 100% [46]. ESS appears to be the most beneficial in these patients as well as those who have anatomic abnormalities which predispose them to PCRS, such as Haller cells, concha bullosa, nasal polyps, and others. Patients with PCRS have been found to have anatomic abnormalities more often when compared to patients with acute bacterial sinusitis [43]

Additionally, in patients with persistent disease it may be possible to manage the remaining symptoms medically following ESS. In a long term follow-up study (6 months – 9 years), 44% of patients experienced persistent mucosal disease but all were able to be managed medically [44]. Only 3 patients out of 115 required revision surgery.

Timing of ESS in terms of symptom duration has also been investigated. No statistically significant difference has been noted in terms of success, although a higher success rate was found in children who underwent ESS with symptom duration between 6 and 12 months when compared to children with symptom duration of less than 6 months or greater than 12 months [45].

ESS is an effective and safe procedure in the treatment of PCRS. The complication rate has been reported to be 1.4% in a review of multiple studies [46]. However, it should be reserved for those patients who have failed medical management, adenoidectomy, or both.

**Special Considerations**

*Cystic Fibrosis*

Involvement of the nose and paranasal sinuses nears 100% in patients with cystic fibrosis. Nasal polyposis in children is considered to be cystic fibrosis until proven otherwise, and indeed two-thirds of patients with CF have nasal polyposis [47]. The treatment of CF associated PCRS involves medical and surgical management that is beyond the scope of this chapter but does deserve some discussion.

Medical management typically involves nasal toilet, intranasal steroids, topical steroids, and nasal saline irrigation. Recombinant enzymes have also been used with some success. Surgical therapy is typically reserved for nasal polyposis or PCRS symptoms not responding to medical management. ESS in CF patient does not improve pulmonary function testing, but do decrease the number of inpatient hospital days and nasal symptoms [48].

## CONCLUSION

Pediatric chronic rhinosinusitis is a complicated disorder but recent literature has helped define clearer diagnostic criteria. The treatment approach should employ a step wise protocol beginning with medical management including antibiotics and adjuvant therapies such as topical steroids and nasal saline irrigation. Surgical management should be employed in those who fail medical therapy. Primary surgical therapy has clearly been defined to be adenoidectomy, followed by endoscopic sinus surgery if necessary. Additional therapies, such as balloon catheter dilation requires further research to determine effectiveness.

## CONFLICT OF INTEREST

The author declares no conflict of interest, financial or otherwise.

## ACKNOWLEDGEMENTS

Declared none.

## REFERENCES

[1]    Brietzke SE, Shin JJ, Choi S, *et al.* Clinical Consensus statement: Pediatric Chronic Rhinosinusitis. Otolaryngol Head Neck Surg 2014; 151(4): 543-54.
[http://dx.doi.org/10.1177/0194599814549302]

[2]    Smart BA. The impact of allergic and non-allergic rhinitis on pediatric sinusitis. Curr Allergy Asthma Rep 2006; 6: 221-7.
[http://dx.doi.org/10.1007/s11882-006-0038-z]

[3]    Larsson M, Hagerhed-Engman L, Sigsgaard T, *et al.* Incidence rates of asthma, rhinitis, eczema symptoms and influential factors in young children in Sweden. Acta Paediatr 2008; 97: 1210-5.
[http://dx.doi.org/10.1111/j.1651-2227.2008.00910.x]

[4]    Deckard NA, Kruper GJ, Bui T, Coticchia J. Comparison of two minimally invasive techniques for treating chronic rhinosinusitis in the pediatric population. Int J Pediatr Otorhinolaryngol 2011; 75: 1296-300.
[http://dx.doi.org/10.1016/j.ijporl.2011.07.015]

[5]    Orb Q, Curtin K, Oakley GM, *et al.* Familial risk of pediatric chronic rhinosinusitis. Laryngoscope 2016; 126: 739-45.
[http://dx.doi.org/10.1002/lary.25469]

[6]    Slack C, Dahn K, Abzug M, *et al.* Antibiotic-resistant bacteria in pediatric chronic sinusitis. Pediatr Infect Dis J 2001; 20: 247-50.
[http://dx.doi.org/10.1097/00006454-200103000-00006]

[7]     Magit A. Pediatric Rhinosinusitis. Otolaryngol Clin North Am 2014; 47: 733-46.
        [http://dx.doi.org/10.1016/j.otc.2014.06.003]

[8]     Leo G, Triulzi F, Consonni D, *et al.* Reappraising the role of radiography in diagnosis of chronic
        rhinosinusitis. Rhinology 2009; 47: 271-4.
        [http://dx.doi.org/10.4193/Rhin08.147]

[9]     Leo G, Triulzi F, Incorvaia C. Sinus imaging for diagnosis of chronic rhinosinusitis in children. Curr
        Allergy Asthma Rep 2012; 12: 136-43.
        [http://dx.doi.org/10.1007/s11882-012-0244-9]

[10]    Bhattacharyya N, Jones DT, Hill M, *et al.* The diagnostic accuracy of computed tomography in
        pediatric chronic rhinosinusitis. Arch Otolaryngol Head Neck Surg 2004; 130: 1029-32.
        [http://dx.doi.org/10.1001/archotol.130.9.1029]

[11]    Cazzavillan A, Castelnuovo P, Berlucchi M, *et al.* Management of chronic rhinosinusitis. Pediatr
        Allergy Immunol 2012; 23: 32-44.
        [http://dx.doi.org/10.1111/j.1399-3038.2012.01322.x]

[12]    Brozek-Madri E, Chmielik LP, Galazka A, *et al.* Chronic rhinosinusitis in children – Bacteriological
        analysis in terms of cytological examination. Int J Pediatr Otorhinolaryngol 2012; 76(4): 512-22.
        [http://dx.doi.org/10.1016/j.ijporl.2012.01.008]

[13]    Perry CM, Scott LJ. Cefdinir: A review of its use in the management of mild-to-moderate bacterial
        infections. Drugs 2004; 64(13): 1433-64.
        [http://dx.doi.org/10.2165/00003495-200464130-00004]

[14]    Don DM, Yellon RF, Casselbrant ML, *et al.* Efficacy of a stepwise protocol that includes intravenous
        antibiotic therapy for the management of chronic rhinosinusitis in children and adolescents. Arch
        Otolaryngol Head Neck Surg 2001; 127: 1093-8.
        [http://dx.doi.org/10.1001/archotol.127.9.1093]

[15]    Tanner SB, Fowler KC. Intravenous antibiotics for chronic rhinosinusitis: are they effective? Curr
        Opin Otolaryngol Head Neck Surg 2004; 12(1): 3-8.
        [http://dx.doi.org/10.1097/00020840-200402000-00003]

[16]    Rose AS, Thorp BD, Zanation AM, *et al.* Chronic Rhinosinusitis in children. Pediatr Clin North Am
        2013; 60: 979-91.
        [http://dx.doi.org/10.1016/j.pcl.2013.04.001]

[17]    Pham V, Sykes K, Wei J. Long-Term Outcome of Once Daily Nasal Irrigation for the Treatment of
        Pediatric Chronic Rhinosinusitis. Laryngoscope 2013; 124(4): 1000-07.
        [http://dx.doi.org/0.1002/lary.24224]

[18]    Hong SD, Kim JH, Kim HY, Jang MS, Dhong HJ, Chung SK. Compliance and efficacy of saline
        irrigation in pediatric chronic rhinosinusitis. Auris Nasus Larynx 2014; 41: 46-9.
        [http://dx.doi.org/10.1016/j.anl.2013.07.008]

[19]    Novembre E, Mori F, Pucci N, *et al.* Systemic treatment of rhinosinusitis in children. Pediatr Allergy
        Immunol 2007; 18 (Suppl. 18): 56-61.
        [http://dx.doi.org/10.1111/j.1399-3038.2007.00636.x]

[20]    Nation J, Kaufman M, Allen M, Sheyn A, Coticchia J. Incidence of gastroesophageal reflux disease
        and positive maxillary antral cultures in children with symptoms of chronic rhinosinusitis. Int J Pediatr
        Otorhinolaryngol 2014; 78: 218-2222.
        [http://dx.doi.org/10.1016/j.ijporl.2013.10.057]

[21]    Ulualp SO, Toohill RJ, Hoffman R, Shaker R. Possible relationship of gastroesophageal reflux with
        pathogenesis of chronic rhinosinusitis. Am J Rhinol 1999; 13: 197-202.
        [http://dx.doi.org/10.2500/105065899781389777]

[22]   Bothwell M, Parsons DS, Talbot R, *et al.* Outcome of reflux therapy on pediatric chronic rhinosinusitis. Otolaryngol Head Neck Surg 1999; 121: 255-62.
[http://dx.doi.org/10.1016/S0194-5998(99)70181-6]

[23]   Phipps CD, Wood WE, Gibson WS, *et al.* Gastroesophageal reflux contributing to chronic sinus disease in children. A prospective analysis. Arch Otolaryngol Head Neck Surg 1999; 121: 255-62.

[24]   Coticchia J, Sheyn A, Nation J. The Role of Biofilms in Otitis Media. Otorinolaryngolgia 2012; 62: 121-30.

[25]   Adappa ND, Coticchia J. Management of Refractory chronic rhinosinusitis in children. Am J Otolararyngol Head Neck Med Surg 2006; 27: 384-9.

[26]   Coticchia J, Zuliani G, Coleman C, *et al.* Biofilm surface area in the pediatric nasopharynx: Chronic rhinosinusitis *vs.* obstructive sleep apnea. Arch Otolaryngol Head Neck Surg 2007; 133: 110-4.
[http://dx.doi.org/10.1001/archotol.133.2.110]

[27]   Neff L, Adil EA. What is the rolde of the adenoid in pediatric chronic rhinosinusitis. Laryngoscope 2015; 125: 1282-3.
[http://dx.doi.org/10.1002/lary.25090]

[28]   Brietzke SE, Brigger MT. Adenoidectomy outcomes in pediatric rhinosinusitis: A meta-analysis. Int J Pediatr Otorhinolaryngol 2008; 72: 1541-5.
[http://dx.doi.org/10.1016/j.ijporl.2008.07.008]

[29]   Rosenfeld RM. Pilot study of outcomes in pediatric rhinosinusitis. Arch Otolaryngol 1995; 121: 729-36.
[http://dx.doi.org/10.1001/archotol.1995.01890070015005]

[30]   Ramadan HH. Adenoidectomy *vs.* endoscopic sinus surgery for the treatment of pediatric sinusitis. Arch Otolaryngol Head Neck Surg 1999; 125: 1208-11.
[http://dx.doi.org/10.1001/archotol.125.11.1208]

[31]   Ramadan HH, Tsiu J. Failures of adenoidectomy for chronic rhinosinusitis in children: For whom and when do they fail? Laryngoscope 2007; 117: 1080-3.
[http://dx.doi.org/10.1097/MLG.0b013e31804154b1]

[32]   Ramadan HH, Cost JL. Outcome of adenoidectomy versus adenoidectomy with maxillary sinus wash for chronic rhinosinusitis in children. Laryngoscope 2008; 118: 871-3.
[http://dx.doi.org/10.1097/MLG.0b013e3181653422]

[33]   Buchman CA, Yellon RF, Bluestone CD. Alternative to endoscopic sinus surgery in the management of Pediatric chronic rhinosinusitis refractory to oral antibiotic therapy. Otolaryngol Head Neck Surg 1999; 120: 219-24.
[http://dx.doi.org/10.1016/S0194-5998(99)70410-9]

[34]   Ramadan HH, Bueller H, Hester ST, *et al.* Sinus balloon catheter dilation after adenoidectomy failure for children with chronic rhinosinusitis. Arch Otolaryngol Head Neck Surg 2012; 138: 635-7.
[http://dx.doi.org/10.1001/archoto.2012.1070]

[35]   Ramadan HH, McLaughlin K, Josephson G, *et al.* Balloon catheter sinuplasty in young children. Am J Rhinol Allergy 2010; 24: E54-6.

[36]   Ramadan HH, Terrell AM. Balloon Catheter Sinuplasty and Adenoidectomy in Children with Chronic Rhinosinusitis. Ann Otol Rhinol Laryngol 2010; 119: 578-82.

[37]   Thottam PJ, Haupert M, Saraiya S, *et al.* Functional endoscopic sinus surgery (FESS) alone versus Balloon catheter sinuplasty (BCS) and ethmoidectomy: A comparative outcome analysis in pediatric chronic rhinosinusitis. Int J Pediatr Otorhinolaryngol 2012; 76: 1355-60.
[http://dx.doi.org/10.1016/j.ijporl.2012.06.006]

[38]   Ference EH, Schroeder JW, Qureshi H, *et al.* Current Utilization of Balloon Dilation versus endoscopic techniques in pediatric sinus surgery. Otolaryngol Head Neck Surg 2014; 151: 852-60.

[http://dx.doi.org/10.1177/0194599814545442]

[39]　Carpenter KM, Graham SM, Smith RJ. Facial skeletal growth after endoscopic sinus surgery in the piglet model. Am J Rhinol 1997; 11: 211-7.
[http://dx.doi.org/10.2500/105065897781751929]

[40]　Senor B, Wirtschafter A, Mai C, *et al.* Quantitative impact of pediatric sinus surgery on facial growth. Laryngoscope 2000; 110: 1210-3.

[41]　Bothwell MR, Piccirillo JF, Lusk RP, *et al.* Long-term outcome of facial after functional endoscopic sinus surgery. Otolaryngol Head Neck Surg 2002; 126: 628-34.
[http://dx.doi.org/10.1067/mhn.2002.125607]

[42]　Peteghem AV, Clement PR. Influence of extensive functional endoscopic sinus surgery (FESS) on facial growth in children with cystic fibrosis. Comparison of 10 cephalometric parameters of the midface for three study groups. Int Otorhinolaryngol 2006; 70S: 1407-13.
[http://dx.doi.org/10.1016/j.ijporl.2006.02.009]

[43]　Stokken J, Gupta A, Krakovitz P, Anne S. Rhinosinusitis in children: A comparison of patients requiring surgery for acute complications versus chronic disease. Am J Otolaryngol Head Neck Med Surg 2014; 35: 641-6.

[44]　Barakate M, Havas T. Surgical management of paediatric chronic rhinosinusitis: review of 10 years experience. JLO 2014; 128: S43-7.
[http://dx.doi.org/10.1017/S0022215114000334]

[45]　Ramadan HH. Timing of Endoscopic Sinus surgery in children: Is there an impact on outcome? Laryngoscope 2001; 111: 1709-11.
[http://dx.doi.org/10.1097/00005537-200110000-00007]

[46]　Makary CA, Ramadan HH. The Role of Sinus Surgery in Children. Laryngoscope 2013; 123: 1348-52.
[http://dx.doi.org/10.1002/lary.23961]

[47]　Feuillet-Fieux MN, Lenoir G, Sermet I, *et al.* Nasal polyposis and cystic fibrosis (CF): review of the literature. Rhinology 2011; 49: 347-55.

[48]　Osborn AJ, Leung R, Ratjen F, James AL. Effect of Endoscopic Sinus Surgery on Pulmonary Function and Microbial Pathogens in a Pediatric Population With Cystic Fibrosis. Arch Otolaryngol Head Neck Surg 2011; 137: 542-7.
[http://dx.doi.org/10.1001/archoto.2011.68]

# CHAPTER 5

# Practical Management of Children with Stridor

Anil Gungor[*]

*Department of Otolaryngology- Head and Neck Surgery, Louisiana State University School of Medicine, Shreveport, LA, USA*

**Abstract:** Stridor is one of the most common reasons for referral to a pediatric ENT subspecialist. This chapter is prepared as technical update for the advanced practitioner (neonatologist, pediatrician, family physician, general ENT) as a supplement to existing classic textbook material. In addition to existing established surgical approaches, newer and more conservative treatment techniques are increasingly successful as the primary or adjunct treatment. Surgical and medical practice continues to be shaped by increased awareness of and demand for conservative procedures and higher risk aversion. Management of stridor now requires a greater variety of updated medical and surgical expertise. Increased collaboration between specialists allows for an extended period of interventions and introduces new challenges and perspectives for all involved. - Practical skills for interview, assessment of the severity and cause of stridor are discussed in detail from the perspective of the pediatric ENT subspecialist collaborating closely with several other subspecialty areas.

**Keywords:** Conservative, Indications, Stridor, Surgical.

## INTRODUCTION

Pediatric stridor management presents challenges that require innovative approaches and comprehensive treatment strategies. Reconstruction of craniofacial malformations, obstructive anomalies of the tongue base, nasal vault and choanae are addressed by subspecialists from various clinical and surgical academic traditions who practice variable levels of required communication. Hypopharyngeal, laryngeal, glottic, subglottic, and tracheobronchial obstructions are solely treated by pediatric otolaryngologists who have additional expertise and/or pediatric ENT fellowship training. The increasing viability of children with multiple levels of obstruction and synchronous airway lesions requires close collaboration for intelligent and effective airway management.

[*] **Corresponding author Anil Gungor**: Department of Otolaryngology- Head and Neck Surgery, Louisiana State University School of Medicine, Shreveport, LA, USA; Tel: 318 6756262; Fax: 318 6756260; Email: entforkids@yahoo.com

Seckin Ulualp (Ed.)

## Definitions

Stridor, simply, is noisy breathing caused by airflow obstruction. In general practice, it is used as a catch all term for all abnormal respiratory noise including stertor, snoring, and mouth-breathing. There may be an academic benefit for a more refined description that distinguishes between stertor (upper nasopharyngeal, palatal), inspiratory (more supraglottic noise), bi-phasic (glottic), and expiratory (more subglottic noise) stridors but these have not become part of the descriptive and diagnostic language use of general practitioners. The same descriptive confusion exists for laryngomalacia (more inspiratory stridor) and tracheomalacia (more expiratory stridor); conditions with very different dynamics and etiology. Many practitioners use tracheomalacia to describe any and all stridor. Since all abnormal respiratory noises require attention, using stridor for all as a starting point is perfectly acceptable for referrals. In addition, stridor, especially in very young babies is not present in classical pure form, nor does it stay the same over time. Feeding, secretion control, reflux, body position, fatigue, intervening respiratory illness as well as growth and maturation all change the quality, phase and, severity of stridor.

## Evaluation of the Stridorous Child

Acute stridor in a child is an airway emergency and needs immediate attention. The differential diagnosis includes foreign body aspiration (FBA), epiglottitis, croup, bacterial tracheitis (Table **1**), among others (seizures, trauma, shaken baby, reflux, aspiration *via* ).

**Table 1. Clinical Diagnosis of Inflammatory Stridor.**

|  | Epiglottitis | Croup | Bacterial Tracheitis |
|---|---|---|---|
| **Microbiology** | H inf type B | Parainfluenza | S Aureus, Strep |
| **Age** | 2-6 yrs | <3 yrs | Wide |
| **Onset** | Rapid (hours) | Slow (days) | Slow (days) |
| **Cough** | Absent | Barking cough | Brassy |
| **Dysphagia** | Severe | None | None |
| **Stridor** | Inspiratory | Biphasic | Variable |
| **Temperature** | Elevated | Elevated | Elevated |
| **Posture** | Sitting forward | Lying back | Lying back |
| **Drooling** | Marked | None | None |
| **Voice** | Muffled | Hoarse | Hoarse |
| **X-ray** | Thumbprint sign | Steeple sign | Narrow tracheal lumen |

All FBA suspects need to have an airway evaluation under anesthesia (AE). Epiglottitis is diagnosed clinically and is best managed conservatively avoiding diagnosis in the operating room if possible. Croup and bacterial tracheitis may need AE if diagnostic uncertainty exists.

Congenital stridor suggests an airway anomaly. Mild stridor can be observed while more clinical information is gathered. Feeding assessment, clinical examination of the palate, tongue, jaw, and their proportionality, features suggestive of syndromic associations (low set ears, webbed neck, limb anomalies *via.*) are important. Meanwhile, cardiac and neuromotor evaluations are conducted. If all is normal, and the stridor remains mild, respiration, voice and feeding are not compromised, no apneas, cyanosis or ALTE's are reported, then careful observation is recommended. Most likely cause of this is mild laryngomalacia. Over time, especially about a month after birth, as the child becomes stronger and is able to command larger and faster air exchange, stridor may increase. Careful assessment of apnea, cyanosis, ALTE's, feeding, weight gain, retractions is performed in the office. Assessment of feeding by a specialist is very helpful especially if uncertain about caregivers' report. Feeding assessment should include an evaluation of protective reflexes (cough, gag, palatal elevation), coordination of sucking, swallowing, breathing, detection of atypical suck/swallow ratio, pacing difficulty, and fatigue. If the length of feedings exceed 30 minutes, and non-nutritive suckling is detected, stridor is no longer considered mild.

At this time, careful auscultation of respiratory sounds in the chest and the neck is performed. Most babies tolerate a distress position that accentuates any pre-existing respiratory compromise and provides important information to the practitioner. This position is obtained by placing baby face up on caregivers' knees and thighs while the examiner sits across, facing the caregiver. The caregiver holds baby tightly on her thighs by his arms and elbows to the side. Gentle traction is applied on the mandible by the examiner, causing extension of the neck and blocking baby's view of the caregiver. This position reduces thoracic volume through abdominal shift, and increases respiratory demand in addition to mild emotional distress due to immobilization and inability to see caregivers' face. Most babies will get agitated and/or start crying in a short while, providing the examiner with valuable time for observation and auscultation. The bell portion of the baby stethoscope is then used to listen to various areas in the neck, (both supra- and subglottic) and chest. Phase of stridor, location, closure (complete, incomplete), ability to clear secretions, ball-valving foreign bodies *via.* can be assessed.

Imaging studies are low yield and may even be risky. Children usually can't cooperate for inhalation-exhalation chest x-rays (for radiolucent FBA), and MRI has to be done under sedation while supine, and both of these conditions increase risk for airway collapse. CT scans do not provide enough detail for treatment planning and may expose the child to unnecessary radiation.

Children who are otherwise healthy but have mild to moderate stridor without displaying signs of respiratory distress can be carefully examined in the office with a flexible trans nasal endoscopy. A nasal spray of xylometazoline and lidocaine is applied. Care is taken to evaluate nasal passages, choanae, nasopharynx, tongue base, vallecula, pyriform sinuses, epiglottis, arytenoid and vocal cord mobility without touching the epiglottis or the laryngeal inlet. The subglottis and the tracheal lumen can't be assessed in office. Any child with an underlying systemic disease, craniofacial anomaly, known cardiac or pulmonary compromise, prematurity, failure to thrive – in short any brittle child is NOT a candidate for in-office endoscopy. These children are at high risk for developing laryngospasm, cardiopulmonary arrest, and may otherwise decompensate during the procedure. These children are evaluated in the OR under general anesthesia with adequate intravenous lines established, their supraglottic larynx adequately anesthetized with topical lidocaine spray and all airway instruments/tools at the ready.

Children with mild laryngomalacia (stridor is mild, supraglottic, inspiratory, no cessation of airflow, no chest or neck retractions) who feed well, gain weight, have a normal voice, who do not have neuromuscular problems, ALTE, cyanosis or apnea, are non-syndromic, without a family history of SIDS will continue to be followed monthly at least another 2 months. Upright feeding and semi-upright nap positions are recommended, as well as increased burping time. Prone positioning during nighttime sleep is a better airway position for babies with laryngomalacia. Caregivers are instructed to return if symptoms change with respect to the above parameters. Watching weight gain on growth charts and assessing feeding status are important parameters [1].

In most children, laryngomalacia is mild enough to be observed until asymptomatic, guided by the principles above. All others will need an airway evaluation in the OR under general anesthesia. This is a dynamic exam, performed with suspension laryngoscopes, flexible and rigid endoscopes while the patient is breathing spontaneously. All airway dynamics during respiratory phases are observed and documented.

If the shape, angle and mucosal condition of the supraglottic structures (epiglottis, arytenoids, aryepiglottic folds, vallecular) appear to be contributing to obstruction during the AE, these can be trimmed, reduced, removed and otherwise adjusted using various techniques (supraglottoplasty, epiglottopexy, arytenoid spot weld *via*.) and tools (LASER, microdebrider, cold instruments, sutures *via*.) and the obstruction relieved.

## Craniofacial Anomalies and Nasal Obstruction

Although there is no universal consensus on the subject, most clinical observations are convincing enough to consider neonates to be obligate nasal breathers for at least the first few weeks of life. Nasal resistance is greatest during infancy, when airways are narrowest [2]. Consequently, any nasal obstruction causes multiple effects on the neonate, amplifying resistance to air-flow and impairing sucking-swallowing responses, with increased risks of aspiration and respiratory distress [3].

The upper airway meets the oropharynx in the supraglottic larynx, where respiration, suckling and swallowing are regulated by the epiglottic switch. In newborn and suckling infants the larynx is positioned very close to the soft palate. The epiglottis forms an anatomic continuum with the uvula. Respiration and sucking functions are mobilized serially during ingestive sequences as breathing is compatible with sucking but not with swallowing [4 - 7].

Respiratory performance may also be dependent on nitric oxide mediation (produced in the nose and sinuses and delivered to the lungs – impeded by nasal obstruction), although relevant research in this age group has not been performed [8].

Bilateral nasal obstruction often presents in the neonatal period leading to serious consequences including respiratory distress, difficulty feeding and failure to thrive. Choanal atresia (the most common congenital nasal anomaly, associated with CHARGE syndrome, also seen with Apert's, Crouzon, and Treacher-Collins syndromes) nasal dermoid, encephalocele, glioma, and CNPAS (congenital nasal pyriform aperture stenosis - isolated or associated with absence of the anterior pituitary, diabetes insipidus, submucous cleft palate, and hypoplastic maxillary sinuses, or as part of the holoprosencephaly sequence), midfacial and nasal hypoplasia, arhinia, single nostril, nasopharyngeal stenosis, nasal duplication, nasolacrimal duct cysts (bilateral in 50%) and various tumors (hemangioma, lymphangioma *via*.) will cause stridor through nasal obstruction.

Other mechanisms of obstruction include cleft palate, cleft lip, severe nasal septal deviation, birth trauma, hormonal (maternal estrogen) or simply narrow anatomy. Some can be treated effectively with decongestants, saline irrigation, and nasal aspiration. Severe obstructions require surgical intervention (CNPAS, choanal atresia). A more moderate category of obstruction responds to temporizing measures such as stents, nasal trumpets, balloon dilations allowing time for the child to both grow (diameter, size) as well as to grow out of (obligate nasal breather status) the compromise.

Narrow nasal passages in a child with Down's syndrome or other craniofacial anomaly can be effectively treated with alternating nasal trumpets used as stents, saline irrigations and decongestants until the child is several weeks old.

A number of children with unilateral or bilateral cleft lips and primary palates but intact secondary palates have been successfully treated with a nasal retainer to keep the nostrils from collapsing. Nasoalveolar molding for presurgical orthodontic treatment of babies with cleft lip and palates is also very effective if the nasal stents are initiated sooner than the usual 3rd week.

Bony narrowing in nasal passages can be dilated with airway balloons under endoscopic guidance and trumpets/stents are inserted without causing mucosal shearing or tearing [9].

Stents, balloons, nostril retainers and in general all nasoalveolar molding procedures in principle, take advantage of the inherent malleability and plasticity of the neonatal cartilage and bone in the presence of transplacental hormonal assistance [10]. Therefore, early application is preferred.

In select cases, the abovementioned temporizing measures and conservative approaches will allow for growth and increased maturity of the child. Exactly when the shift from an obligate to preferential nasal breather status happens is not known and therefore needs to be determined by the clinician for each child.

### *Choanal Atresia-Stenosis and CNPAS (Congenital Nasal Piriform Aperture Stenosis)*

Bilateral choanal atresia presents as an airway emergency in the first week of life. Feeding difficulties are always associated and may prompt diagnostic evaluations. Unilateral and bilateral complete atresias are usually easy to diagnose, since passing a nasal suction tube (8Fr) through both nasal passages and aspirating the airway have become a routine part of the newborn management in nurseries. More problematic is the diagnosis of choanal stenosis or, narrow nasal or choanal anatomy. This includes CNPAS. Although in the majority of cases nasal catheters can be passed through a narrow anatomy, nasal breathing is nevertheless compromised. Diagnosis is performed by nasal endoscopy and CT imaging. It is important to educate staff to refrain from repeated blind attempts at passing catheters once an initial difficulty is verified. Repeat attempts only help make matters worse by creating circumferential injury and subsequent scarring that is very difficult to treat. In all cases, mucosal injury should be avoided and prompt endoscopic evaluation and imaging initiated.

Unilateral atresia and stenosis usually are managed conservatively by keeping the contralateral passage patent through the use of decongestants, suctioning and, saline irrigations until the child is older and more refined surgical treatment with higher success rates can be employed [11]. In bilateral cases, treatment should be prompt, since babies are obligate nasal breathers. Variety of surgical techniques are described and success depends on the skill and experience of the surgeon.

Bilateral Membranous Choanal Atresia is best managed by endoscopic surgery that includes excision of the membranous atretic plate and removal of the posterior part of the vomerine bone converting the posterior nasal cavity into a common opening [12, 13]. Lateral mucosal injury should be avoided to prevent scarring. Lasers and stents are unnecessary and will increase scarring [14 - 16]. Adverse effects from applying Mitomycin C to prevent scarring are not studied in neonates and are not recommended [17].

Bilateral Bony Choanal Atresia is difficult to treat. The aggressive trans-palatal approach is reserved for severe and recurrent stenosis; initial approach should be endoscopic trans-nasal.

The atretic plate can be too thick to safely penetrate and enlarge. Endoscopic high speed drills are used to enlarge the posterior nasal vault and create a common cavity. This procedure carries a high risk of vascular injury in the sphenopalatine region and requires preparation for transfusion as well as experience [18]. Long-term stenting may be required since a large denuded area will be created. In children with multiple co-morbidities (CHARGE association, holoprosencephaly *via*.) surgical success is limited and a tracheotomy should be considered instead [19].

CNPAS and mid-nasal stenosis can be treated conservatively by balloon dilation and/or stenting with nasal trumpets [9]. This procedure utilizes endoscopic placement of rigid sinus (or airway) dilation balloons and stenting the dilated passage with nasal trumpets that are sutured in place for 4-6 weeks. When feasible, trumpets are exchanged with a larger size to. Mucosal injury-avulsion is avoided with careful technique. The alternative is the traditional aggressive sublabial-transnasal degloving approach to the piriform aperture, using drills to enlarge the stenotic bone.

In milder stenoses, a temporizing approach may work and alternating nasal trumpets (without suturing), positioning, decongestants, saline irrigations, supplemental O2, BiPAP (Bi-level Positive Airway Pressure), and even short term intubation (especially when there is high surgical risk) can all be used in combination to buy time and allow the child to grow. Close monitoring is required to assess adequacy of these methods.

## *Mandibular Glossopexy for Tongue Base Obstruction*

Craniofacial malformations including anomalies of the size, position and geometry of the mandible usually are associated with anomalies of the size and position of the tongue as well as primary or associated deficiencies of motor control and muscle tone. The obstruction caused by these anomalies is evident in the first days of life and have to be managed with primacy. Among the techniques used, the Tongue-Lip Adhesion (TLA) procedure has as many proponents as it has opponents. The disagreements between accomplished surgeons over the effectiveness of the procedure can be traced to semantics.

When this procedure is performed as a soft tissue adhesion between the lower lip and the tongue (tip and/or floor of mouth) as the literal reading of the name of the procedure suggest, the results are unsatisfactory. Many surgeons who have reviewed and used such interventions have concluded (sarcastically) that the TLA only works in children who don't need them. More than 80% of institutions have abandoned standard TLA with or without sub periosteal release [20, 21] citing morbidities caused by tethering the tongue. (Exacerbation of dysphagia, prolonged nasogastric tube feeding, gastrostomy tube placement, second surgery for release of the adhesion). The concept and justification of sub periosteal release also is problematic.

The reason for the failure of the simple soft tissue adhesion TLA in relieving the obstruction is its inability to control the tongue base. Soft tissue flaps between the tongue and the lower lip will inevitably str*via*h and relax the tongue base, even if at the time of surgery, relatively adequate forward pull of the tongue base is achieved/observed. When TLA is modified to include a sturdy loop-stitch around the base of tongue that is anchored anteriorly to the mandible, excluding soft tissue flaps between the tongue and lower lip, the technique helps achieve remarkable results. The technique involves a 2.0 nylon suture inserted around the tongue base and both ends are threaded under the tongue through the floor of the mouth, (avoiding submandibular ducts and vessels) and looped around or through the mandible briefly surfacing in the gingivolabial sulcus, to be tied together and buried in the floor of mouth or gingival sulcus anteriorly. Threading the suture through the mandible is done with an 18G needle close to mandibular rim (avoiding tooth germs and neurovascular bundle). In the first few weeks of life, going through the mandibular bone with a sharp needle is possible without the use of drills. This is a permanent stitch and will hold the tongue base forward with a mild protrusion of the tongue. The tongue protrusion usually resolves within weeks but the tongue base stays in its anterior position. There are variations of the technique; some surgeons continue to perform the tongue-lip mucosal flaps in addition to the tongue base stitch, but in this author's opinion, this is not necessary and creates a cosmetic disruption as well as the additional morbidities described previously. Mann *et al* have described the tongue base stitch in a weaving pattern [22]. However, in an infant, this proves difficult and in our experience, does not provide better control of the tongue base when compared with a well-placed single (depth 2-3 mm) tongue base suture. Adding a trans-mandibular K-Wire to a soft tissue TLA also does not seem to provide adequate tongue base mobilization [23]. Argamaso describes a variation of standard TLA using a circum-mandibular suture to anchor the anterior tongue to the mandible [24], which also deviates from the principle of tongue base control. The simple tongue base suspension altogether helps avoid the pitfalls of the standard TLA and should ideally not be referred to as a TLA. We need a better term to describe tongue-base suspension with a soft tissue-to-bone anchor. I propose using the term **mandibular glossopexy (MGP).** Successful MGP as described, provides immediate and lasting relief from tongue base obstruction, does not exacerbate or cause dysphagia, and is well tolerated by the baby who needs additional positioning and feeding support. If neurological compromise is present, or aspiration is a major problem, gastrostomy tubes and tracheotomy should be considered instead of MGP.

## Synchronous Airway Lesions (SAL)

Craniofacial anomalies, syndromic or not, are usually present with predictable sites of obstruction apparent from clinical exam and respiratory behavior during the first few days of life. In practice however, up to 15% of children with craniofacial anomalies presenting with respiratory distress have multiple airway problems that need to be addressed in order to achieve satisfactory results [25]. The false belief in the predictability of a 'single' problem 'single site' is likely showing up in reports of varying success levels addressing 'single site' or 'single' problems.

SAL's are diagnosed in more than 50% of otherwise normal children scheduled for adenoidectomy to treat upper airway obstruction causing OSA. These children, all under 18 months of age, were diagnosed with a variety of additional airway anomalies including laryngeal edema, laryngomalacia, tracheal vascular compression, subglottic stenosis, vocal fold lesions, bronchial stenosis, and vocal cord paralysis. Of these, 30% had laryngopharyngeal reflux disease and 13% also had eosinophilic esophagitis diagnosed with esophageal biopsy [25]. Similar findings including tracheal cobble-stoning (usually considered to be a sign of aspiration of reflux), subglottic stenosis, laryngomalacia, tracheobronchomalacia, external vascular compression, subglottic cysts, laryngeal clefts, vocal cord paresis, subglottic nodule and trapped first tracheal ring were reported in 67% of children up to 3 years of age who were scheduled to undergo tonsillectomy and adenoidectomy for obstructive sleep apnea (OSA). When tracheal cobble stoning, the most frequent finding, was removed from the analysis, 65% of children in the series still had at least one SAL. Moreover, the severity of OSA as measured by PSG did not predict the presence of a SAL [26].

In 27% of a heterogeneous group of children with laryngomalacia, airway evaluation helped diagnose epiglottic and vallecular cysts, subglottic stenosis, laryngotracheal cleft, tracheomalacia and vocal cord dysfunction [27].

When a known syndromic association with airway anomalies was investigated such as the 22q11 deletion syndrome, additional findings of subglottic stenosis, glottic web, vocal nodules, laryngomalacia, laryngeal paralysis and bronchial malposition were reported in 14% of the series [28]. The most commonly known association of a syndrome with airway compromise is in children with Down Syndrome: multiple anomalies of the upper airway including large retro-positioned tongue, small anteroposterior craniofacial distances, short neck, poor muscle tone and, sometimes a cleft palate accompanying a high incidence of SAL's including laryngomalacia, tracheal bronchus, subglottic stenosis, tracheomalacia in up to 70% of children evaluated [29, 30],

The examples can be extended to include the majority of craniofacial syndromes as well as otherwise healthy children with respiratory compromise.

## Premature Babies

Apart from the effects of premature birth on the cardiorespiratory anatomy and physiology, there are additional risk factors for stridor in premature babies. Many premature babies require ventilation support through endotracheal intubation. The subsequent injury at the narrowest portion of the airway may be severe enough to cause concentric scarring and subglottic stenosis. Even when trauma and scarring are minimal, mucus gland outflow may be obstructed by scar and may lead to formation of single or multiple subglottic cysts. These cysts grow slowly and present as progressive stridor and failure to thrive, several weeks after discharge from hospital. Any endotracheal intubation history is important, regardless of the duration of the intubation or excellence of NICU care. A history of multiple self-extubations while in the NICU also should alert the physician to the possibility of severe subglottic injury.

## CONCLUSION

Stridorous breathing in a child requires prompt management that is organized, collaborative and comprehensive. Clinical assessments through history, careful observation and examination are crucial for management planning, diagnosis and treatment. Possibilities in the diagnostic repertoire are exhaustive and indirect methods often inadequate. Physicians should not solely rely on initial, subjective clinical presentations of stridor and respiratory distress. When feasible, a detailed airway evaluation including flexible laryngeal, nasal and nasopharyngeal endoscopy and rigid bronchoscopy should be performed with the possibility of surgical therapeutic intervention based on pathology discovered.

## CONFLICT OF INTEREST

The authors declare no conflict of interest, financial or otherwise.

## ACKNOWLEDGEMENTS

Declared none.

## REFERENCES

[1]     Neiner J, Gungor A. Evaluation of growth curves in children after Supraglottoplasty. Am J Otolaryngol 2016; 37(2): 128-31.
[http://dx.doi.org/10.1016/j.amjoto.2015.11.003]

[2]     Dunagan D, Georgitis J. Intranasal disease and provocation Diagnostic Testing of Allergic Disease. New York, NY, USA 2000; pp. 151-73.

[3]     Harding R, Jakubowska JE, McCrabb GJ. Postnatal development of responses to airflow obstruction. Clin Exp Pharmacol Physiol 1995; 22(8): 537-43.
[http://dx.doi.org/10.1111/j.1440-1681.1995.tb02063.x]

[4]     Goldfield EC, Richardson MJ, Lee KG, Margetts S. Coordination of sucking, swallowing, and breathing and oxygen saturation during early infant breast-feeding and bottle feeding. Pediatr Res 2006; 60(4): 450-5.
[http://dx.doi.org/10.1203/01.pdr.0000238378.24238.9d]

[5]     Kelly B, Huckabee ML, Jones R, Frampton C. The first year of human life: coordinating respiration and nutritive swallowing. Dysphagia 2007; 22(1): 37-43.
[http://dx.doi.org/10.1007/s00455-006-9038-3]

[6]     Paul K, Dittrichova J, Papousek H. Infant feeding behavior: development in patterns and motivation. Dev Psychobiol 1996; 29: 563-76.
[http://dx.doi.org/10.1002/(SICI)1098-2302(199611)29:7<563::AID-DEV2>3.0.CO;2-S]

[7]     Wolff PH. The serial organization of sucking in the young infant. Pediatrics 1968; 42(6): 943-57.

[8]     Gungor AA. The aerodynamics of the sinonasal interface: the nose takes wing-a paradigm shift for our time. Int Forum Allergy Rhinol 2013; 3(4): 299-306.
[http://dx.doi.org/10.1002/alr.21105]

[9]     Gungor AA, Reiersen DA. Balloon dilatation for congenital nasal piriform aperture stenosis (CNPAS): a novel conservative technique. Am J Otolaryngol 2014; 35(3): 439-42.
[http://dx.doi.org/10.1016/j.amjoto.2013.12.016]

[10]    Taylor TD. Clinical maxillofacial prosthetics Quintessence. Chicago 2000; pp. 63-84.

[11]    Newman JR, Harmon P, Shirley WP, Hill JS, Woolley AL, Wiatrak BJ. Operative management of choanal atresia: a 15-year experience. JAMA Otolaryngol Head Neck Surg 2013; 139(1): 71-5.
[http://dx.doi.org/10.1001/jamaoto.2013.1111]

[12]    Ibrahim AA, Magdy EA, Hassab MH. Endoscopic choanoplasty without stenting for congenital choanal atresia repair. Int J Pediatr Otorhinolaryngol 2010; 74(2): 144-50.
[http://dx.doi.org/10.1016/j.ijporl.2009.10.027]

[13]    Rodríguez H, Cuestas G, Passali DA. 20-year experience in microsurgical treatment of choanal atresia. Acta Otorrinolaringol Esp 2014; 65(2): 85-92.
[http://dx.doi.org/10.1016/j.otoeng.2013.09.001]

[14]    Schoem SR. Trans nasal endoscopic repair of choanal atresia: why stent? Otolaryngol Head Neck Surg 2004; 131(4): 362-6.
[http://dx.doi.org/10.1016/j.otohns.2004.03.036]

[15]    Yuan HB, Poon KS, Chan KH, Lee TY, Lin CY. Fatal gas embolism as a complication of Nd-YAG laser surgery during treatment of bilateral choanal stenosis. Int J Pediatr Otorhinolaryngol 1993; 27(2): 193-9.
[http://dx.doi.org/10.1016/0165-5876(93)90136-Q]

[16]    Ramsden JD, Campisi P, Forte V. Choanal atresia and choanal stenosis. Otolaryngol Clin North Am 2009; 42(2): 339-52.
[http://dx.doi.org/10.1016/j.otc.2009.01.001]

[17]    Carter JM, Lawlor C, Guarisco JL. The efficacy of mitomycin and stenting in choanal atresia repair: a 20 year experience. Int J Pediatr Otorhinolaryngol 2014; 78(2): 307-11.
[http://dx.doi.org/10.1016/j.ijporl.2013.11.031]

[18]    Gujrathi CS, Daniel SJ, James AL, Forte V. Management of bilateral choanal atresia in the neonate: an institutional review. Int J Pediatr Otorhinolaryngol 2004; 68(4): 399-407.
[http://dx.doi.org/10.1016/j.ijporl.2003.10.006]

[19]    Asher BF, McGill TJ, Kaplan L, Friedman EM, Healy GB. Airway complications in CHARGE association. Arch Otolaryngol Head Neck Surg 1990; 116(5): 594-5.
[http://dx.doi.org/10.1001/archotol.1990.01870050094014]

[20]    Myer CM, Reed JM, Cotton RT, *et al.* Airway management in Pierre Robin Sequence. Otolaryngol Head and Neck Surgery 1998; 118(5): 630-5.
[http://dx.doi.org/10.1177/019459989811800511]

[21]    Scott AR, Tibesar RJ, Sidman JD. Pierre Robin Sequence: evaluation, management, indications for surgery, and pitfalls. Otolaryngol Clin North Am 2012; 45(3): 695-710.
[http://dx.doi.org/10.1016/j.otc.2012.03.007]

[22]    Mann RJ, Neaman KC, Hill B, Bajnrauh R, Martin MD. A novel technique for performing a tongue-lip adhesion-the tongue suspension technique. Cleft Palate Craniofac J 2012; 49(1): 27-31.
[http://dx.doi.org/10.1597/10-036]

[23]    Rawashdeh, Ma'amon A. Trans mandibular K-Wire in the Management of Airway Obstruction in Pierre Robin Sequence. J Craniofac Surg 2004; 15(3): 447-50.
[http://dx.doi.org/10.1097/00001665-200405000-00020]

[24]    Argamaso RV. Glossopexy for upper airway obstruction in Robin sequence. Cleft Palate Craniofac J 1992; 29(3): 232-8.
[http://dx.doi.org/10.1597/1545-1569(1992)029<0232:GFUAOI>2.3.CO;2]

[25]    Mandell DL, Yellon RF. Synchronous airway lesions and esophagitis in young patients undergoing adenoidectomy. Arch Otolaryngol Head Neck Surg 2007; 133(4): 375-8.
[http://dx.doi.org/10.1001/archotol.133.4.375]

[26]   Rastatter JC, Schroeder JW Jr, French A, Holinger L. Synchronous airway lesions in children younger than age 3 years undergoing adenotonsillectomy. Otolaryngol Head Neck Surg 2011; 145(2): 309-13.
[http://dx.doi.org/10.1177/0194599811403071]

[27]   Yuen HW, Tan HK, Balakrishnan A. Synchronous airway lesions and associated anomalies in children with laryngomalacia evaluated with rigid endoscopy. Int J Pediatr Otorhinolaryngol 2006; 70(10): 1779-84.
[http://dx.doi.org/10.1016/j.ijporl.2006.06.003]

[28]   Leopold C, De Barros A, Cellier C, Drouin-Garraud V, Dehesdin D, Marie JP. Laryngeal abnormalities are frequent in the 22q11 deletion syndrome. Int J Pediatr Otorhinolaryngol 2012; 76(1): 36-40.
[http://dx.doi.org/10.1016/j.ijporl.2011.09.025]

[29]   Pravit J. Bronchoscopic findings in Down syndrome children with respiratory problems. J Med Assoc Thai 2014; 97 (Suppl. 6): S159-63.

[30]   Bertrand P, Navarro H, Caussade S, Holmgren N, Sánchez I. Airway anomalies in children with Down syndrome: endoscopic findings. Pediatr Pulmonol 2003; 36(2): 137-41.
[http://dx.doi.org/10.1002/ppul.10332]

# CHAPTER 6

# Update on the Management of Laryngomalacia

**Mohamed Akkari**[*], **Catherine Blanchet** and **Michel Mondain**

*Department of E.N.T. and Head and Neck Surgery, University Hospital Gui de Chauliac, University of Montpellier, 80 avenue Augustin Fliche 34295 Montpellier Cedex 5, France*

**Abstract:** Laryngomalacia (LM) is the most common cause of stridor in children. It presents during the first days of life with inspiratory stridor often associated with feeding difficulties. Diagnosis must be confirmed by performing a flexible fiberoptic laryngoscopy. LM is classified in mild, moderate and severe LM depending on respiratory and feeding severity symptoms. LM usually goes with gastroesophageal reflux disease, and can also be associated to synchronous airway lesions, neurological disorders, heart disease and congenital syndromes. Identification and management of co-morbidities using appropriate complementary examinations are essential as they influence LM severity and treatment outcomes. Medical management of LM includes lifestyle/dietary measures and anti-acid treatment. Supraglottoplasty, including several technique variants, is the mainstay of severe LM treatment, with numerous studies reporting high success and low complications rates. Tracheotomy and non-invasive ventilation are indicated in case of supraglottoplasty failure, most of the time due to associated neurological disorder and congenital syndromes.

**Keywords :** Gastroesophageal reflux disease, Inspiratory supraglottic collapse, Laryngomalacia, Lifestyle/dietary measures, Neonates and infants, Non-invasive ventilation, Stridor, Tracheotomy, Trans-oral supraglottoplasty.

## INTRODUCTION

Laryngomalacia (LM) is defined as an inspiratory supraglottic collapse causing stridor. It typically presents during the first 10 days of life with inspiratory high-pitched stridor worsening with feeding, agitation, crying and supine positioning [1]. Feeding difficulties are often associated.

The pathophysiological mechanisms involved in LM are the infant's specific laryngeal anatomy [2], an abnormally integrated peripheral and central nervous system mechanism of laryngeal function and tone involving the superior laryngeal nerve [3], and the occurrence of mucosal posterior oedema induced by

[*] **Corresponding author Mohamed Akkari**: Department of E.N.T. and Head and Neck Surgery, University Hospital Gui de Chauliac, University of Montpellier, 80 avenue Augustin Fliche 34295 Montpellier Cedex 5, France; Tel: +33 4 67 33 68 25; Fax: +33 4 67 33 67 28; Email: m-mondain@chu-montpellier.fr

**Seckin Ulualp (Ed.)**

gastroesophageal reflux disease (GERD) and mucosal trauma during inspiration [4]. Consequently, the increased airflow through an area of obstruction creates turbulence and vibrations of supraglottic structures leading to stridor. LM is responsible for 60-70% of all congenital stridors [5].

After a peak at 6-8 months, it is commonly admitted that in most of the cases, spontaneous resolution of LM and its symptoms occurs after 24 months old [6, 7]. In a recent review of the literature, Isaac *et al* [8] have highlighted the paucity of the literature regarding the natural history of LM, with an uncertainty concerning the rate and time to resolution, and suggested caution when informing parents about the evolution of the symptoms.

In 10-20% of cases, LM is associated with respiratory and/or feeding signs of severity that require a more specific management. These cases need an early identification in order to provide the most appropriate treatment, including surgical procedures. LM Consensus recommendations have recently been published by the International Pediatric ORL Group (IPOG) [9].

The aim of this chapter is to present an update on the diagnostic and therapeutic management of LM according to the most recent literature.

## DIAGNOSTIC MANAGEMENT

All children with stridor must benefit from an ENT evaluation. The objectives are to confirm the diagnosis of LM, to determine its severity and to identify potential associated lesions.

### History

Medical history must be detailed: birth term, obstetrical and neonatal medical events, associated congenital diseases. Parents questioning will specify the timing and circumstances of stridor appearance, stridor characteristics and aggravating factors. Feeding difficulties, usually due to swallowing dysfunction (trouble to coordinate the suck swallow breath sequence) [10] or association with GERD (regurgitation, emesis, cough, and slow feedings) must be sought-after, and their intensity needs to be evaluated: milk rations, meal frequency, and above all weight gain.

### Physical Examination

A complete pediatric clinical examination must be performed, including height and weight measurement, respiratory sound and rate evaluation, chest movements and deformation analysis, lung auscultation, and search for associated morbidities.

As stridor is not a specific symptom of LM [11], direct visualization of the larynx using flexible fiberoptic laryngoscopy (FFL) is essential to confirm the diagnosis and eliminate others causes of inspiratory stridor [12, 13]. Nasal FFL is easily performed in the office with the help of a caregiver, usually without local anesthesia. In children with cardiorespiratory fragility, this exam must be performed in a medical environment including resuscitation equipment [4].

Olney *et al* [14] have proposed a classification of LM based on FFL usual endoscopic findings:

-Type 1 (57%): anterior prolapse of mucosa and corniculate cartilages overlying the arytenoid cartilages. This prolapse will be favored in case of mucosal oedema induced by GERD and mucosal trauma during inspiration.
-Type 2 (15%): foreshortened aryepiglottic folds
-Type 3 (13%): posterior displacement of the epiglottis which is usually omega-shaped.
-Combined types (15%)

## Severity Classification

LM can be classified into mild, moderate and severe categories [9], which are not based on the intensity of the stridor but rather on the associated respiratory and feeding symptoms [15].

Mild LM accounts for 40% of cases at the time of presentation. Symptoms are an inspiratory stridor with occasional feeding symptoms (cough, chocking and regurgitation) without swallowing dysfunction. According to Landry *et al* [15], approximatively 30% of the children presenting mild LM will progress to the moderate category, mainly due to the evolution of the GERD symptoms.

Moderate LM accounts for 40% of cases at the time of presentation. Children present stridor with frequent and additional more intense feeding symptoms (slow feeding, swallowing dysfunction). Approximatively 30% of the children presenting moderate LM will progress to the severe category despite an appropriate medical treatment [15].

Severe LM accounts for 20% of cases at the time of presentation and will require surgical treatment [16]. Respiratory signs of severity are: episodes of respiratory distress, malaise, recurrent cyanosis, permanent inter or subcostal retraction that can lead to pectus excavatum, obstructive sleep apnea, chronic respiratory failure with pulmonary artery hypertension, cor pulmonale and heart failure. Feeding signs of severity are: iterative suffocation during feeding, failure to thrive due to insufficient caloric intake and heightened metabolic expenditure, major swallowing disorders with aspiration responsible for pneumonia.

## Associated Diseases

### Gastroesophageal Reflux Disease (GERD)

According to Thompson *et al* [16] GERD is associated in 65 to 100% of infants with LM. It is favored by the negative intrathoracic pressure generated by the airway obstruction. Gastric acid reflux favors posterior laryngeal mucosal edema, which increases the airway obstruction, thus creating a self-perpetuating vicious process. Moreover, acid exposure decreases laryngeal sensation [16], favoring choking during feedings, and influences the vagal reflex, that is also responsible for lower esophageal sphincter tone and esophageal motility, thus favoring GERD in a second way [15].

### Synchronous Airway Lesions (SAL)

The incidence of SAL associated with LM in the literature ranges from 7.5 to 64% [17 - 19]. A higher prevalence of SAL has been reported in case of severe LM [17], even if some authors relate this association to a selection bias in the studied cohorts [20]. Indeed the increased risk for SAL in these patients might rather be related to other causes (cardiac/large-vessel malformations, prematurity, repeated or prolonged intubations, acute infections, or prior airway surgery).

Tracheomalacia and subglottic stenosis are the most frequent SAL. The other reported laryngo-tracheal lesions are vocal cord paralysis, anterior glottis web, laryngeal diastema, oesotracheal fistula, and laryngeal dyskinesia. Pharyngeal lesions may also be observed, such as microretrognathism, glossoptosis, vallecular cyst, palatal anomaly, choanal atresia [4].

### Neurological Disorders (ND)

Congenital ND such as hypotonia, psychomotor retardation, cerebral palsy, microcephaly, quadriparesis, Chiari malformation, epilepsy can be associated to LM, especially severe cases, with a prevalence ranging from 20 to 45% [15]. Acquired ND such as stroke, degenerative disease, brain tumour can also lead to a LM of late onset. When associated to a neurological disease, LM can be a part of a broader condition described as pharyngo-laryngomalacia (PLM), where sleep disordered breathing and swallowing dysfunction are at the forefront [21]. Association of LM with ND leads to a significant reduction of supraglottoplasty success rate [22].

## Heart Disease

Association with congenital heart disease is reported in 10% of children with LM [15]. It influences LM severity [16] as it is an additive cause of hypoxemia and malaise, and complicates the surgical management as it increases the perioperative risk.

## Congenital Syndrome

Association with a multiple malformation syndrome (Down syndrome, CHARGE association, Pierre Robin sequence, 22q11 microdeletion syndrome) is reported in 8 to 50% of children with LM [19, 23]. The most frequent is Down syndrome. As for ND, association with a congenital syndrome leads to a significant reduction of supraglottoplasty success rate [22]. This is partly explained by the multilevel airway obstruction, especially when micrognathia and retrodisplacement of the tongue base are associated, such as in CHARGE and Pierre Robin sequence [15]. Another explanation is the presence within the syndrome of the other associated lesions listed above. Consequently, those patients are more likely to require tracheotomy [9].

## Atypical Laryngomalacias

As recently highlighted by Camacho and Lee [24, 25], atypical laryngomalacia are a non-homogenous group of unusual presentations including:

- late onset laryngomalacia, defined by symptoms appearance after 2 years old in infants free of prior disease [26, 27],
- occult laryngomalacia, defined by a stridor limited to sleep or exercise [28],
- state dependent laryngomalacia, which approximates the occult laryngomalacia related to sleep, but with a correlation between the intensity and the level of consciousness [29].

Management of these atypical presentations is not clearly defined, but tend to be the same as for congenital LM, *i.e.* a correct diagnosis and a therapeutic management dictated by the severity of the disease. Isaac *et al* question the fact that these entities are distinct from typical congenital LM, or might in fact be a continuum of a single disease process [8].

## Complementary Examinations

They will be dictated by the need for severity evaluation and the suspicion for associated diseases.

## Measurement of PO2 and PCO2

Easily performed during hospital surveillance, it evaluates the consequences on gas exchange in severe LM, and contribute to the surgical decision. In Thorn's severity scale [1], a resting SaO2 of 86% or under at time of presentation is a severity criteria.

## Chest X-ray

They are indicated in patients who may be aspirating and/or have pulmonary disease [9].

## Rigid Laryngotracheal Endoscopy under General Anaesthesia

This examination will be systematically performed when surgery is indicated, prior to supraglottoplasty during the same procedure, in order to seek for a SAL. The other indications are [4, 9]:

- stridor without the FFL signs described above
- discrepancy between the severity of the symptoms and the benignity of the FFL findings
- symptoms suggestive of an associated SAL.

## Polysomnography (PSG)

This examination is useful when obstructive sleep apnea associated to LM is suspected. In a recent meta-analysis, Camacho *et al* [30] have assessed PSG results before and after supraglottoplasty, and highlighted a significant improvement of the apnea hypopnea index (IAH) after surgery. Tanphaichitr *et al* [31] have reported an increased rate of central sleep apneas associated with laryngomalacia. Besides, PSG can be useful in case of associated neurological or cardiac disorders as it will help distinguish the actual repercussions of LM and guide the therapeutic decision. It is not routinely performed in the work-up strategy of LM. Indeed, the difficult access to PSG due to the rarity of sleep laboratories and the difficulties to perform this examination on an infant is rarely compatible with the potential emergency of the surgical decision in case of severe LM. Besides, its prohibitive cost is also a restraint to a wide ruse.

## Drug Induced Sleep Endoscopy (DISE)

DISE has been recently assessed in children for site of obstruction identification in obstructive sleep apnea [32]. It is useful to disclose an occult LM related to sleep [28] or a state-dependant LM [29]. In the surgery room, FFL is performed after sleep induction by Propofol under anaesthetic supervision.

## Swallow Studies

Barium or video fluoroscopic swallow study evaluates reflux, aspiration and looks for an associated malformation such as laryngeal diastema and oesotracheal fistula. Esophagram will provide further information about potential containment gastrointestinal disorders such as pyloric stenosis in case of severe GERD. Functional endoscopic swallow study can also be useful, but might be more complicated to perform in neonates.

## Twenty Four-hour PH Study

This examination is indicated in case of severe GERD despite acid suppression therapy in view of fundoplication surgery.

## Echocardiogram

This examination is indicated in case of congenital heart disease, in order to assess the perioperative cardiac risk, and evaluate the part of hypoxemia unrelated to LM that is expected to linger post operatively.

## Polymalformative Assessment

According to the clinical presentation, other complementary examinations might be performed, such as cerebral MRI, thoracic and abdominal CT scan, kidney ultrasound ophthalmological assessment, genetic tests…

## THERAPEUTIC MANAGEMENT

### Mild Laryngomalacia

Simple observation is usually sufficient, in association with lifestyle/dietary measures: use of thickened milk, high-caloric formula, upright positioning during and after feeding, use of bottles that minimize aerophagia, head of bed elevation.

A one month symptom check is recommended, and if stable or improving the follow-up can be extended to a 3 to 6 month check [9]. Parents' reassurance is also important, as loudness of the stridor can be overwhelming to them despite the mildness of the presentation. Indeed, LM has been shown to have a negative emotional impact on parents, and to be associated with a lower quality of life [33, 34].

### Moderate Laryngomalacia

In addition to the previous measures, acid suppression therapy is indicated. The main molecules available are histamine type 2 receptor antagonists (H2RA) that can be used at 3mg/kg/day, and proton pump inhibitors (PPI) that can be used at 1 to 2 mg/kg/day. Therapy can be started with both H2RA and PPI and then weaned to a single therapy when symptoms improve, or started with a single molecule, and switched to a double therapy if symptoms are not controlled [9]. Efficacy of PPI in infants is controversial in the literature [35], and it still doesn't benefit from FDA approval for patients under 1 year old. Prokinetic agents such as erythromycin ethylsuccinate, which influence gastrointestinal motility, can be used in addition to acid suppression therapy. The IPOG recommend to maintain treatment for at least 3 months [9]; the average time of therapy reported in the literature is 9 months [16].

## Severe Laryngomalacia

In patients presenting signs of severity and who failed to respond to conservative treatment, a more aggressive treatment is indicated.

### *Transoral Supraglottoplasty*

The aim of this procedure is to prevent inspiratory collapse by stabilizing and/or reducing supraglottic tissues. It is currently the mainstay of severe LM treatment.

### ***Surgical Technique***

Preceded by a systematic rigid laryngotracheal endoscopy, surgery is performed using an operating microscope after suspension of the larynx. Spontaneous breathing anesthesia is usually used, as endotracheal intubation may interfere with the procedure. Jet ventilation and intermittent apnea have also been proposed but are not the mainstay procedure.

Supraglottoplasty actually includes several surgical techniques than can be performed individually or combined. The endoscopic analysis of the supraglottic obstruction will influence the choice of the technique: aryepiglottic fold division in type 2 LM, removal of redundant mucosal arytenoid tissue in type 1 LM, epiglottopexy and epiglottic suture or partial epiglottectomy in type 3 LM [36, 37].

The most common first-line procedure is bilateral aryepiglottic fold division associated with bilateral removal of redundant mucosal arytenoid tissue [38]. The posterior inter arytenoid zone should be spared, in order to avoid post-operative supraglottic stenosis. Compresses soaked in adrenaline saline (1mg in 10ml) can be used for hemostasis. Several surgical tools are available: microlaryngeal cold-steel instruments, $CO_2$ laser (1 Watt), Thulium laser (1.5 Watt) [39], microdebrider (2.9 or 3.5 mm laryngeal blade, 800 rotation per minute in oscillating mode without irrigation) [40]. Laser and micro-debrider allow a lower intraoperative bleeding, while cold-steel instruments are more cost-effective. Laser is associated with a risk of fire if misused, and an increased risk of oedema due to the burn of mucosa. As literature data show similar success rates between these tools [41 - 43], the choice of the instrumentation should be guided by the surgeons habits and training. Unilateral and staged aryepiglottic fold division and removal of redundant mucosal arytenoid tissue have been proposed as initial surgical procedure to avoid supraglottic stenosis and post-operative aspiration [44, 45]. Recently, supraglottoplasty under 3-Dimensional endoscopy has been assessed to improve visualization of complex airway anatomy and allow a more precise tissue removal [46].

Epiglottopexy, epiglottic suture and partial epiglottectomy have been proposed, mainly when type 3 LM is involved, but also by some authors regardless of the anatomical abnormality [36, 47]. Those 3 techniques can be performed separately or combined. Epiglottopexy consists in laser vaporisation of the lingual surface of epiglottis and tongue base allowing stabilization of the epiglottis [36]. Epiglottic suture consists in placing a resorbable suture to unfold the folded epiglottis and shift apart the adjacent aryepiglottic folds [36]. Partial C-shaped suprahyoid epiglottectomy, or simple excision of epiglottic mucosa using microscissors or laser have also been described. Caution should be taken when operating on the epiglottis considering potential post-operative swallowing dysfunction; nonetheless, teams familiar with these techniques do not report an increased risk of post-operative aspiration [36, 47].

## *Post-operative Care*

A course of systemic corticosteroids (methylprednisolone 2mg/kg) is administered during the surgical procedure in order to minimize post-operative oedema [7].

Children may require a 24 hours post-operative intubation depending on the anaesthesia settings. If no intubation is necessary, they are still usually admitted in an intensive care unit (ICU). Some authors recently suggested that ICU monitoring may not be necessary if using cold steel instruments [48]. Nevertheless, this suggestion should be taken with caution, as the child's post-operative respiratory behavior is unpredictable, especially in the case of a misdiagnosed underlying disease.

Lifestyle/dietary measures and acid suppression therapy must be continued after surgery, in order to lower the risk of granuloma formation from exposure of the surgical site to gastric acid, provider of supraglottic stenosis.

An early FFL must be performed a few days after surgery to eliminate any early synechiae or granuloma, and 1 month after surgery to assess mucosal surface healing.

## *Surgical Outcomes-complications*

Improvement of symptoms after supraglottoplasty are reported in 70 to 100% of cases in several cohorts [14, 45, 49, 50]. In Van der Heijden *et al* study [51], supraglottoplasty led to statistically significant faster complete improvement than wait-and-see policy (5 *vs* 29 weeks). Nonetheless, Faria *et al* [52] found no difference in weight gain between surgery and medical treatment (acid suppression, speech and swallowing therapy, high-calorie formula), suggesting exclusive medical management for appropriately selected severe LM. Respiratory improvement is usually based on subjective criteria: reduction of stridor, resolution of apneic and cyanotic episodes, FFL findings. Ideally, supraglottoplasty respiratory efficacy should be evaluated by objective criteria such as PSG results [53, 54], but its limited access and cost avoid is routine use. Concerning feeding improvement assessment after supraglottoplasty, clinical objective criteria such as height and weight gain are monitored. Several authors reported a significant weight gain within 6 months of surgery, with normalization of the growth curve 3 years after the surgery [55, 56].

Supraglottoplasty failure, resulting in persistent respiratory and feeding difficulties, occurs in approximatively 30% of cases according to the most recent literature [22, 57]. Treatment options are revision supraglottoplasty, tracheotomy or non-invasive ventilation. The main risk factor for failure is the association with congenital syndrome and neurological anomalies [43, 57, 58]. Another identified risk factor is the presence of severe pre-operative reflux symptoms [43, 59]. Hoff *et al* [60] found a higher rate of revision supraglottoplasty in children undergoing surgery at less than 2 months age compared to those operated between 2 and 10 months (36.4% *vs* 5.3%, p<0.05). It has been shown that prematurity is neither a risk factor for LM [4, 19], nor a risk factor for supraglottoplasty failure [61].

## *Tracheotomy*

The aim of this procedure is to bypass the laryngeal obstruction. It is nowadays rarely performed in this indication, and is reserved for supraglottoplasty failures, presence of SAL and syndromic patients presenting multilevel airway obstruction and/or combining neurological, cardiac and airway diseases. Despite its efficiency to treat airway obstruction, tracheotomy in infants requires a complex management, and is associated with a significant post-operative complications rate around 20%, and a mortality related to the procedure of 1% [62, 63].

## Noninvasive Ventilation (NIV)

The aim of this technique is to decrease the respiratory work of patients with upper airway obstruction such as LM [64, 65]. It is used in cases of severe LM in the context of awaiting surgery, when surgery is not possible, or in case of supraglottoplasty failure, as an alternative to tracheotomy. As no consensus guidelines are available for NIV indications in LM, comparison of risk/benefit ratio to tracheotomy is essential for therapeutic decision. Continuous Positive Airway Pressure (CPAP) is usually used [64], with an interface adapted to the infant's face (commercially or handmade nasal mask). Bilevel Positive Airway Pressure (BPAP) has also shown its efficacy [65], but can be responsible for a respiratory asynchronism in case of unadapted inspiratory trigger sensitivity [66]. Side effects of NIV comprise skin lesions, maxillary retrusion and global flattening of the face [67]. Because this equipment requires a high level of expertise, it must be managed by an experienced multidisciplinary team.

## CONCLUSION

Diagnosis of LM must be systematically confirmed by performing a FFL. Severity symptoms must be thoroughly assessed in order to determine the best therapeutic options and follow-up schedule. Identification and management of co-morbidities are essential as they influence LM severity and treatment outcomes. Supraglottoplasty, including aryepiglottic fold division, removal of redundant mucosal arytenoid tissue, epiglottopexy, epiglottic suture, partial epiglottectomy, is the mainstay of severe LM treatment, with high success and low complications rates. It must be performed by an experienced team in a medical center equipped with an ICU. Tracheotomy and NIV are second line treatments, mainly indicated in case of supraglottoplasty failure, SAL and neurological and syndromic comorbidities.

## CONFLICT OF INTEREST

The authors declare no conflict of interest, financial or otherwise.

## ACKNOWLEDGEMENTS

Declared none.

## REFERENCES

[1]    Thorne MC, Garetz SL. Laryngomalacia: Review and Summary of Current Clinical Practice in 2015. Paediatr Respir Rev 2016; 17: 3-8.
[http://dx.doi.org/10.1016/j.prrv.2015.02.002]

[2]    Manning SC, Inglis AF, Mouzakes J, Carron J, Perkins JA. Laryngeal anatomic differences in pediatric patients with severe laryngomalacia. Arch Otolaryngol Head Neck Surg 2005; 131(4): 340-3.

[http://dx.doi.org/10.1001/archotol.131.4.340]

[3] Thompson DM. Abnormal sensorimotor integrative function of the larynx in congenital laryngomalacia: a new of etiology. Laryngoscope 2007; 117 (6 Pt 2 Suppl 114): 1-33.
[http://dx.doi.org/10.1097/MLG.0b013e31804a5750]

[4] Ayari S, Aubertin G, Girschig H, Van Den Abbeele T, Mondain M. Pathophysiology and diagnostic approach to laryngomalacia in infants. Eur Ann Otorhinolaryngol Head Neck Dis 2012; 129(5): 257-63.
[http://dx.doi.org/10.1016/j.anorl.2012.03.005]

[5] Daniel SJ. The upper airway: congenital malformations. Paediatr Respir Rev 2006; 7 (Suppl. 1): S260-3.
[http://dx.doi.org/10.1016/j.prrv.2006.04.227]

[6] Wright CT, Goudy SL. Congenital laryngomalacia: symptom duration and need for surgical intervention. Ann Otol Rhinol Laryngol 2012; 121(1): 57-60.
[http://dx.doi.org/10.1177/000348941212100110]

[7] Richter GT, Thompson DM. The surgical management of laryngomalacia. Otolaryngol Clin North Am 2008; 41(5): 837-64. [vii.].
[http://dx.doi.org/10.1016/j.otc.2008.04.011]

[8] Isaac A, Zhang H, Soon SR, Campbell S, El-Hakim H. A systematic review of the evidence on spontaneous resolution of laryngomalacia and its symptoms. Int J Pediatr Otorhinolaryngol 2016; 83: 78-83.
[http://dx.doi.org/10.1016/j.ijporl.2016.01.028]

[9] Carter J, Rahbar R, Brigger M, Chan K, Cheng A, Daniel SJ, *et al.* International Pediatric ORL Group (IPOG) laryngomalacia consensus recommendations. Int J Pediatr Otorhinolaryngol 2016.
[http://dx.doi.org/10.1016/j.ijporl.2016.04.007]

[10] Simons JP, Greenberg LL, Mehta DK, Fabio A, Maguire RC, Mandell DL. Laryngomalacia and swallowing function in children. Laryngoscope 2016; 126(2): 478-84.
[http://dx.doi.org/10.1002/lary.25440]

[11] Zwartenkot JW, Hoeve HL, Borgstein J. Inter-observer reliability of localization of recorded stridor sounds in children. Int J Pediatr Otorhinolaryngol 2010; 74(10): 1184-8.
[http://dx.doi.org/10.1016/j.ijporl.2010.07.011]

[12] Mondain M, Blanchet C. Arch Pediatr 2010; 17(6): 602-3. [Stridor or not stridor].
[http://dx.doi.org/10.1016/S0929-693X(10)70018-X]

[13] Cheng J, Smith LP. Endoscopic surgical management of inspiratory stridor in newborns and infants. Am J Otolaryngol 2015; 36(5): 697-700.
[http://dx.doi.org/10.1016/j.amjoto.2015.05.009]

[14] Olney DR, Greinwald JH Jr, Smith RJ, Bauman NM. Laryngomalacia and its treatment. Laryngoscope 1999; 109(11): 1770-5.
[http://dx.doi.org/10.1097/00005537-199911000-00009]

[15] Landry AM, Thompson DM. Laryngomalacia: disease presentation, spectrum, and . Int J Pediatr 2012; 2012: 753526.

[16] Thompson DM. Laryngomalacia: factors that influence disease severity and outcomes of management. Curr Opin Otolaryngol Head Neck Surg 2010; 18(6): 564-70.
[http://dx.doi.org/10.1097/MOO.0b013e3283405e48]

[17] Dickson JM, Richter GT, Meinzen-Derr J, Rutter MJ, Thompson DM. Secondary airway lesions in infants with laryngomalacia. Ann Otol Rhinol Laryngol 2009; 118(1): 37-43.
[http://dx.doi.org/10.1177/000348940911800107]

[18] Krashin E, Ben-Ari J, Springer C, Derowe A, Avital A, Sivan Y. Synchronous airway lesions in

laryngomalacia. Int J Pediatr Otorhinolaryngol 2008; 72(4): 501-7.
[http://dx.doi.org/10.1016/j.ijporl.2008.01.002]

[19]   Schroeder JW Jr, Bhandarkar ND, Holinger LD. Synchronous airway lesions and outcomes in infants with severe laryngomalacia requiring supraglottoplasty. Arch Otolaryngol Head Neck Surg 2009; 135(7): 647-51.
[http://dx.doi.org/10.1001/archoto.2009.73]

[20]   Rifai HA, Benoit M, El-Hakim H. Secondary airway lesions in laryngomalacia: a different perspective. Otolaryngol Head Neck Surg 2011; 144(2): 268-73.
[http://dx.doi.org/10.1177/0194599810391600]

[21]   Froehlich P, Seid AB, Denoyelle F, Pransky SM, Kearns DB, Garabedian EN, *et al.* Discoordinate pharyngolaryngomalacia. Int J Pediatr Otorhinolaryngol 1997; 39(1): 9-18.
[http://dx.doi.org/10.1016/S0165-5876(96)01454-1]

[22]   Durvasula VS, Lawson BR, Bower CM, Richter GT. Supraglottoplasty outcomes in neurologically affected and syndromic children. JAMA Otolaryngol Head Neck Surg 2014; 140(8): 704-11.
[http://dx.doi.org/10.1001/jamaoto.2014.983]

[23]   Masters IB, Chang AB, Patterson L, Wainwright C, Buntain H, Dean BW, *et al.* Series of laryngomalacia, tracheomalacia, and bronchomalacia disorders and their associations with other conditions in children. Pediatr Pulmonol 2002; 34(3): 189-95.
[http://dx.doi.org/10.1002/ppul.10156]

[24]   Camacho M, Song SA, Cable BB. In response to supraglottoplasty for laryngomalacia with obstructive sleep apnea: A systematic review and meta-analysis. Laryngoscope 2016.

[25]   Lee CF, Lee CH, Kang KT, Hsu WC. In reference to supraglottoplasty for laryngomalacia with obstructive sleep apnea: A systematic review and meta-analysis. Laryngoscope 2016.
[http://dx.doi.org/10.1002/lary.25950]

[26]   Richter GT, Rutter MJ, deAlarcon A, Orvidas LJ, Thompson DM. Late-onset laryngomalacia: a variant of disease. Arch Otolaryngol Head Neck Surg 2008; 134(1): 75-80.
[http://dx.doi.org/10.1001/archoto.2007.17]

[27]   Digoy GP, Burge SD. Laryngomalacia in the older child: clinical presentations and management. Curr Opin Otolaryngol Head Neck Surg 2014; 22(6): 501-5.
[http://dx.doi.org/10.1097/MOO.0000000000000111]

[28]   Oomen KP, Modi VK. Occult laryngomalacia resulting in obstructive sleep apnea in an infant. Int J Pediatr Otorhinolaryngol 2013; 77(9): 1617-9.
[http://dx.doi.org/10.1016/j.ijporl.2013.07.006]

[29]   Amin MR, Isaacson G. State-dependent laryngomalacia. Ann Otol Rhinol Laryngol 1997; 106(11): 887-90.
[http://dx.doi.org/10.1177/000348949710601101]

[30]   Camacho M, Dunn B, Torre C, Sasaki J, Gonzales R, Liu SY, *et al.* Supraglottoplasty for laryngomalacia with obstructive sleep apnea: A systematic review and meta-analysis. Laryngoscope 2015.

[31]   Tanphaichitr A, Tanphaichitr P, Apiwattanasawee P, Brockbank J, Rutter MJ, Simakajornboon N. Prevalence and risk factors for central sleep apnea in infants with laryngomalacia. Otolaryngol Head Neck Surg 2014; 150(4): 677-83.
[http://dx.doi.org/10.1177/0194599814521379]

[32]   Manickam PV, Shott SR, Boss EF, Cohen AP, Meinzen-Derr JK, Amin RS, *et al.* Systematic review of site of obstruction identification and non-CPAP treatment options for children with persistent pediatric obstructive sleep apnea. Laryngoscope 2016; 126(2): 491-500.
[http://dx.doi.org/10.1002/lary.25459]

[33]   Kilpatrick LA, Boyette JR, Hartzell LD, Norton JA, Boswell JB, Bower CM, *et al.* Prospective quality

of life assessment in congenital laryngomalacia. Int J Pediatr Otorhinolaryngol 2014; 78(4): 583-7.
[http://dx.doi.org/10.1016/j.ijporl.2014.01.001]

[34]    Thottam PJ, Simons JP, Choi S, Maguire R, Mehta DK. Clinical relevance of quality of life in laryngomalacia. Laryngoscope 2015.

[35]    Winter H, Gunasekaran T, Tolia V, Gottrand F, Barker PN, Illueca M. Esomeprazole for the Treatment of GERD in Infants Ages 1-11 Months. J Pediatr Gastroenterol Nutr 2015; 60 (Suppl. 1): S9-S15.
[http://dx.doi.org/10.1097/MPG.0b013e3182496b35]

[36]    Baljosevic I, Minic P, Trajkovic G, Markovic-Sovtic G, Radojicic B, Sovtic A. Surgical treatment of severe laryngomalacia: Six month follow up. Pediatr Int 2015; 57(6): 1159-63.
[http://dx.doi.org/10.1111/ped.12706]

[37]    Dias R, Deshmukh CT, Tullu MS, Divecha C, Karande S. Rare treatment option for a common pediatric airway problem. Indian J Crit Care Med 2015; 19(11): 681-3.
[http://dx.doi.org/10.4103/0972-5229.169355]

[38]    Ayari S, Aubertin G, Girschig H, Van Den Abbeele T, Denoyelle F, Couloignier V, *et al.* Management of laryngomalacia. Eur Ann Otorhinolaryngol Head Neck Dis 2013; 130(1): 15-21.
[http://dx.doi.org/10.1016/j.anorl.2012.04.003]

[39]    Ayari-Khalfallah S, Fuchsmann C, Froehlich P. Thulium laser in airway diseases in children. Curr Opin Otolaryngol Head Neck Surg 2008; 16(1): 55-9.
[http://dx.doi.org/10.1097/MOO.0b013e3282f43419]

[40]    Groblewski JC, Shah RK, Zalzal GH. Microdebrider-assisted supraglottoplasty for laryngomalacia. Ann Otol Rhinol Laryngol 2009; 118(8): 592-7.

[41]    Denoyelle F, Mondain M, Gresillon N, Roger G, Chaudre F, Garabedian EN. Failures and complications of supraglottoplasty in children. Arch Otolaryngol Head Neck Surg 2003; 129(10): 1077-80.
[http://dx.doi.org/10.1001/archotol.129.10.1077]

[42]    Rastatter JC, Schroeder JW, Hoff SR, Holinger LD. Aspiration before and after Supraglottoplasty regardless of Technique. Int J Otolaryngol 2010; 2010: 912814.
[http://dx.doi.org/10.1155/2010/912814]

[43]    Douglas CM, Shafi A, Higgins G, *et al.* Risk factors for failure of supraglottoplasty. Int J Pediatr Otorhinolaryngol 2014; 78(9): 1485-8.
[http://dx.doi.org/10.1016/j.ijporl.2014.06.014]

[44]    Walner DL, Neumann DB, Hamming KK, Miller RP. Supraglottoplasty in Infants: A Staged Approach. Ann Otol Rhinol Laryngol 2015; 124(10): 803-7.
[http://dx.doi.org/10.1177/0003489415585869]

[45]    Reddy DK, Matt BH. Unilateral *vs.* bilateral supraglottoplasty for severe laryngomalacia in children. Arch Otolaryngol Head Neck Surg 2001; 127(6): 694-9.
[http://dx.doi.org/10.1001/archotol.127.6.694]

[46]    Gaudreau P, Fordham MT, Dong T, Liu X, Kang S, Preciado D, *et al.* Visualization of the Supraglottis in Laryngomalacia With 3-Dimensional Pediatric Endoscopy. JAMA Otolaryngol Head Neck Surg 2016; 142(3): 258-62.
[http://dx.doi.org/10.1001/jamaoto.2015.3370]

[47]    Whymark AD, Clement WA, Kubba H, Geddes NK. Laser epiglottopexy for laryngomalacia: 10 years' experience in the west of Scotland. Arch Otolaryngol Head Neck Surg 2006; 132(9): 978-82.
[http://dx.doi.org/10.1001/archotol.132.9.978]

[48]    Fordham MT, Potter SM, White DR. Postoperative management following supraglottoplasty for severe laryngomalacia. Laryngoscope 2013; 123(12): 3206-10.
[http://dx.doi.org/10.1002/lary.24108]

[49]   O'Donnell S, Murphy J, Bew S, Knight LC. Aryepiglottoplasty for laryngomalacia: results and recommendations following a case series of 84. Int J Pediatr Otorhinolaryngol 2007; 71(8): 1271-5.
       [http://dx.doi.org/10.1016/j.ijporl.2007.05.001]

[50]   Roger G, Denoyelle F, Triglia JM, Garabedian EN. Severe laryngomalacia: surgical indications and results in 115 patients. Laryngoscope 1995; 105(10): 1111-7.
       [http://dx.doi.org/10.1288/00005537-199510000-00018]

[51]   van der Heijden M, Dikkers FG, Halmos GB. Treatment outcome of supraglottoplasty *vs.* wait-and-see policy in patients with laryngomalacia. Eur Arch Otorhinolaryngol 2016.
       [http://dx.doi.org/10.1007/s00405-016-3943-3]

[52]   Faria J, Behar P. Medical and surgical management of congenital laryngomalacia: a case-control study. Otolaryngol Head Neck Surg 2014; 151(5): 845-51.
       [http://dx.doi.org/10.1177/0194599814541921]

[53]   O'Connor TE, Bumbak P, Vijayasekaran S. Objective assessment of supraglottoplasty outcomes using polysomnography. Int J Pediatr Otorhinolaryngol 2009; 73(9): 1211-6.
       [http://dx.doi.org/10.1016/j.ijporl.2009.05.007]

[54]   Sesterhenn AM, Zimmermann AP, Bernhard M, Kussin A, Timmesfeld N, Stiller S, *et al.* Polysomnography outcomes following transoral $CO_2$ laser microsurgery in pediatric patients with laryngomalacia. Int J Pediatr Otorhinolaryngol 2009; 73(10): 1339-43.
       [http://dx.doi.org/10.1016/j.ijporl.2009.06.002]

[55]   Czechowicz JA, Chang KW. Catch-up growth in infants with laryngomalacia after supraglottoplasty. Int J Pediatr Otorhinolaryngol 2015; 79(8): 1333-6.
       [http://dx.doi.org/10.1016/j.ijporl.2015.06.005]

[56]   Neiner J, Gungor A. Evaluation of growth curves in children after supraglottoplasty. Am J Otolaryngol 2016; 37(2): 128-31.
       [http://dx.doi.org/10.1016/j.amjoto.2015.11.003]

[57]   Escher A, Probst R, Gysin C. Management of laryngomalacia in children with congenital syndrome: the role of supraglottoplasty. J Pediatr Surg 2015; 50(4): 519-23.
       [http://dx.doi.org/10.1016/j.jpedsurg.2014.05.035]

[58]   Hwang E, Chung J, MacCormick J, Bromwich M, Vaccani JP. Success of supraglottoplasty for severe laryngomalacia: the experience from Northeastern Ontario, Canada. Int J Pediatr Otorhinolaryngol 2013; 77(7): 1103-6.
       [http://dx.doi.org/10.1016/j.ijporl.2013.04.010]

[59]   Preciado D, Zalzal G. A systematic review of supraglottoplasty outcomes. Arch Otolaryngol Head Neck Surg 2012; 138(8): 718-21.
       [http://dx.doi.org/10.1001/archoto.2012.1251]

[60]   Hoff SR, Schroeder JW Jr, Rastatter JC, Holinger LD. Supraglottoplasty outcomes in relation to age and comorbid conditions. Int J Pediatr Otorhinolaryngol 2010; 74(3): 245-9.
       [http://dx.doi.org/10.1016/j.ijporl.2009.11.012]

[61]   Durvasula VS, Lawson BR, Bower CM, Richter GT. Supraglottoplasty in premature infants with laryngomalacia: does gestation age at birth influence outcomes? Otolaryngol Head Neck Surg 2014; 150(2): 292-9.
       [http://dx.doi.org/10.1177/0194599813514370]

[62]   Ozmen S, Ozmen OA, Unal OF. Pediatric tracheotomies: a 37-year experience in 282 children. Int J Pediatr Otorhinolaryngol 2009; 73(7): 959-61.
       [http://dx.doi.org/10.1016/j.ijporl.2009.03.020]

[63]   D'Souza JN, Levi JR, Park D, Shah UK. Complications Following Pediatric Tracheotomy. JAMA Otolaryngol Head Neck Surg 2016.
       [http://dx.doi.org/10.1001/jamaoto.2016.0173]

[64]    Essouri S, Nicot F, Clement A, *et al.* Noninvasive positive pressure ventilation in infants with upper airway obstruction: comparison of continuous and bilevel positive pressure. Intensive Care Med 2005; 31(4): 574-80.
[http://dx.doi.org/10.1007/s00134-005-2568-6]

[65]    Fauroux B, Pigeot J, Polkey MI, *et al.* Chronic stridor caused by laryngomalacia in children: work of breathing and effects of noninvasive ventilatory assistance. Am J Respir Crit Care Med 2001; 164(10 Pt 1): 1874-8.
[http://dx.doi.org/10.1164/ajrccm.164.10.2012141]

[66]    Fauroux B, Leroux K, Desmarais G, *et al.* Performance of ventilators for noninvasive positive-pressure ventilation in children. Eur Respir J 2008; 31(6): 1300-7.
[http://dx.doi.org/10.1183/09031936.00144807]

[67]    Fauroux B, Lavis JF, Nicot F, *et al.* Facial side effects during noninvasive positive pressure ventilation in children. Intensive Care Med 2005; 31(7): 965-9.
[http://dx.doi.org/10.1007/s00134-005-2669-2]

# CHAPTER 7

# Synopsis of Management of Diabetes Mellitus Types 1 and 2

Eric Velazquez and Bethany A. Auble[*]

*Medical College of Wisconsin, Children's Hospital of Wisconsin, Milwaukee, Wisconsin, USA*

**Abstract:** Diabetes involves pancreatic dysfunction due to autoimmune destruction of the beta cells and insulin deficiency. The prevalence and incidence of Type 1 and Type 2 are increasing in the general population. Type 1 Diabetes often begins in childhood and requires lifelong insulin replacement therapy and monitoring of blood glucose levels. Long and short-acting insulin allows for adjustment of therapies around patients' lives, but close medical observation and a good patient-provider relationship is necessary for optimal management. Type 2 Diabetes is characterized by severe insulin resistance and partial deficiency that has become more prevalent in pediatric patients, often occurring around puberty. Therapy involves lifestyle changes to promote active weight loss, healthy eating habits, and exercise. Few pharmacological therapies are approved, but many are being studied for pediatric use.

**Keywords:** Artificial Pancreas, Bariatric Surgery, Closed Loop Control, Continuous Glucose Monitoring, Continuous Subcutaneous Insulin Injection, Glucagon, Insulin, Lifestyle Changes, Metformin, Multiple Daily Insulin Injections, Type 1 Diabetes, Type 2 Diabetes.

## INTRODUCTION

Diabetes Mellitus is a life-altering diagnosis, requiring adjustment of a patient's life and schedule. In pediatric patients, it also changes the entire family's focus. Loss of insulin-secreting beta cells results in loss of glycemic control with subsequent hyperglycemia in Type 1 diabetes. Insulin replacement therapy remains the mainstay of current therapy. Advances in insulin pumps, continuous glucose monitors, and closed loop control systems have resulted in long-term improved glycemic control. New advancements in pancreatic transplant, stem cell therapy, biomarker screenings, and prevention strategies are being published yearly. Type 2 Diabetes requires an alternative approach to management with a

[*] **Corresponding author Bethany A. Auble**: Medical College of Wisconsin, Children's Hospital of Wisconsin, Milwaukee, Wisconsin, USA; Tel: 414-337-8717; Fax: 414-266-6749; Email: bauble@mcw.edu

**Seckin Ulualp (Ed.)**

strong emphasis placed on diet, exercise, and lifestyle modifications. The medical therapies for the treatment of Type 2 Diabetes are a growing field of research, but pharmacotherapy must be combined with lifestyle changes if lasting health improvements are to be achieved.

## Epidemiology

In the United States, the prevalence of Type 1 Diabetes is estimated for 0.25% of the population [1]. From 2001–2009, prevalence of Type 1 diabetes increased by nearly 20%, with projections suggesting that from 2010 to 2050, the number of youth with Type 1 diabetes may triple. In this same time period, the prevalence of Type 2 diabetes increased by nearly 30% and accounts for 45% of newly diagnosed cases of diabetes in the pediatric population. Projections suggest that from 2010 to 2050, a nearly 4-fold increase might occur of patients with Type 2 diabetes. While still relatively uncommon, the rates of new cases of type 2 diabetes were greater among peripubertal individuals aged 10–19 years than in younger children, with higher rates among U.S. minority populations than in non-Hispanic whites.

## Physiology

The pancreas is both an exocrine gland and an endocrine gland. Endocrine cells are located within scattered Islets of Langerhans and divided into three categories: alpha-cells (produce glucagon), beta-cells (produce insulin and amylin) and delta-cells (produce somatostatin). Insulin stimulates cells to uptake free glucose, glycogenesis in the liver, and uptake amino acids, proteins and fat from the bloodstream. Humans are born with a varying amount of beta-cells, and even within these cells, there is variation to susceptibility to auto-immune attack [2]. In Type 1 Diabetes, autoimmune destruction of beta-cells produces gradual dysregulation of glucose and its symptoms develop after >80-90% of cells are lost. Type 2 Diabetes is caused by the relative deficiency of insulin due to severe peripheral tissue resistance.

Glucagon works primarily in the liver to convert glycogen into glucose to raise blood glucose. Its function becomes dysregulated in type 2 diabetes, leading to postprandial hypersecretion, worsening overall hyperglycemia. Amylin is a neuroendocrine peptide hormone that is co-secreted with insulin, uses the same processing enzymes, and works to suppress release of glucagon, slows digestion and slows rate of insulin entering the bloodstream. The benefit of delayed gastric emptying is creating a slower rise, and overall lower peak level of blood glucose [3]. Somatostatin is a peptide hormone that has many GI effects but is active in slowing gastric emptying, suppressing insulin and glucagon release, and suppressing exocrine pancreatic secretions. Incretins are small hormones released by intestinal mucosa that stimulate insulin release, delay gastric emptying and inhibit glucagon release. While native molecules have short half-lives, synthetic versions last much longer and are being looked at as therapeutic alternatives.

## TYPE 1 DIABETES MELLITUS

The "event" of stage II most likely is not a single event but some combination of environmental and genetic triggers. The time period of stage III-IV is highly variable, the reasons for why are being closely studied [2]. Patients most often present with classic symptoms of onset: polyuria, polydipsia, hyperglycemia and ketonuria during Stage V (some present in full diabetic ketoacidosis). The "honeymoon period" between Stage V and VI is called such as very low supplemental insulin is required to maintain normoglycemia Fig. (**1**).

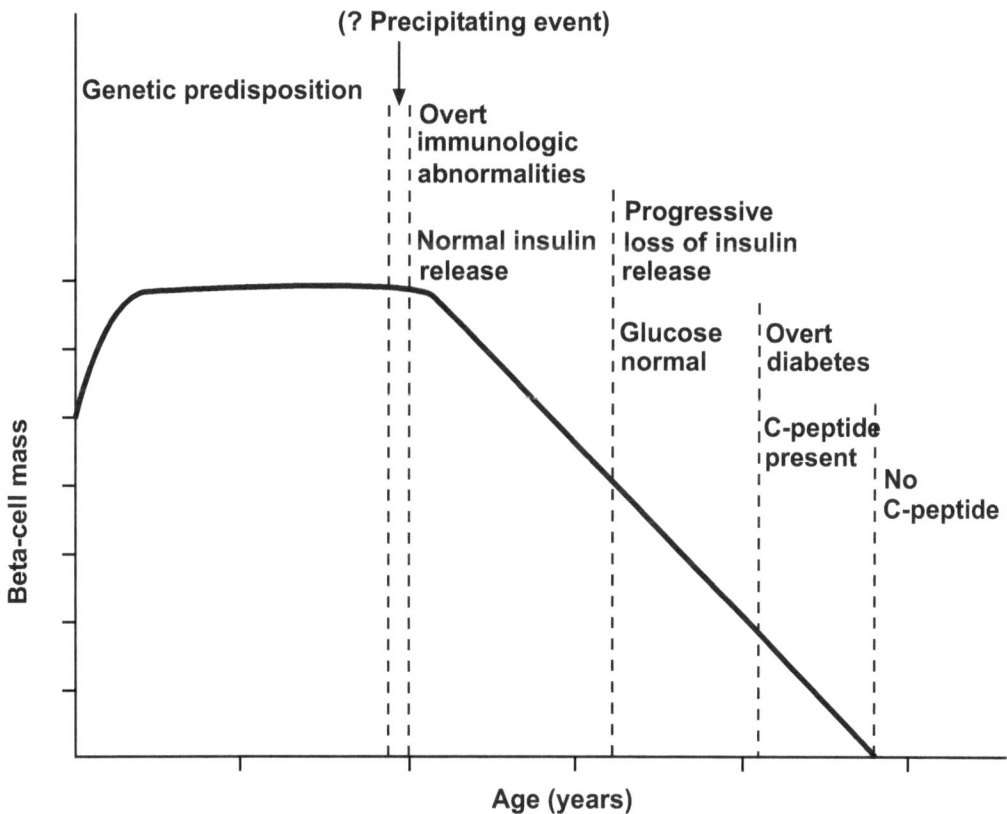

**Fig. (1).** The Eisenbarth model for the development of Type 1 Diabetes is divided into six stages: 1. Genetic Predisposition, 2. Triggering "Event," 3. Activation of Autoimmune Response, 4. Immunologic Response with progressive loss of insulin secretion with maintenance of normal blood sugar level, 5. Symptoms develop, but residual insulin secretion is maintained, 6. Loss of residual insulin secretion to a point of glucose dysregulation [4].

Hemoglobin A1c is the form of hemoglobin produced through nonenzymatic glycation within red blood cells. Production varies directly with plasma glucose levels. Monitoring concentration allows for idea of average glucose levels over the life span of the red blood cells (roughly 2-3 months). The ADA treatment guidelines recommend: HbA1C <7.5% in pediatrics, <7% in adults (lower for pregnant women), reduction in hypoglycemic events and prevention of long-term complications of poor glycemic control. Most adults are not meeting the ADA HbA1c goal, and patients 13-25 years old actually have the worst control based on HbA1c levels [5].

## Multiple Daily Injection Insulin Regimens

Multiple Daily Injection (MDI) insulin regimen is the standard therapeutic approach of Type 1 Diabetes and involves calculating daily insulin requirement, basal insulin amount, carbohydrate coverage dosing, and meal-time sliding-scale bolus doses. Total daily insulin dose is highly variable, but is generally determined by the patient's pubertal status (Table **1**).

Table 1. Types of Insulin.

| Insulin Type | Examples | Onset of Action | Peak Effect | Duration of Action |
|---|---|---|---|---|
| Rapid-Acting | Insulin Lispro (Humalog), Insulin Aspart (NovoLog) Insulin Glulisine (Apidra) | 15-20 minutes | 30-90 minutes | 1-4 hours |
| Regular-Acting | Novolin R and Humulin R | 30-45 minutes | 2-3 hours | 5-8 hours |
| Intermediate-Acting | NPH (Humulin N, Novolin N) | 2-4 hours | 4-10 hours | 4-12 hours |
| Long-Acting | Insulin glargine (Lantus) Insulin detemir (Levemir) | 2-4 hours | No peak 8-10 hours | 20-24 hours Dose-related |

Use of a basal/bolus dosing regiment attempts to establish patterns that most closely approximate normal human physiologic release of insulin. Advantages for this style of dosing include: improved glycemic control, lower HbA1c, and may reduce hypoglycemic events overnight. Pre-meal injections allows for a more flexible meal-time schedule to accommodate lifestyle. The addition of carbohydrate coverage dosing allows for freedom of meal choice (*e.g.* high-carbohydrate meal will need more insulin; a low-carbohydrate meal will need less). Disadvantage of basal-bolus dosing of insulin is that multiple injections throughout the day are needed, and frequent glucose checks are also required. The number of fingerstick blood glucose checks and injections can be distressing to some patients. With the advent of insulin pump therapy, new basal-bolus approaches became possible (Table **2**).

**Table 2. Calculation of Insulin Requirements.**

|  | Insulin | Dose Calculation | Calculation for 20 kg Child | Dose |
|---|---|---|---|---|
| Total Daily Insulin Dose |  | 0.5 – 1.0 units/kg/day | 0.5 x 20 = 10 units/day | 10 Units |
| Basal Dose | Glargine | 50% of total | 50% x 10 = 5 units | 5 Units |
|  | Detemir | 50% of total divided into twice a day dosing |  |  |
| Meal-time Glucose Correction | Lispro, Aspart | 1800 / Daily Dose | 1800 / 10 = 180 | 1 unit for every 180 mg/dL > ideal glucose |
|  |  | 1500/ Daily Dose | 1500 / 10 = 150 | 1 U for every 150 mg/dL > ideal glucose |
|  | Regular |  |  |  |
| Carbohydrate Coverage Ratio | Lispro, Aspart | 400 / Daily Dose | 400 / 10 = 40 | 1 unit for every 40 g carbs |
|  |  | 500 / Daily Dose | 500 / 10 = 50 | 1 unit for every 50 g carbs |
|  | Regular |  |  |  |

## Continuous Subcutaneous Insulin Injection (Insulin Pumps)

Compact insulin pumps were first introduced in the 1990s, being attractive to patients due to less daily injections and overall less medical equipment to carry. The introduction of smart pumps in the 2000's saw benefits such as incremental dose adjustments possible, alternative basal patterns, and temporary basal rate options. Better physiologic understanding of insulin effect in the body, coupled with dosing technology, allowed for matching of basal insulin to circadian variations in hormones that affect insulin sensitivity. Disadvantages of insulin pumps include, the cost of the unit, and the need for pump to be constantly attached to body. Because there is no long-acting insulin, if an insulin pump is accidently disconnected, the patient is not receiving insulin infusion.

Insulin pumps may be an attractive option for patients, and current studies have shown that pumps result in no increase in rate of DKA [6], no differences in severe hypoglycemia, no lasting differences in A1c in small children [7], and only some improvement in older children with high baseline A1c [8]. There is however, a modest improvement in quality of life. A "standard" bolus combines continuous basal insulin infusion with short-acting pre-meal bolus dosing. It is useful as a basic insulin regimen. An "extended" bolus combines continuous basal insulin with a meal-time bolus. The bolus, however, is given over a prolonged period of time. This type of dosing is useful for patients with gastroparesis, meals high in fat or protein but lower in carbohydrates, or if patient is eating small amounts of carbohydrates over a long period of time (*i.e.* movie popcorn, party appetizers). A "combination" bolus functions similar to extended dosing but also includes an immediate bolus with the extended bolus. This can be useful for meals high in fat, protein and carbohydrates to address fast but sustained elevation in blood glucose (*i.e.* pizza). A "super" bolus combines basal and bolus dosing but either stops or partially reduces basal dosing prior to a meal. The amount of insulin not given is combined with bolus to give a "super bolus." This is useful for very high glycemic index foods, large intake of carbohydrates, or situations where more insulin is needed quickly.

## Continuous Glucose Monitors

The introduction, and subsequent newer models, of continuous glucose monitors (CGM) opens up new doors for management of type 1 diabetes. This technology involves a subcutaneous monitor of interstitial glucose concentration multiple times per hour, allowing for analysis of trends and warnings of future hypoglycemia as well as monitoring for asymptomatic nocturnal hypoglycemia, an often under-recognized problem in patients with diabetes. Initial studies found that benefit of CGM, including improved HbA1c, was only seen in adult populations [9]. More recent studies have shown benefit in pediatric patients. The Endocrine Society recommends CGM for persons >8 years of age with Type 1 Diabetes, if they are able to wear it on a near-daily basis. Continued innovation is resulting in shorter lag time between readings and improved accuracy of glucose levels. The technology requires close contact with medical providers, consistent use, and an understanding that it will not reduce efforts in diabetes management by families with improvement of knowledge of blood glucose levels [10].

## New Advances in Technology

Attempts to connect insulin pump technology with continuous glucose monitoring to function as similarly to a pancreas are showing promise. This combination involves computer module constructs called "closed loop control." The primary goal of these systems is to maintain normal range glucose levels with real time microadjustments in insulin infusion volumes without increasing frequency of hypoglycemia. Newer and more sophisticated systems and algorithms are being developed continuously [11]. Uses of amylin or glucagon daily injections to augment or balance out insulin are also being researched. Subcutaneous glucagon injections, when linked to continuous glucose monitoring and delivered in pulse fashion, may significantly decrease time spent in hypoglycemia. Many studies are looking into the feasibility of glucagon pumps. Since glucagon does not last long in solution and must be reconstituted prior to usage in emergency hypoglycemia events, studies are looking for stable long-term formulations and at physiologic activity of "aged" glucagon [12]. Amylin injections have been shown to improve glycemic control, reduce degree of postprandial glucose elevations, and decrease marked swings in blood glucose levels [3].

## Family Questions you may be asked

a. "When will they invent an artificial pancreas/will a transplant be an option?" - The answer is complicated, however progress is being made from three fundamentally separate but interrelated pathways: use of current medical equipment in new novel combinations, bio-artificial beta-islet cell sheets for implantation, and genetic therapy with DNA viruses to stimulate cells to become insulin-producing. Much research is going into each of these areas, with advancements slowly being worked into current practice guidelines even now.

b. "Is there a way to prevent the disease from occurring in my other children, or reverse its activity currently?" - In the recent decades, more dedicated focus has been placed on considering what roles aging, diet, geographic location, immune cell metabolism, microbiomes, viral and microbial pathogens and even epigenetics might play on disease development. Even with new papers and studies being released and started every year, much remains unknown with regards to prevention.

c. "Is there genetic testing available for those at risk for developing type 1 diabetes?" - The classic biomarkers that "predict" type 1 diabetes are serum autoantibodies, with four major targets: Insulin, GAD65, IA-2 and zinc transporter 8. However, despite identifying these genes, constructing strong predictive algorithms based around genetics remains unable to be successfully performed. Attempts to use autoreactive T-cells, biomarkers of beta cell stress, metabolomics and proteomics have all had yet to identify validated predictors of Type 1 Diabetes [13].

d. "What about the new inhaled insulin that just came out?" Afrezza is an inhaled, rapid-acting insulin, which was released in 2015 but met with poor initial sales. Onset of action is within 15-20 minutes, peak activity achieved by 30 minutes after inhalation, and remains in system for only 180 minutes. More studies are needed to look at safety and efficacy in children as well assessing clinical use in patient care.

## TYPE 2 DIABETES MELLITUS

Patients with Type 2 diabetes often present with insidious onset of symptoms, and there can be chronic behavioral and lifestyle habits that may worsen disease progression. Type 2 Diabetes occurs more commonly in adults, but has been increasingly diagnosed in pediatric patients. It is associated with obesity and a strong familial predisposition, with many first- and second-degree relatives often having Type 2 Diabetes. In addition, there can be high rates of patients lost to follow up. A sharp increase in prevalence of Type 2 diabetes has prompted new research into pathophysiology and therapeutic options to decrease, reverse, or prevent complications of insulin resistance and beta-cell dysfunction [14]. While the disease prevalence among pediatric patients is increasing, therapeutic modalities continue to be limited. An absence of data concerning the various medication subclasses efficacy and safety in pediatric patients prevents using various adult Type 2 diabetes medication options. Therapy must address blood glucose control, but also needs to address the increased risks of comorbidities such as hypertension, dyslipidemia and renal disease. Treatment goals of Type 2 Diabetes include: weight management, increasing physical activity, achieving glycemic control with normalization of HbA1c, and managing comorbidities such as dyslipidemia and hypertension [14].

### Lifestyle Modifications

The most impactful aspect of care for Type 2 Diabetes is family-based behavioral lifestyle interventions. Type 2 diabetes is a disease involving, and worsened by, obesity, so prevention of weight gain and/or weight loss are key parts of care. The importance of family-centered modifications is based on concerns that most pediatric patients do not often purchase their own food, so lifestyle changes can be limited by parental choice. Proper dietary counseling is critical as exercise without dietary changes often limits full results. This includes, eliminate sugar-containing beverages and high-fat high-calorie foods, portion control, improved food choices, and regular meal schedule. Exercise goals include decreasing amounts of time spent being sedentary (*e.g.* television, other screen time, video games) and promoting reasonable health goals.

### Pharmacotherapy in Type 2 Diabetes

Metformin is the only current FDA-approved oral treatment for youth with Type 2 Diabetes. HbA1c is lowered and fasting plasma glucose is improved in studies. Nonsignificant decreases in LDL cholesterol were also noted. Side effects notable from metformin use included abdominal pain, diarrhea, nausea/vomiting and headache, but all symptoms are improved with appropriate dosing and passage of time [15].

Insulin is the only additional pharmacological agent used to treat uncontrolled Type 2 Diabetes in pediatric patients, often with HbA1c levels >9%. A 16-week study in adolescents showed that use of premixed insulin can improve HbA1c without significant changes in BMI or hypoglycemia. Dose-adjustment in response to target blood glucose levels even resulted in many patients requiring even shorter courses of therapy. The effects observed were also noted to persist for 12 months after stopping the 16-week trial [16]. A major issue with insulin therapy is that while the goal is to keep/get patients off of insulin, only a limited number of patients are able to discontinue insulin therapy, and many being restarted due to poor glycemic control.

Use of Thiazolidinediones and insulin secretagogues is widely debated by pediatric endocrinologists due to absence of good literature to support safety and efficacy. A study comparing glimepiride (sulfonylurea) *versus* metformin usage over 26 weeks showed comparable HbA1c reduction and relative safety profile. Patients receiving glimepiride had more weight gain and higher BMI compared to metformin users, but this is a known side effect of sulfonylurea agents [17]. Limited studies exist for use of TZD in adolescent patients, what is present shows moderate HbA1c reduction but significant concern exists over the medications safety profile in the adult literature.

Glinides and Glucosidase inhibitors (Acarbose) are currently being examined for use in adolescent patients. The need for medication usage prior to every meal may make adherence to regimen a concern for patients.

Exenatide, an incretin-mimetic agent, has been used as an adjunctive therapy in adults due to its glucagon-like peptide (GLP-1) properties. It decreases glucose-dependent insulin secretion, slows gastric emptying, increases satiety, has been found to reduce body weight, and improves some cardiovascular risk factors. A recent study in adolescents used low-dose Exenatide and observed pharmacokinetics and dynamics to see if agents are safe for adolescent usage. Minimal side effects and reduced postprandial glucose levels were noted, encouraging further testing with higher dosing to observe effects. While reassuring, further research needs to be performed before this agent can be more strongly recommended for therapy [18].

## Bariatric Surgery

Eligibility criteria for adolescents include BMI >35 kg/m2, if a serious comorbidity, like Type 2 Diabetes, is present. Patient must be Tanner stage IV or V, having achieved skeletal maturity. Small studies exist that show favorable results post-surgery with regard to BMI, diabetic control, hyperlipidemia, and hypertension [19]. Caution should be applied before considering this as a recommended therapy until larger, longer and better-controlled studies exist.

## Comorbidities and Complications

Microalbuminuria is more prevalent in Type 2 diabetic youth compared to Type 1 diabetics. A few studies have shown that presence of microalbuminuria in adolescent Type 2 diabetics is associated with a higher rate of end stage renal disease compared to adult-onset type 2 diabetics with microalbuminuria. The rate of progression of microalbuminuria to renal disease tends to be more rapid in adolescents as well [20].

Recommendations exist for treatment of hypertension based on systolic and diastolic pressures by height [21], since no absolute cutoff for elevated blood pressure exists for pediatrics. The recommendation is aggressive treatment to delay progression to end stage renal disease. ACE-inhibitors, or if not tolerated, angiotensin receptor blockers (ARBSs) should be used.

Dyslipidemia exists in approximately 18-61% of youth with type 2 diabetes. The combination of these risk factors has been associated with early signs of cardiovascular disease. Goal LDL for patients with diabetes is less than 100 mg/dl, triglycerides <150 mg/dL, and HDL >35 mg/dL. Pharmacotherapy should be started for patients with an LDL >160 mg/dL, and should be considered 130-159 mg/dL, if other risk factors are present. Statin therapy usage in adolescents has been found to be safe and effective [22], fibric acid and Omega-3 fatty acids can be considered if triglycerides are >1000 mg/dL, given the risk for pancreatitis.

## CONCLUSION

The care of the patient with diabetes can be challenging. Patients and their families require significant education, lifestyle changes, medication adjustment, frequent clinic visits, and often benefit from an external support system. The diagnosis of Type 1 Diabetes tasks children and their families to learn the importance of diet, exercise, and personal control of health. A good working relationship with health care providers and family is necessary to navigate the changes of adolescence to allow for greater independence. A diagnosis of Type 2 Diabetes is also significantly challenging to manage. The patient's underlying health issues, including obesity, hypertension, renal disease, and hyperlipidemia often exist prior to the development of overt diabetes. The family must actively commit to lifestyle changes, which may be difficult in many patients. A high degree of loss to follow-up is observed in many studies of children and adolescents with Type 2 diabetes, highlighting the challenge of treatment. A strong personal relationship with patients and their families is ideal to improve the health outcomes.

## CONFLICT OF INTEREST

The authors declare no conflict of interest, financial or otherwise.

## ACKNOWLEDGEMENTS

Declared none.

## REFERENCES

[1]　Dabelea D, Mayer-Davis EJ, Saydah S, *et al.* Prevalence of type 1 and type 2 diabetes among children and adolescents from 2001 to 2009. JAMA 2014; 311(17): 1778-86.
[http://dx.doi.org/10.1001/jama.2014.3201]

[2]　Atkinson MA, von Herrath M, Powers AC, Clare-Salzler M. Current concepts on the pathogenesis of type 1 diabetes--considerations for attempts to prevent and reverse the disease. Diabetes Care 2015; 38(6): 979-88.
[http://dx.doi.org/10.2337/dc15-0144]

[3]　Schmitz O, Brock B, Rungby J. Amylin agonists: a novel approach in the treatment of diabetes. Diabetes 2004; 53 (Suppl. 3): S233-8.
[http://dx.doi.org/10.2337/diabetes.53.suppl_3.S233]

[4]　Eisenbarth GS. Type I diabetes mellitus. A chronic autoimmune disease. N Engl J Med 1986; 314(21): 1360-8.
[http://dx.doi.org/10.1056/NEJM198605223142106]

[5]　Miller KM, Foster NC, Beck RW, *et al.* Current state of type 1 diabetes treatment in the U.S.: updated data from the T1D Exchange clinic registry. Diabetes Care 2015; 38(6): 971-8.
[http://dx.doi.org/10.2337/dc15-0078]

[6]　Weinzimer SA, Ahern JH, Doyle EA, *et al.* Persistence of benefits of continuous subcutaneous insulin infusion in very young children with type 1 diabetes: a follow-up report. Pediatrics 2004; 114(6): 1601-5.
[http://dx.doi.org/10.1542/peds.2004-0092]

[7]　DiMeglio LA, Pottorff TM, Boyd SR, France L, Fineberg N, Eugster EA. A randomized, controlled study of insulin pump therapy in diabetic preschoolers. J Pediatr 2004; 145(3): 380-4.
[http://dx.doi.org/10.1016/j.jpeds.2004.06.022]

[8]　Mameli C, Scaramuzza AE, Ho J, Cardona-Hernandez R, Suarez-Ortega L, Zuccotti GV. A 7-year follow-up retrospective, international, multicenter study of insulin pump therapy in children and adolescents with type 1 diabetes. Acta Diabetol 2014; 51(2): 205-10.
[http://dx.doi.org/10.1007/s00592-013-0481-y]

[9]　Juvenile Diabetes Research Foundation Continuous Glucose Monitoring Study Group. Continuous glucose monitoring and intensive treatment of type 1 diabetes. N Engl J Med 2008; 359(14): 1464-76.
[http://dx.doi.org/10.1056/NEJMoa0805017]

[10]　Larson NS, Pinsker JE. The role of continuous glucose monitoring in the care of children with type 1 diabetes. Int J Pediatr Endocrinol 2013 Mar 26; 2013(1): 8-9856-2013-8.
[http://dx.doi.org/10.1186/1687-9856-2013-8]

[11]　Breton M, Farret A, Bruttomesso D, *et al.* Fully integrated artificial pancreas in type 1 diabetes: modular closed-loop glucose control maintains near normoglycemia. Diabetes 2012; 61(9): 2230-7.
[http://dx.doi.org/10.2337/db11-1445]

[12]　Castle JR, Engle JM, El Youssef J, *et al.* Novel use of glucagon in a closed-loop system for prevention of hypoglycemia in type 1 diabetes. Diabetes Care 2010; 33(6): 1282-7.
[http://dx.doi.org/10.2337/dc09-2254]

[13]    Bonifacio E. Predicting type 1 diabetes using biomarkers. Diabetes Care 2015; 38(6): 989-96.
[http://dx.doi.org/10.2337/dc15-0101]

[14]    Weigensberg MJ, Goran MI. Type 2 diabetes in children and adolescents. Lancet 2009; 373(9677): 1743-4.
[http://dx.doi.org/10.1016/S0140-6736(09)60961-2]

[15]    Jones KL, Arslanian S, Peterokova VA, Park JS, Tomlinson MJ. Effect of metformin in pediatric patients with type 2 diabetes: a randomized controlled trial. Diabetes Care 2002; 25(1): 89-94.
[http://dx.doi.org/10.2337/diacare.25.1.89]

[16]    Sellers EA, Dean HJ. Short-term insulin therapy in adolescents with type 2 diabetes mellitus. J Pediatr Endocrinol Metab 2004; 17(11): 1561-4.
[http://dx.doi.org/10.1515/JPEM.2004.17.11.1561]

[17]    Gottschalk M, Danne T, Vlajnic A, Cara JF. Glimepiride *versus* metformin as monotherapy in pediatric patients with type 2 diabetes: a randomized, single-blind comparative study. Diabetes Care 2007; 30(4): 790-4.
[http://dx.doi.org/10.2337/dc06-1554]

[18]    Malloy J, Capparelli E, Gottschalk M, Guan X, Kothare P, Fineman M. Pharmacology and tolerability of a single dose of exenatide in adolescent patients with type 2 diabetes mellitus being treated with metformin: a randomized, placebo-controlled, single-blind, dose-escalation, crossover study. Clin Ther 2009; 31(4): 806-15.
[http://dx.doi.org/10.1016/j.clinthera.2009.04.005]

[19]    Inge TH, Miyano G, Bean J, *et al.* Reversal of type 2 diabetes mellitus and improvements in cardiovascular risk factors after surgical weight loss in adolescents. Pediatrics 2009; 123(1): 214-22.
[http://dx.doi.org/10.1542/peds.2008-0522]

[20]    Pavkov ME, Bennett PH, Knowler WC, Krakoff J, Sievers ML, Nelson RG. Effect of youth-onset type 2 diabetes mellitus on incidence of end-stage renal disease and mortality in young and middle-aged Pima Indians. JAMA 2006; 296(4): 421-6.
[http://dx.doi.org/10.1001/jama.296.4.421]

[21]    National High Blood Pressure Education Program Working Group on High Blood Pressure in Children and Adolescents. The fourth report on the diagnosis, evaluation, and treatment of high blood pressure in children and adolescents. Pediatrics 2004 Aug; 114(2 Suppl 4th Report): 555-76.

[22]    Rosenbloom AL, Silverstein JH, Amemiya S, Zeitler P, Klingensmith GJ. Type 2 diabetes in children and adolescents. Pediatr Diabetes 2009; 10 (Suppl. 12): 17-32.
[http://dx.doi.org/10.1111/j.1399-5448.2009.00584.x]

# CHAPTER 8

# Pediatric Type 2 Diabetes Mellitus

**Carisse Orsi***, **Maria Rayas, Jessica Hutchins** and **Elia Escaname**

*Department of Pediatrics, University of Texas San Antonio Health Science Center, San Antonio, TX, USA*

**Abstract:** Pediatric Type 2 Diabetes Mellitus (T2DM) is an increasing medical concern for the pediatric community. It is most commonly diagnosed in adolescents but has also been seen in patients as young as 5 years of age. Presentation of T2DM can range from mild symptoms of polyuria, polydipsia and nocturia to diabetic ketoacidosis. Guidelines by the American Diabetes Association are used to diagnose and treat children with diabetes. Early diagnosis and aggressive treatment is critical in delaying complications of diabetes. Poorly controlled diabetes can lead to significant increase in morbidity and mortality with development of hypertension, nephropathy and retinopathy. In this chapter, a review of the epidemiology of Type 2 diabetes, diagnosis and treatment options will be discussed.

**Keywords:** A1c, Acanthosis nigricans, Hypertension, Insulin resistance, Metformin, Nephropathy, OGTT, Pediatric, Pediatrics, Rosiglitazone, T2DM.

## INTRODUCTION

When diabetes is discussed in the pediatric setting, one primarily thinks of Type 1 diabetes mellitus (T1DM). In the past decade, more physicians caring for pediatric patients are encountering an increase in the number of overweight and obese patients. These subset of patients bring along co-morbidities that are considered uncommon in general pediatrics. Now the pediatric provider must be able to identify patients at risk for not only Type 2 diabetes mellitus (T2DM), but also conditions such as hypertension, dyslipidemia and non-alcoholic fatty liver disease.

## EPIDEMIOLOGY

Although initially referred to as adult onset diabetes, T2DM is now commonly diagnosed by physicians in the pediatric population. The increase in T2DM in

* **Corresponding author Carisse Orsi**: Department of Pediatrics, University of Texas San Antonio Health Science Center, San Antonio, TX, USA; Tel: 210-567-5283; Fax: 210-567-0492; Email: orsic@uthscsa.edu

Seckin Ulualp (Ed.)

children coincides with the rising childhood obesity rate. In a study conducted through Yale Pediatric Obesity clinic, impaired glucose tolerance (prediabetes) was reported in 25% of children and 21% of adolescents with a BMI >95% for age and sex [1]. The worrisome concern in this particular population is that the progression from impaired glucose tolerance to overt T2DM seems to occur at an accelerated pace in children compared to adults [2]. Additional factors that may contribute to the increase in childhood T2DM are exposure to diabetes in utero and endocrine disrupting chemicals, such as organophosphates and nicotine [3].

The SEARCH study is the largest to date registry for diabetes in youth <20 years of age. This study evaluated the prevalence of T1DM, T2DM, maturity onset diabetes (MODY) and "uncertain type". Ten years ago, T2DM accounted for less than 3% of all new cases of diabetes in adolescents, but now accounts for 20-50%. Comparing data from 2001 and 2009 reveals a 30.5% increase in T2DM diagnosed in children <20 years of age [4].

The prevalence of T2DM by race is highest in American Indians, followed by blacks, Hispanics, Asian Pacific Islanders and lastly whites [4]. The prevalence is higher in ages 15-19 years compared to ages 10-14 due to the increase in insulin resistance appreciated during puberty [2]. Females are more likely to be diagnosed with T2DM than males. Of the children diagnosed with T2DM, 75% have a first or second degree relative with T2DM [2].

## DIAGNOSIS

With the increasing number of T2DM cases, it is imperative that the pediatric provider identifies children at risk for T2DM in hope to prevent or at least delay the diagnosis. A thorough family history is important to determine risks factors, as well as, distinguish risks for other types of diabetes like MODY. Based on the 2016 ADA diabetes guidelines, screening for T2DM in the pediatric population is indicated in patients that have a BMI >85% for age and sex plus two other additional risk factors (Table **1**) [5]. Screening should begin at 10 years of age or earlier depending on the onset of puberty. The timing of puberty is important given its association with increased insulin resistance. Patients at risk should be screened every 3 years. They may be screened more often if they exhibit symptoms consistent with T2DM, such as polyuria or polydipsia.

Another risk factor includes the presence of acanthosis nigricans (AN). AN refers to darkening of the skin associated with insulin resistance that is usually appreciated on the back of the neck or other skin folds. It is a helpful physical finding that health care providers may use to identify children at risk for diabetes. It is also a non-invasive tool utilized in the school setting to increase the screening of children that may not be receiving regular health care. It can be graded on a scale described by Burke *et al*. (Table **2**) [6]. Its regression can be a sign of improved glycemic control and insulin resistance. There does not appear to be any correlation between the degree of AN and the development of T2DM.

**Table 1. Risk factor for diabetes.**

| **Testing for Type 2 Diabetes or Prediabetes in Asymptomatic Children (<18 years)** |
|---|
| **Criteria:** <br> ☐ Overweight (BMI >85% for age and sex, weight for height >85%, or weight >120% of ideal for height) |
| **Plus any two of the following risk factors:** <br> ☐ Family history of T2DM in fort or second degree relative <br> ☐ Race/ethnicity (Native American, African American, Latino, Asian American, Pacific Islander) <br> ☐ Signs of insulin resistance or condition associated with insulin resistance (acanthosis, hypertension, dyslipidemia, polycystic ovarian syndrome, SGA birth weight) <br> ☐ Maternal History of diabetes or GDM during the child's gestation |

**Table 2. Grading system for Acanthosis Nigricans.**

| **Acanthosis Nigricans Score** | **Acanthosis Nigricans Description** |
|---|---|
| 0 | Absent |
| 1 | Present on close visual inspection |
| 2 (mild) | Present at the base of the skull (does not extend to lateral neck)or axillae |
| 3 (moderate) | Extends to lateral margins of the neck; in axillae it is visible only with arms raised |
| 4 (severe) | Extends to anterior neck; in axillae it is visible without arms raised |

Once a child is identified as being at risk for developing T2DM, then screening for diabetes using fasting plasma glucose levels, 2 hour oral glucose tolerance test (OGTT) or hemoglobin A1c (A1c) can be performed. There is debate as to whether the A1c is a reliable screening tool in the pediatric population. Given the variability of fasting glucoses and the convenience of obtaining an A1c when compared to an OGTT, many health care providers prefer to use an A1c. A provider should be aware of medical conditions that can interfere with the accuracy of the A1c. In conditions such as sickle cell anemia, hemoglobinopathies and cystic fibrosis, the A1c can be falsely low and therefore an unreliable tool. Table **3** is adapted from the 2016 ADA Standards of Medical Care in Diabetes and discusses the criteria for the diagnosis of both T1DM and T2DM.

Without a clear diagnosis of diabetes mellitus then a repeat test should be performed that same day with a new blood sample to confirm a diagnosis [5]. For example, if the initial A1c is 6.5%, then a repeat A1c should be done on a new blood sample to confirm the diagnosis. If different tests are used and one does not confirm the diagnosis, then the test result that did meet diagnostic criteria should be repeated. The diagnosis is then based on that confirmatory test result [5]. Providers also need to be aware that patients with T1DM can present with obesity and AN. Until autoantibodies for T1DM are confirmed negative, the diagnosis cannot be excluded. The most commonly tested autoantibodies are islet cell, insulin and glutamic acid decarboxylase (GAD) autoantibodies [5]. With the many complications seen in these patients, once a diagnosis is suspected or confirmed for T2DM, an immediate referral should be made to a pediatric endocrinologist.

Table 3. Criteria for the diagnosis of diabetes.

| Lab Test | Diagnostic Value |
|---|---|
| Fasting plasma glucose | $\geq 126$ mg/dL |
| 2 hour glucose post OGTT | $\geq 200$ mg/dL |
| A1C | $\geq 6.5\%$ |
| Random plasma glucose with hyperglycemia symptoms | $\geq 200$ mg/dL |

*OGTT- oral glucose tolerance test with 75 gram carb load.

In autoantibody negative patients, other secondary types of diabetes should be considered. Patients with medical conditions such as cancer, rheumatologic disorders, or pulmonary disease that require high-dose steroids may present with complications of prolonged hyperglycemia and insulin resistance, commonly referred to as steroid-induced diabetes. These patients do not usually have positive antibodies, but do tend to present with insulin resistance. Treatment of patients with steroid-induced diabetes differs from T2DM, therefore identification of these patients is important.

**TREATMENT**

Treatment of T2DM in adolescents and children should be aimed at reducing the risk of long-term complications. In adults, using lower A1c targets has been shown to reduce microvascular and macrovascular disease [7]. In particular, these patients are at risk for diabetic retinopathy, neuropathy and nephropathy. An A1c of less than 6.5% should be the glycemic goal of initial treatment. Treatment of T2DM in children and adolescents is first dictated by the severity of hyperglycemia and presence or absence of ketosis/ketoacidosis [8]. Nevertheless, lifestyle modifications should be initiated at the time of diagnosis of T2DM [8, 9].

The success of lifestyle modification depends on a patients and families readiness to change and should include strategies used in evidence based obesity prevention including elimination of sugar-sweetened beverages, consumption of ≥5 servings of fruits and vegetables per day, limiting screen time to ≤2 hours per day with no television where the child sleeps, and engaging in >1 hour of daily physical activity [10]. It is also recommended that management of youth with T2DM include incorporation of the Pediatric Nutritional Guidelines set forth by the Academy of Nutrition and Dietetics. Treatment with a ketogenic very-low calorie diet in obese adolescents with poorly controlled T2DM has been shown to be effective in reducing A1c, although it is often unrealistic to sustain [11].

The International Society for Pediatric and Adolescent Diabetes (ISPAD) recommends initial pharmacological treatment with metformin, insulin alone or in combination for youth diagnosed with T2DM [8]. It is recommended that at the time of diagnosis asymptomatic patients with no acidosis and an A1c of less than 9% be started on metformin monotherapy with lifestyle changes, while symptomatic patients with an A1c greater than 9% and acidosis should be started on insulin. Additionally, starting metformin can be considered at the same time as insulin in symptomatic children with an A1c greater than 9%, if there is no evidence of acidosis present [8].

Metformin is in the biguanide class of drugs and it is approved in children down to age 10. Currently, only metformin and insulin are FDA approved in the treatment of T2DM in children and adolescents (Table **4**). Metformin has been shown to work primarily through the actions of adenosine monophosphate (AMP) kinase with actions including reduction of hepatic gluconeogenesis and increased glucose uptake at the level of the myocyte, however the mechanism of action remains to be fully elucidated and newer studies suggest that the intestine may be an important site of action of the glucose lowering effects of metformin [12 - 14]. Typically, metformin is started at a dose of 500 mg twice a day. It is taken with food, ideally with breakfast and dinner, to avoid or diminish any gastrointestinal side-effects. If the medication is tolerated, the dose should be increased to 1000 mg twice a day, which is the maximum dose. Higher doses are rarely associated with hypoglycemia. Liver and kidney function tests should be evaluated before and after starting metformin. Generally, if the AST and ALT are >2.5 times the upper limit of normal, this could increase risk of lactic acidosis and insulin should be considered as first-line therapy. Non-alcoholic fatty liver disease (NAFLD) is often present at the time of diagnosis and can be the cause of the abnormal liver function. Improved glycemic control and insulin sensitizers such as metformin may actually improve NAFLD and may be considered as insulin is transitioned off with continued close monitoring of liver enzymes [8]. If insulin is used with metformin, a long-acting insulin is used as a second-line therapy. If there is continued poor control with the combination therapy, a fast-acting insulin can be added. A sliding scale can be used based on the degree of hyperglycemia. If more aggressive therapy is needed, the pre-meal insulin dose can be increased by adding a carbohydrate scale. Initiation doses can vary by the age and weight of the child and insulin is typically started by an endocrinologist.

**Table 4. Medications used to treat T2DM.**

| Drug Name | Lantus/Levemir and NPH | Metformin | Glimepiride/ Glyburide | Rosiglitazone/ Pioglitazone | Exenatide/ Liraglutide |
|---|---|---|---|---|---|
| Drug Class | Long Acting Basal Insulin and Intermediate-Acting Insulin Analogues | Biguanide | Sulfonylureas | Thiazolidinediones | Glucagon-like peptide-1 (GLP-1) receptor agonists |
| FDA Approved for T2DM | Yes | Immediate release: FDA approved in those ≥10 years of age. | Not FDA approved for those < 18 years of age. | Not FDA approved for those < 18 years of age. | Not FDA approved for those < 18 years of age. |
| Mechanism of Action | Act through specific membrane bound insulin receptors in various tissues. Pharmacokinetics varies depending on formulation. | Actions of adenosine monophosphate (AMP) kinase in liver, muscle and fat tissue including, reduction of hepatic gluconeogenesis, and insulin stimulated glucose uptake in muscle/fat. | Bind to receptors on the K+/ATP channel complex causing K+ channels to close resulting in insulin secretion. | Bind to nuclear peroxisome proliferator activator receptors (PPAR gamma) and increase insulin sensitivity in muscle, adipose, and liver tissue by a variety of mechanisms. | Increases insulin secretion proportionate to BG concentrations, suppresses glucagon, increases B-cell growth/replication, prolongs gastric emptying and promotes satiety. |
| Main Side Effects | Hypoglycemia, weight gain. | Gastrointestinal side effects, risk of lactic acidosis | Hypoglycemia, weight gain. | Weight gain, anemia, fluid retention (including congestive heart failure), and liver toxicity. | Hypoglycemia, nausea, vomiting, diarrhea, infrequent dizziness, headache and dyspepsia. |

*Note.* Data for medications used in T2DM from references 3 and 8.

In adults, there are several drug options with varying mechanism of actions. Few of these medications have been studied in children. Findings from the Treatment Options for Type 2 Diabetes in Adolescents and Youth (TODAY) study, a large multicenter trial study, demonstrated that metformin plus rosiglitazone was superior to metformin alone or in combination with lifestyle intervention in sustained reduction of glycemic control as defined by maintaining an A1c of at least 8% for a 6 month period or an inability to wean from insulin after metabolic decompensation [9, 15]. Other pharmacological agents are generally not approved for use in children and adolescents given the limited amount of studies of use of these medications in children (Table **4**). Data related to the safety and tolerability of metformin and rosiglitazone was acquired as part of the TODAY trial [16]. Most of the side effects were related to GI upset; however anemia, abnormal liver transaminases, excessive weight gain, psychological events, lactic acidosis, diabetic ketoacidosis and severe hypoglycemia were also reported [16]. Other treatment options include incretin mimetics such as GLP-1 receptor agonists which are promising agents for future treatment but have not yet been approved for use in those under the age of 18.

Data from the TODAY trial suggest that not only do these children and adolescents experience similar complications and co-morbidities as seen in adults, but that it occurs on an accelerated timeline [9]. Therefore, care for these high risk youth should also involve the assessment and management of co-morbidities and complications.

## LONG-TERM COMPLICATIONS

Long-term outcomes of T2DM in youth include both microvascular and macrovascular complications. Progression to complications appears to occur at a more accelerated pace when compared to T1DM and is precipitated by poor glycemic control. In contrast to those with T1DM, complications such as hypertension and microalbuminuria are common at the time of presentation; therefore screening typically begins at the time of diagnosis. General guidelines regarding screening and treatment provided below were adapted from the American Academy of Pediatrics recommendations for managing newly diagnosed T2DM in children and adolescents [17].

### Hypertension

Hypertension is defined as a blood pressure ≥ 95% for height, age, and gender obtained on three separate occasions using an appropriately sized blood pressure cuff. Screening should be performed at each clinic visit starting at the time of diagnosis. A review article highlighting T2DM complications in youth reports that the prevalence of hypertension at diagnosis is estimated to be eight times more frequent in children with T2DM when compared to those with T1DM and varies between 10-32% [18]. In the TODAY cohort (N = 699), hypertension was appreciated in 11.9% of adolescents at baseline and increased to almost 34% at follow-up nearly four years later [19]. A low-salt diet, physical activity, and weight loss should be encouraged as initial interventions. An angiotensin-converting enzyme inhibitor (ACE-I) is used as first line pharmacological treatment to prevent the progression to diabetic nephropathy. The goal of treatment is to consistently achieve systolic and diastolic blood pressures < 90th percentile. Angiotensin receptor blockers may be used if an ACE-I is not tolerated (*i.e.*, chronic cough). Referral to nephrology is indicated if hypertension is not adequately controlled with medication and lifestyle modifications.

## Nephropathy

Screening for diabetic nephropathy includes testing for microalbuminuria with a random morning urine microalbumin-to-creatinine ratio. Screening should begin at the time of diagnosis and then repeated annually. Two of three consecutive urine samples collected over a 3 to 6 month period with a ratio ≥ 30 μg/mg is representative of persistent microalbuminuria. A study following Pima Indians noted 22% prevalence of microalbuminuria at diagnosis that increased to nearly 60% after 10 years [20]. In the TODAY cohort, the prevalence was 6.3% at baseline, 10.3% at the 4 year follow-up, and 16.6% at the end of the study [19]. A cross-sectional study performed in Australia reported that despite having a shorter duration of diabetes (1.3 vs. 6.8 years) youth with T2DM had a significantly higher rate of microalbuminuria when compared to youth with T1DM (28% vs. 6%) [21]. Similarly, a multicenter trial in New Zealand reported an increased rate of microalbuminuria in those with T2DM (72%) when compared to T1DM (17%) despite shorter diagnosis of diabetes (3 vs. 6 years) [22]. In a normotensive adolescent, persistent microalbuminuria is managed by optimizing glycemic control. A hypertensive adolescent warrants treatment with an ACE-I. Medication should be titrated to ideally normalize microalbumin excretion without causing hypotension. Referral to a nephrologist is indicated if proper control is not achieved. Microalbuminuria may progress to macroalbuminuria (≥ 300mcg/mg creatinine), proteinuria (≥ 1,000mcg/mg creatinine), and end-stage renal disease requiring dialysis and renal transplantation.

## Retinopathy

Retinopathy is diagnosed by an ophthalmologist using a slit-examination through dilated pupils. Screening should be performed at the time of diagnosis and repeated annually. Severity ranges from mild nonproliferative retinopathy to proliferative retinopathy. Data obtained on 517 subjects in the final year of the TODAY study revealed that 27% had some form of retinopathy ranging from early, mild retinopathy to nonproliferative retinopathy with microaneurysms or cotton wool infarcts [19]. Although studies demonstrate the prevalence of retinopathy is more common in adolescents with T1DM, the duration of diabetes to progress to retinopathy is shorter in those with T2DM [21, 22]. Progressive microvascular retinal changes result in vision impairment and eventual blindness. Treatment for retinopathy includes laser therapy, injection of corticosteroids, and vitrectomy.

## Dyslipidemia

Even though criteria used to define fasting dyslipidemia are not consistent across studies, the presence of lipid abnormalities in adolescents with T2DM at diagnosis is common and varies between 18-61% [18]. In the TODAY study, 4.5% of subjects at baseline either had an elevated low-density lipoprotein (LDL) $\geq$ 130mg/dl or were taking lipid-lowering medications. At three years (N=264), the percentage increased to 10.7%. Authors of the TODAY study report that many components of the lipid panel increased over time (*i.e.*, LDL, triglycerides, and non high-density lipoprotein) regardless of the treatment arm [19]. Screening includes a fasting lipid panel at the time of diagnosis and annually thereafter. Non-pharmacologic management includes optimizing glycemic and blood pressure control. For LDL levels persistently $\geq$ 130 mg/dl, treatment with a HMG Co-A reductase inhibitor (statin therapy) is recommended. The treatment goal is to achieve an LDL < 130 mg/dl with an ideal target of <100 mg/dl. Fenofibrate or niacin therapy can be considered if triglycerides are > 700 mg/dl despite genuine efforts to minimize the intake of simple sugars. Type 2 diabetes and dyslipidemia are major risk factors for the development of cardiovascular disease.

## Non-alcoholic Fatty Liver Disease

Fatty infiltration of the liver resulting in elevated liver enzymes is appreciated in children with T2DM. Screening includes the measurement of alanine aminotransferase (ALT) and aspartate aminotransferase (AST) at diagnosis and then annually. In patients with fatty liver, AST and ALT levels may be greater than two or three times the upper limit of normal. Some patients with fatty liver may have normal liver function tests. A liver ultrasound may be helpful in the diagnosis. Treatment options are limited to lifestyle modifications. Referral to a gastroenterologist may be warranted if liver enzymes are worsening despite improvements in weight, nutrition, and glycemic control. The progression from fatty liver to cirrhosis necessitating liver transplantation is not well understood, but is a definite concern given the increasing prevalence of obesity and T2DM in youth. Many medications commonly used in T2DM are contraindicated in patients with elevated liver function tests (*i.e.*, statins), therefore monitoring liver enzymes may be imperative when managing youth with T2DM.

## Depression

Although studies are limited, clinical depression appears to be more common in youth with T2DM than those with T1DM [21]. Questionnaires completed by the participants of TODAY study (N=687) revealed that at baseline, 14.8% self-reported symptoms were consistent with clinically significant depression [19]. Validated tools to screen for depression are available to general practitioners, but patients with positive screens should generally be referred to psychiatry.

## Neuropathy

The true incidence of diabetic neuropathy in the type 2 pediatric population is largely unknown and likely not common, given that information available is limited to a few case reports. Screening includes questioning about symptoms consistent with neuropathy such as numbing and tingling of the extremities or erectile dysfunction. Screening techniques on physical exam include testing for intact ankle reflexes, light touch sensation using monofilaments, and vibration.

## CONCLUSION

With the rise in number of children who are overweight and obese, health care providers are seeing and treating more patients at risk for developing T2DM. Proper screening of and early identification of these patients can delay the diagnosis of T2DM by implementing lifestyle modifications and therapies. Accurate diagnosis is critical for appropriately managing these patients, especially since the diagnosis of T1DM can be missed if the patient is overweight or obese. Therapy should be focused on achieving glycemic control with the monitoring A1c levels at scheduled visits. With appropriate therapy, long-term complications of T2DM can be delayed or prevented. While adults with T2DM have many therapeutic options, these medications have not been approved for pediatric patients. Additional studies are needed on children to test the safety and efficacy of these diabetic medications to provide improved medical management of patients with T2DM.

## CONFLICT OF INTEREST

The authors declare no conflict of interest, financial or otherwise.

## ACKOWLEDGEMENTS

Declared none.

## REFERENCES

[1]     Sinha R, Fisch G, Teague B, *et al.* Prevalence of impaired glucose tolerance among children and

adolescents with marked obesity. N Engl J Med 2002; 346(11): 802-10.
[http://dx.doi.org/10.1056/NEJMoa012578]

[2]     D'Adamo E, Caprio S. Type 2 diabetes in youth: Epidemiology and pathophysiology. Diabetes Care 2011; 34 (Suppl. 2): S161-5.
[http://dx.doi.org/10.2337/dc11-s212]

[3]     Thayer KA, Heindel JJ, Bucher JR, Gallo MA. Role of environmental chemicals in diabetes and obesity: A national toxicology program workshop review. Environ Health Perspect 2012; 120(6): 779-89.
[http://dx.doi.org/10.1289/ehp.1104597]

[4]     Dabelea D, Mayer-Davis EJ, Saydah S, *et al.* Prevalence of type 1 and type 2 diabetes among children and adolescents from 2001 to 2009. JAMA 2014; 311(17): 1778-86.
[http://dx.doi.org/10.1001/jama.2014.3201]

[5]     Chamberlain JJ, Rhinehart AS, Shaefer CF Jr, Neuman A. Diagnosis and management of diabetes: Synopsis of the 2016 American diabetes association standards of medical care in diabetes. Ann Intern Med 2016.
[http://dx.doi.org/10.7326/M15-3016]

[6]     Burke JP, Hale DE, Hazuda HP, Stern MP. A quantitative scale of acanthosis nigricans. Diabetes Care 1999; 22(10): 1655-9.
[http://dx.doi.org/10.2337/diacare.22.10.1655]

[7]     American Diabetes Association. Standards of medical care in diabetes-2016 Abridged for primary care providers. Clinical diabetes : a publication of the American Diabetes Association 2016; 34(1): 3-21.
[http://dx.doi.org/10.2337/diaclin.34.1.3]

[8]     Zeitler P, *et al.* ISPAD Clinical Practice Consensus Guidelines 2014. Type 2 Diabetes in the Child and Adolescent. Pediatr Diabetes 2014; 15 (Suppl. 20): 26-46.
[http://dx.doi.org/10.1111/pedi.12179]

[9]     George MM, Copeland KC. Current treatment options for type 2 diabetes mellitus in youth: today's realities and lessons from the TODAY Study. Curr Diab Rep 2013; 13(1): 72-80.
[http://dx.doi.org/10.1007/s11892-012-0334-z]

[10]    Barlow S E. Expert committee recommendations regarding the prevention, assessment, and treatment of child and adolescent overweight and obesity: Summary report. Pediatrics 2007; 120 (Suppl. 4): S164-92.
[http://dx.doi.org/10.1542/peds.2007-2329C]

[11]    McGavock J, Dart A, Wicklow B. Lifestyle therapy for the treatment of youth with type 2 diabetes. Current Diabetes Reports 2015; 15(1): 568,014-0568-z.
[http://dx.doi.org/10.1007/s11892-014-0568-z]

[12]    Buse JB, DeFronzo RA, Rosenstock J, *et al.* The primary glucose-lowering effect of metformin resides in the gut, not the circulation: results from short-term pharmacokinetic and 12-week dose-ranging studies. Diabetes Care 2016; 39(2): 198-205.
[http://dx.doi.org/10.2337/dc15-0488]

[13]    Pernicova I, Korbonits M. Metformin-Mode of action and clinical implications for diabetes and cancer. Nat Rev Endocrinol 2014; 10(3): 143-56.
[http://dx.doi.org/10.1038/nrendo.2013.256]

[14]    Zhou G, *et al.* Role of AMP-activated protein kinase in mechanism of metformin action. J Clin Invest 2001; 108(8): 1167-74.
[http://dx.doi.org/10.1172/JCI13505]

[15]    TODAY Study Group. Effects of metformin, metformin plus rosiglitazone, and metformin plus lifestyle on insulin sensitivity and beta-cell function in TODAY. Diabetes Care 2013; 36(6): 1749-57.
[http://dx.doi.org/10.2337/dc12-2393]

[16]    TODAY Study Group. Safety and tolerability of the treatment of youth-onset type 2 diabetes: The TODAY experience. Diabetes Care 2013; 36(6): 1765-71.
[http://dx.doi.org/10.2337/dc12-2390]

[17]    Copeland K, Silverstein J, Moore K, *et al.* Management of newly diagnosed type 2 diabetes mellitus (T2DM) in children and adolescents. Pediatrics 2013; 131(2): 364-82.
[http://dx.doi.org/10.1542/peds.2012-3494]

[18]    Pinhas-Hamiel O, Zeitler P. Acute and chronic complications of type 2 diabetes mellitus in children and adolescents. Lancet 2007; 369(9575): 1823-31.
[http://dx.doi.org/10.1016/S0140-6736(07)60821-6]

[19]    Tryggestad J, Willi S. Complications and comorbidities of T2DM in adolescents: findings from the TODAY clinical trial. J Diabetes Complications 2015; 29(2): 307-12.
[http://dx.doi.org/10.1016/j.jdiacomp.2014.10.009]

[20]    Fagot-Campagna A, Knowler W, Pettit D. Type 2 Diabetes in Pima Indian children: cardiovascular risk factors at diagnosis and 10 years later. Diabetes 1998; 47 (Suppl.): A155.

[21]    Eppens MC, Craig ME, Cusumano J, *et al.* Prevalence of diabetes complications in adolescents with type 2 compared with type 1diabetes. Diabetes Care 2006; 29: 1300-6.
[http://dx.doi.org/10.2337/dc05-2470]

[22]    Scott A, Toomath R, Bouchier D, *et al.* First national audit of the outcomes of care in young people with diabetes in New Zealand: high prevalence of nephropathy in Maori and Pacific Islanders. N Z Med J 2006; 119: U2015.

# CHAPTER 9

# Practical Guide for Management of Children with Obesity

**Neslihan Gungor**[*]

*Department of Pediatrics Division of Endocrinology, Louisiana State University-Health Sciences Center/University Health, Shreveport, Louisiana, USA*

**Abstract:** The worldwide prevalence of pediatric obesity has increased remarkably over the past three decades turning pediatric obesity into a serious and challenging public health concern. One in three children and adolescents in the US are overweight or obese. Pediatric obesity is associated with numerous comorbidities, cardiovascular risk factors, and adulthood obesity. Obesity has been a major contributor to increasing healthcare expenses. Increasing awareness of pediatric obesity in the public as well as the healthcare platform is essential to tackle the problem and plan primary and secondary prevention. Given the limited pharmacotherapy options for pediatric obesity, a multifaceted approach of lifestyle changes involving nutrition, physical activity and behavior modification is needed. In order to make a meaningful impact, collaboration among the government, employers, schools, healthcare and other organizations from the community is required. This chapter intends to provide a comprehensive yet concise review of evaluation and management of pediatric obesity.

**Keywords:** Adolescent, Cardiovascular risk, Child, Diabetes, Dyslipidemia, Lifestyle modification, Obesity, Overweight, Pediatric, Prevention, Type 2 diabetes mellitus, Weight management.

## INTRODUCTION

The prevalence of pediatric obesity has increased substantially in the past three decades turning it into a major public health problem [1, 2]. Childhood obesity is a multifactorial condition which can adversely affect nearly every organ system. It has been associated with serious physical and psychosocial comorbidities [1 - 3]. This chapter intends to review the definition, determinants, epidemiology and comorbidities of pediatric obesity and provide a practical approach to clinical evaluation and treatment.

---

[*] **Corresponding author Neslihan Gungor**: Department of Pediatrics Division of Endocrinology, Louisiana State University-Health Sciences Center/University Health, Shreveport, Louisiana, USA; Tel: (318) 675-6076; Email: ngungo@lsuhsc.edu

## DEFINITION

The term obesity refers to excess of body fat or adiposity. However, the methods used to directly measure body fat are not available in routine clinical practice. In clinical practice and population health surveillance systems, obesity is defined by the body mass index (BMI), a mathematical formula of weight-for-height index. The BMI is calculated by weight in kilograms divided by height in meters squared ($kg/m^2$). The BMI has a high correlation with adiposity and excess weight at the population level. However, the BMI does neither quantify total body adiposity, nor distinguish between fat and muscle on an individual basis. Furthermore, the BMI does not predict body fat distribution. Therefore it may overestimate adiposity in a child with increased muscle mass (*e.g.*, an athlete) and underestimate adiposity in a child with reduced muscle mass (*e.g.* sedentary child) [3 - 5]. In the pediatric age group gender-specific BMI-for-age, percentile charts are used to define overweight and obesity. Children and adolescents with a BMI over the 85th but less than the 95th percentile for age and gender are considered overweight, and those with a BMI equal to or greater than the 95th percentile are considered obese. The term "severely obese" has been used to refer to children and adolescents with a BMI greater than the 99th percentile [3, 6]. In the United States (US), the gender-specific Growth Charts, released in May 2000 by the Centers for Disease Control are available to assess Body Mass Index for children 2 to 20 years of age [6]. The International Obesity Task Force (IOTF) has developed an international standard growth chart which enables comparison of prevalence globally [7]. The World Health Organization has published growth standards for infants and children from birth to 5 years of age [8] and growth reference curves for BMI for children 5–19 years of age [9]. However, many countries have elected to use country-specific growth charts.

## ETIOLOGY AND RISK FACTORS

In broad terms, obesity is the result of a chronic imbalance between energy intake and expenditure, with more calories being consumed than expended. In general a lack of physical activity in the presence of unhealthy eating patterns result in excess energy intake. Obesity is a complex, multi-factorial condition affected by genetic and non-genetic factors and interactions between these [1, 5, 10, 11]. Due to the extensive nature of this topic and space restrictions, the reader is referred to additional references. Energy consumption and expenditure are impacted upon by epigenetic programming, environmental and social factors. Specific causes for the increase in prevalence of childhood obesity are not clear. To date, the effects of a single factor has not been identified. (Fig. **1**) provides a general overview of the determinants [1, 5, 10, 11] of pediatric overweight/obesity (Fig. **1**).

As seen in the figure, there are multiple social, environmental, behavioral and biological determinants. There are interindividual differences in susceptibility or resistance to the obesogenic environment [5, 10, 12]. Genetic variation plays a major role in this. Various hormones, most of which originate from the gastrointestinal tract, play role in appetite regulation and energy homeostasis [5, 10, 12 - 15]. For example ghrelin is currently the only known appetite-stimulating (orexigenic) gut hormone, secreted by the oxyntic glands of the stomach. Ghrelin levels rise shortly before mealtimes. Peptide tyrosine tyrosine (PYY), pancreatic polypeptide, oxyntomodulin, amylin, glucagon, glucagon-like peptide-1 (GLP-1), and GLP-2 are the anorexigenic gut hormones which decrease appetite and food intake.

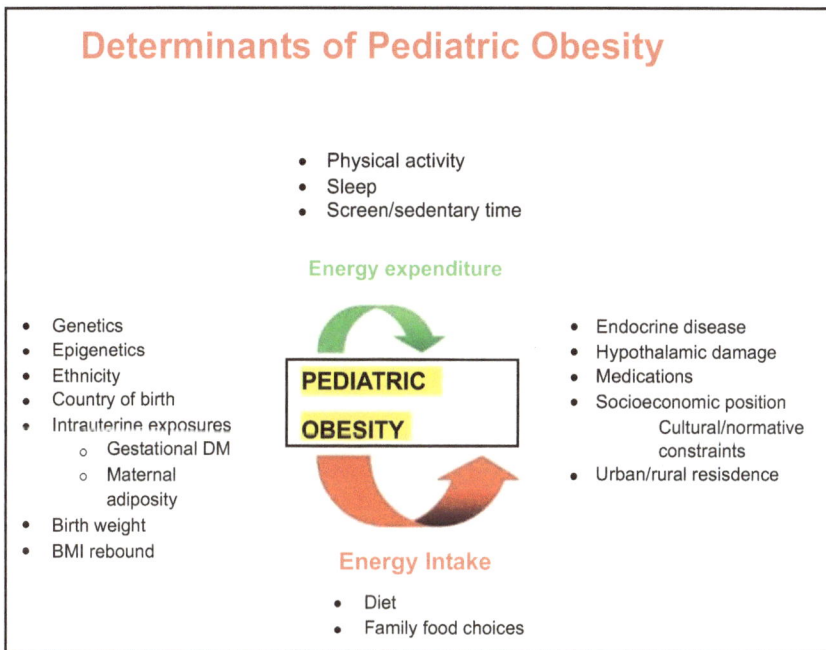

**Fig. (1).** Determinants of pediatric obesity. Pediatric obesity is a multifactorial condition of positive energy balance, stemming from both genetic and non-genetic factors, as well as complex interactions among these (Adopted from Reference 11, with permission).

Endocrine causes of obesity account for less than 1% of obesity in the pediatric age group. Hypothyroidism (primary or central), growth hormone deficiency or resistance and cortisol excess are the potential endocrine conditions leading to obesity. Polycystic ovarian syndrome (PCOS) is closely associated with obesity. Obesity may also be seen in pseudohypoparathyroidism (caused by Gsα inactivating mutation) [1, 5, 11]. Albright hereditary osteodystrophy (AHO) is an autosomal dominant disorder due to germline mutations in GNAS1 which decrease expression or function of Gsalpha (Gsα) protein. Maternal transmission of GNAS1 mutations results with AHO (with features of short stature, obesity, skeletal defects and impaired olfaction) and resistance to several hormones (*e.g.* parathyroid hormone) that activate Gsα in their target tissues. Paternal transmission leads only to the AHO phenotype.

## PREVALENCE AND EPIDEMIOLOGY

There has been a significant increase in the worldwide prevalence of childhood obesity in recent decades [1]. In the US the incidence of pediatric obesity has increased from less than 5% to approximately 20% in the past 30 years [2, 16]. Prevalence estimates of obesity are derived from surveys or population studies. In the US, The National Center for Health Statistics of the CDC, National Health and Nutrition Examination Survey (NHANES) program provides national estimates of overweight for adults, adolescents, and children. Based on the 2011-2012 NHANES data [2], the prevalence of obesity in the United States was 16.9% in youth and 34.9% in adults. The overall prevalence of obesity among youth remained unchanged compared with that in 2009-2010 (16.9%) [16], and there was no significant change since 2003-2004.

## COMORBIDITIES AND COMPLICATIONS

Obesity is a proinflammatory state. Pediatric obesity can have a negative impact on almost every organ system and lead to serious physical and psychosocial comorbidities [1, 5, 10, 11, 17]. The increasing prevalence of pediatric obesity has brought multiple chronic illnesses and risk factors historically seen only in adults, to the consideration of the pediatrician. Table **1** summarizes the comorbidities and complications of childhood obesity.

**Table 1. Comorbidities and complications of childhood obesity.**

| 1- Endocrine: |
|---|
| a) Glucose tolerance problems: |
| - Insulin resistance |
| - Prediabetes (impaired fasting glucose/ impaired glucose tolerance) |
| - Type 2 diabetes mellitus |
| - Metabolic syndrome |
| b) Growth and puberty related issues |
| Girls: |
| - Hyperandrogenism/Polycystic ovarian syndrome |

*(Table 1) contd.....*

| |
|---|
| -Earlier menarche |
| Boys: |
| -Later pubertal onset |
| -Pseudo-micropenis (hidden penis) |
| -Reduced circulating androgens |
| c) Thyroid function aberrations |
| 2- Cardiovascular |
| - Hypertension |
| - Left ventricular hypertrophy |
| - Dyslipidemia |
| - Other cardiovascular risks |
| -Adult coronary heart disease |
| 3- Gastrointestinal |
| - Non alcoholic fatty liver disease (NAFLD) |
| - Steatohepatitis |
| - Cholestasis/cholelithiasis |
| - Gastroesophageal reflux disease |
| 4-Pulmonary |
| -Asthma |
| - Obstructive sleep apnea |
| -Obesity hypoventilation syndrome (Pickwickian syndrome) |
| 5- Orthopedic |
| -Coxa vara |
| - Slipped capital femoral epiphysis (SCFE) |
| - Tibia vara (Blount disease) |
| - Fractures |
| -Legg-Calve-Perthes disease |
| 6-Neurologic |
| - Idiopathic intracranial hypertension (pseudotumor cerebri) |
| 7- Dermatologic |
| -Acanthosis nigricans |
| -Intertrigo |
| -Furunculosis |
| 8- Psychosocial |
| -Low self-esteem |

*(Table 1) contd.....*

| -Depression |
| -Decreased health-related quality of life |
| [References 5, 11, 44] |

## 1- Endocrine

**a) Glucose-Tolerance And Related Consequences:** Insulin resistance is the common denominator for many of the metabolic and cardiovascular complications of obesity. Hyperinsulinemia is the most common biochemical abnormality seen in obesity. Insulin resistance and compensatory hyperinsulinemia are the early steps in this 2DM pathogenesis. The next step is impaired early insulin secretion paving the way post-prandial and fasting hyperglycemia, respectively. Diabetes becomes clinically-manifest with this progression [19 - 21]. Impaired glucose tolerance is a relatively common condition in obese children and adolescents, with a reported prevalence ranging from 15% to greater than 20% [22 - 24]. The progressive increase in rates of pediatric obesity since late 1980's has transformed T2DM from a historically adult-only disease, to a serious pediatric public health problem [19, 25]. The SEARCH for Diabetes in Youth Study [26], the largest surveillance effort of diabetes in youth in the US, has depicted remarkably increased rates of T2DM in 10-19 year-old minority adolescents. Among youth in 10-19 year age group, the proportion of type 2 diabetes ranged from 6% (0.19 cases per 1000 youth for non-Hispanic white youth) to 76% (1.74 cases per 1000 youth for American Indian youth). The reported prevalence of T2DM were 22% in Mexican American youths, 33% in African American youths, and 40% in Asian/Pacific Islander youths [26]. Prediabetes (impaired fasting glucose and/or impaired glucose tolerance) requires attention from a secondary prevention perspective to offset conversion to T2DM.

Certain metabolic disturbances have been noted to cluster together since the beginning of the past century. Insulin resistance has been proposed as a common etiologic factor for the group of metabolic disturbances collectively referred to Syndrome X or the metabolic syndrome (MetS). Current definitions of MetS comprise the following key features: hyperinsulinemia or insulin resistance, dyslipidemia, hypertension, and obesity, with a particular emphasis on central adiposity. Pediatric MetS represents a group of risk factors linked to cardiovascular disease, which include insulin resistance, obesity, hyperlipidemia, and hypertension. Currently there is no consensus on the definition of MetS in youth; however, identification of children at risk for developing MetS remains an important task given the presence of multiple cardiovascular risks and the evidence that the clustering of these conditions persists in adulthood [27]. Early stages of the atherosclerotic process are detectable in obese children. Endothelial dysfunction represents the key early step in the development of atherosclerosis [28]. Intima media thickness (IMT) of the peripheral arterial vessels is a surrogate marker for atherosclerosis and increased IMT has been documented in obese children and adolescents [29]. Cardiovascular risk factors present in childhood are predictive of coronary artery disease in adulthood, as demonstrated by the Bogalusa Heart study [30]. Low density lipoprotein cholesterol (LDL) and BMI measured in childhood were identified as the risk factors which predicted IMT in young adults. In a follow up study of childhood participants of the Bogalusa Heart Study as adults, children who had metabolically healthy overweight/obesity were noted to have favorable cardiometabolic profiles in adulthood. Metabolically healthy overweight/obesity was defined as having a body mass index in the top quartile, with LDL, triglycerides, mean arterial pressure, and glucose in the bottom 3 quartiles, and high density lipoprotein cholesterol (HDL) in the top 3 quartiles. No difference was found in carotid intima-media thickness in adulthood between metabolically healthy children and non-overweight/obese children [31].

**b) Growth and Puberty Related Concerns:** Polycystic ovarian syndrome (PCOS) is a noteworthy condition in females of reproductive age group and characterized by hyperandrogenism and oligo/anovulation in adolescents [32]. A recent Endocrine Society Clinical Practice Guideline [32] recommends using the Rotterdam criteria for diagnosing PCOS (presence of two of the following criteria: androgen excess, ovulatory dysfunction, or polycystic ovaries). Establishing a diagnosis of PCOS is not straightforward in adolescents. Hyperandrogenism is central to the presentation in adolescents. Evaluation of adolescents with PCOS should exclude alternate androgen-excess disorders. Overweight and obesity are common findings among adolescent girls with PCOS, particularly in the US population [33]. There is a high prevalence of insulin resistance, prediabetes and T2DM among adolescent girls and adult women with PCOS and screening is recommended [33].

Obesity results with changes in other hormonal systems. Age of onset of puberty continues to decrease, particularly in African Americans. This has been attributed, in part, to increase in overnutrition and BMI in this population [34]. Excessive aromatization of androgen to estrogen by peripheral adipose tissue may promote gynecomastia in males. Obstructive sleep apnea is among the pulmonary complications of obesity and the hypercapnia associated with this can suppress hypothalamic GnRH function and lead to delayed puberty [35]. Obesity accelerates statural growth and causes advancement of the bone age.

**c) Thyroid Function Aberrations:** It is a common practice to screen overweight/obese children for thyroid function [36]. Elevated TSH concentrations in association with normal or slightly elevated free T4 and/or free T3 levels have been consistently found in obese subjects, but the mechanisms underlying these changes are still unclear. It is also notable that most of the weight gain in hypothyroid individuals is due to accumulation of salt and water, so hypothyroidism rarely causes substantial weight gain.

## 2-Cardiovascular Comorbidities

These involve hypertension, dyslipidemia, as well as risks for adult coronary heart disease. Cardiovascular disease is the leading cause of adult mortality and morbidity. Longitudinal epidemiologic studies have demonstrated that risk factors in childhood, such as obesity and dyslipidemia, predict adult cardiovascular disease. The Bogalusa Heart Study [37] depicted increased prevalence of clinically recognized hypertension and dyslipidemia in overweight *versus* lean adolescents (8.5-fold and 3.1- to 8.3-fold, respectively). Excess weight in adolescence persists into young adulthood, and has a strong adverse impact on multiple cardiovascular risk factors, necessitating primary prevention early in life [37].

## 3-Gastrointestinal Problems

These encompass nonalcoholic fatty liver disease (NAFLD), nonalcoholic steatohepatitis (NASH), cirrhosis and cholelithiasis [18]. NAFLD has turned into the most common etiology of chronic liver disease in children in the United States, along with the increasing frequency of obesity [18, 38]. NAFLD represents fatty infiltration of the liver in the absence of alcohol consumption. NAFLD has a spectrum of severity ranging from steatosis to NASH that may ultimately result in advanced fibrosis, cirrhosis, and hepatocellular carcinoma. Because NAFLD is usually asymptomatic, screening is required for detection. Non-invasive evaluation can be used to make the diagnosis of NAFLD; detection of markers of liver injury (elevated liver enzymes) or fibrosis and/or fatty infiltration on ultrasound or magnetic resonance imaging. These diagnostic methods are suboptimal in sensitivity and specificity for NAFLD and other causes of liver disease must be ruled out. The differential diagnosis of elevated transaminases in overweight/obese children should include viral hepatitis (such as hepatitis B, hepatitis C), autoimmune hepatitis, α1-antitrypsin deficiency, and, in older children, Wilson disease. It is notable that NASH is the progressive form of NAFLD, associated with progression to cirrhosis [38]. Liver biopsy is required for staging and grading of NAFLD. Insulin resistance frequently coexists in both adults and children with NAFLD [39].

## 4-Pulmonary Comorbidities

These consist of obstructive sleep apnea (OSA) and obesity hypoventilation syndrome [5, 40, 41]. Obese children are up to six times more likely than lean children to have OSA. OSA syndrome is a disorder of breathing characterized by prolonged partial upper airway obstruction and/or intermittent complete obstruction (obstructive apnea) that interferes with normal ventilation during sleep and normal sleep patterns. Symptoms include habitual (nightly) snoring (frequently with intermittent pauses, snorts, or gasps), disturbed sleep, and daytime neurobehavioral problems. Daytime sleepiness may occur [41]. The prevalence of asthma is also increased in obese children.

## 5-Orthopedic Complications

These include slipped capital femoral epiphysis (SCFE), genu valga, tibia vara (Blount disease) and fractures. SCFE presents with hip/knee pain and decreased internal rotation of hip. Blount disease presents with pain at the medial aspect of knee. The clinician should have a low threshold for suspicion of SCFE in the obese child with knee, thigh, or hip pain with or without history of trauma. Overweight children have a higher incidence of fractures [42].

## 6-Neurologic Complications

Idiopathic intracranial hypertension is a disorder which typically presents with headache and blurred vision. The diagnosis is made by the detection of papilledema and elevated intracranial pressure in the absence of infectious, vascular, or structural causes. It can lead to blindness in up to 10% of patients, particularly if not recognized or treated promptly [43, 44].

## 7-Dermatologic Complications

Obesity can alter the skin barrier, induce skin manifestations, and worsen existing skin diseases like psoriasis. Cutaneous manifestations of obesity include acanthosis nigricans (AN), fibroma pendulans (skin tags, fibroepithelial polyps) and striae distensae [45]. AN is a dermatologic condition which is associated with obesity, Type 2 diabetes mellitus and insulin resistance [19, 46, 47] (Fig. **2**).

Histologically, it is characterized by the proliferation of epidermal keratinocytes and fibroblasts. AN is a velvety thickening of the epidermis that primarily affects the axillae, posterior cervical skinfold, flexor skin areas, and umbilicus. Clinically, the lesions appear as dark-brown thickened plaques. It is an important cutaneous marker of insulin resistance. Clinicians can quantify the severity of AN [47]. Obesity is also associated with hyperandrogenism in women and girls, promoting acne vulgaris, hirsutism, and androgenic alopecia. An association between the severity of psoriasis and the body mass index has been noted. Obesity increases risk for skin infections like erysipelas and intertrigo [45].

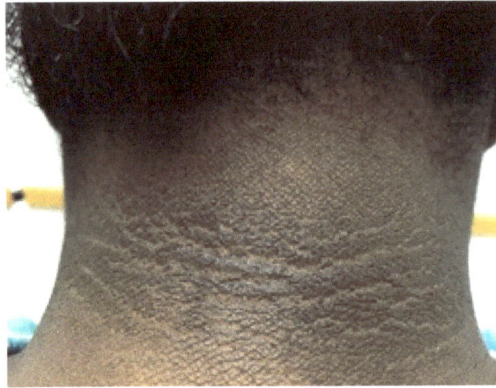

**Fig. (2).** 15 year old African American female with obesity and acanthosis nigricans at the posterior cervical skinfold (Photo courtesy of Neslihan Gungor, M.D. (author), obtained after informed consent).

## 8-Psychosocial Complications

These represent a wide spectrum. Body dissatisfaction, depression, loss-of-control eating, unhealthy and extreme weight control behaviors, impaired social relationships, obesity stigma, and decreased health-related quality of life are conditions with small to moderate associations with child and adolescent obesity. Complications with insignificant to small associations include low self-esteem, clinically significant depression (of diagnostic severity, linked to significant distress and/or impairment, or involving serious symptomatology), suicide, and full-syndrome eating disorders [48 - 51]. As the clinical setting is often the first point of contact for families, pediatricians are instrumental in the identification and referral of children with psychological complications [48 - 51]. Motivational interviewing, patient talking points, brief screening measures, and referral resources are important tools in this process.

## CLINICAL EVALUATION

The evaluation of the overweight/obese child should start with a comprehensive history and physical examination which will help the clinician assess severity and comorbid conditions [47]. Accurate anthropometric measurements (weight and height) and vital signs are required. Laboratory and radiologic studies may be obtained if indicated [44]. Certain screening tests are recommended for a general metabolic assessment in all patients and a more detailed evaluation should be planned if indicated by the case-specific characteristics.

Nutrition and physical activity history, environmental and social supports and barriers, opinions on cause and effect of the problems, as well as self-efficacy and readiness to change should be evaluated.

## Diagnosis

All children older than two years should have their BMI calculated at least annually from measured height and weight. The data should be plotted on an appropriate growth curve. Weight, height and BMI growth charts are not only diagnostic tools but also essential for patient and family education. Not only the BMI percentile but also the trend of the BMI percentile for age and sex require attention. Early detection of an increasing BMI trend (more than three to four units (kg/m$^2$) per year and starting to cross percentile lines) should prompt early intervention.

## History

The history should include the age of onset of overweight and information about the child's eating and exercise habits. The age of onset is helpful in distinguishing overfeeding from genetic causes of overweight since syndromic obesity often has onset before two years of age (Table **2A**). It is also important to keep in mind the single gene defects associated with obesity which present with early onset obesity (Table **2B**). The clues from the dietary and activity history may help determine potential areas for intervention. History of uncontrolled consumption of large amounts of food may be indicative of an eating disorder. An association has been shown between skipping meals, particularly breakfast, and overweight/obesity. It must be noted that this is not a causal relationship [52]. The medical history should include review of all medications, particularly those that are known to accelerate weight gain [53, 54] (Table **3**).

**Table 2A. Genetic syndromes associated with obesity.**

| |
|---|
| 1-Albright hereditary osteodystrophy (Pseudohypoparathyroidism type 1 a) |
| 2-Alström syndrome |
| 3-Bardet-Biedl syndrome |
| 4-Beckwith-Wiedemann syndrome |
| 5-Carpenter syndrome |
| 6-Cohen syndrome |
| 7-Prader Willi syndrome |

**Table 2B. Single gene defects associated with obesity.**

| |
|---|
| 1. Leptin deficiency (LEP) |
| 2. Pro-opiomelanocortin deficiency (POMC) |
| 3. Proprotein convertase 1 (PCSK1, also known as prohormone convertase 1) |
| 4. Melanocortin receptor 4 haploinsufficiency (MC4R) |
| 5. Leptin receptor deficiency (LEPR) |
| [References 5, 11, 15] |

**Table 3. Drugs that promote weight gain.**

| |
|---|
| 1- Insulin, insulinotropic agents |
| 2- Beta-blockers |
| 3- Corticosteroids |
| 4- Cyproheptadine |
| 5- Antipsychotics (thioridazine, risperidone and lithium carbonate) |
| 6- Antiepileptic drugs (sodium valproate, carbamazepine, gabapentin) |
| 7- Tricyclic antidepressants (such as amitriptyline |
| [References 53, 54] |

## Review of Systems

The review of systems should try to identify underlying etiologies and co-existing problems. For example an abrupt onset of obesity with rapid weight gain should prompt investigation of medication-induced weight gain, a major psychosocial trigger (such as depression), endocrine causes of obesity (*e.g.,* Cushing disease, hypothalamic tumor), or some obesity syndromes (Prader-Willi syndrome, or rapid-onset obesity with hypothalamic dysfunction, hypoventilation, autonomic dysregulation, and neural crest tumor (ROHHADNET syndrome) [55].

## Family History

Obesity in one or both parents is an important predictor for a child's prospective obesity risk extending to adulthood [56 - 58]. The family history should inquire about obesity in first-degree relatives, and common comorbidities of obesity, such as cardiovascular disease, hypertension, diabetes, liver or gallbladder disease, and respiratory insufficiency in first- and second-degree relatives [56 - 59].

## Psychosocial History

The psychosocial history should encompass; (1) Depression (2) Information about school and social environment (3) Tobacco use. A careful and considerate approach should be taken while discussing the topics of weight and mental health [48]. It has been noted that even health care professionals hold biased attitudes toward adult patients that may be extended to patients in the pediatric age group [60]. This may include a tendency to blame parents for their children's weight status, negative comments on the parents' or child's weight, or failure to listen to parents. Parents may feel guilt, anger, and frustration because they do not know how to help their children [61]. Parents are instrumental in the provision of their children's physical and social environments and a positive working relationship is essential to their children's physical and mental health [48, 61, 62]. A family-centered approach is recommended.

**Physical Examination**

The physical examination should look for underlying etiologies, comorbidities and help the clinician with management [5, 47]. Highlighting certain findings in the exam room may be instrumental in engaging the families and help them understand the concerns.

Assessment of general appearance should include evaluation for dysmorphic features (which may suggest a genetic syndrome), assessment of affect, and assessment of fat distribution which may help to distinguish the etiology of obesity. The excess fat in exogenous obesity usually has a generalized distribution in the trunk and periphery. In contrast, the centripetal distribution of body fat (concentrated in the interscapular area, face, neck, and trunk) is suggestive of Cushing syndrome. Abdominal obesity (also referred to as central, visceral, android, or male-type obesity) is associated with certain comorbidities, including the MetS, PCOS, and insulin resistance. Measurement of the waist circumference, along with calculation of the body mass index (BMI), may help identify patients at risk for these comorbidities. Waist circumference standards for American children of various ethnic groups are available [63].

A careful blood pressure measurement should be obtained with a proper sized cuff. Hypertension increases the long-term cardiovascular risk in overweight / obese children. Hypertension may be a sign of Cushing syndrome [5, 47]. Hypertension is defined as a blood pressure greater than the 95th percentile for gender, age and height on three separate occasions. Age-, gender- and height-specific blood pressure percentile references should be used [64].

Assessment of height and height velocity is useful in distinguishing exogenous obesity from obesity that is secondary to genetic or endocrine etiologies, including hypothalamic-pituitary lesions. Because exogenous obesity drives linear height, most obese children are tall for their age. On the contrary, short stature is a manifestation of most endocrine and genetic causes of obesity [5, 44]. Growth velocity may decelerate in children with endocrine causes of obesity. Children with Prader-Willi syndrome are often short for their genetic potential and/or fail to have a pubertal growth spurt.

Examination of the head, eyes, and throat may provide clues to the etiology of obesity and/or comorbidities [5, 47, 65]. For example microcephaly is a feature of Cohen syndrome. Blurred disc margins may indicate pseudotumor cerebri [43, 47]. Nystagmus or visual complaints raise the concern for a hypothalamic-pituitary lesion [66]. Other findings that support this possibility are rapid onset of obesity or hyperphagia, decrease in growth velocity, precocious puberty, or neurologic symptoms. Clumps of pigment in the peripheral retina may indicate retinitis pigmentosa, which occurs in Bardet-Biedl syndrome [67]. Enlarged tonsils may indicate obstructive sleep apnea.

Dry, coarse, or brittle hair may be present in hypothyroidism. Striae and ecchymoses may be manifestations of Cushing syndrome. Striae in general result from rapid accumulation of subcutaneous fat. Further evaluation on width and color (such as violet-colored, wide stretch marks) may provide clues for likely association with Cushing disease Acanthosis nigricans may point to insulin resistance and risk of T2DM. Hirsutism may accompany polycystic ovarian syndrome (PCOS) or Cushing syndrome [45, 47, 65].

Abdominal tenderness may be a sign of gallbladder disease. Right upper quadrant pain and/or hepatomegaly may be a clue to NAFLD [18, 47, 65].

The musculoskeletal examination may provide important clues on underlying etiology or comorbidities of pediatric overweight: Nonpitting edema may suggest hypothyroidism. Postaxial polydactyly (an extra digit next to the fifth digit) may be seen in Bardet-Biedl syndrome, and small hands and feet may be present in Prader-Willi syndrome [67]. Physical exam is instrumental in diagnosing slipped capital femoral epiphysis (limited range of motion at the hip, gait abnormality) or Blount disease (bowing of the lower legs).

The genitourinary examination and evaluation of pubertal stage may also provide additional input regarding genetic or endocrine causes of obesity [68]. Undescended testicles, small penis, and scrotal hypoplasia may point to Prader-Willi syndrome. Small testes may suggest Prader-Willi or Bardet-Biedl syndrome [5, 67]. Delayed or absent puberty may be a component of hypothalamic-pituitary tumors, Prader-Willi syndrome, Bardet-Biedl syndrome, leptin deficiency, or leptin receptor deficiency [5, 67] Precocious puberty occasionally is a presenting symptom of a hypothalamic-pituitary lesion.

The syndromic causes of overweight in children are frequently associated with cognitive or developmental delay (Table **2A-B**) [5, 12]. Severe hypotonia during infancy and delayed development of gross motor skills are features of Prader-Willi syndrome.

Psychological complications are frequently seen in obese children. Health care providers managing obesity in children and adolescents are in a crucial position to help screen and identify depression to facilitate proper assessment and care of patients. Use of standardized screening tools such as Patient Health Questionnaire (PHQ-9) should be considered for adolescent depression screening [47, 69].

## LABORATORY STUDIES

The laboratory evaluation for overweight and obesity in children is not fully standardized and must be tailored to the patient. In our clinics, if the child is not fasting at the time of initial clinical evaluation a comprehensive metabolic profile, thyroid screening (free T4 and TSH), and hemoglobin A1c level are considered. The metabolic panel provides a random glucose, serum alanine aminotransferase (ALT), and aspartate aminotransferase (AST). Hemoglobin A1C is a useful marker of the average blood glucose concentration over the preceding 8 to 12 weeks and has gained more emphasis as a screening tool for diabetes mellitus in the past decade. In year 2010, the American Diabetes Association (ADA) authorized the use of HbA1c as a diagnostic criterion for diabetes and other glucose abnormalities with the prerequisite of using an assay certified by the National Glycohemoglobin Standardization Program (NGSP) [70]. The prediabetic range was defined as HbA1c $\geq$ 5.7% and <6.5% in adults. Diseases such as iron deficiency anemia, cystic fibrosis, sickle cell disease, thalassemia, and other hemoglobinopathies alter HbA1c results. Therefore clinical judgment should be used [71]. A follow up laboratory evaluation may be scheduled as a fasting blood draw and include a lipid panel (total cholesterol, triglycerides, LDL- and HDL-cholesterol), and fasting glucose. In our clinics we try to coordinate this with a lifestyle counseling session with specialty nurse educator. A fasting insulin level may be considered for purposes of counseling rather than screening as also recommended by an international consensus report on pediatric insulin resistance in 2010 [72]. It is important to stress that routine fasting insulin screening is not recommended.

The ADA Consensus Panel Guidelines recommend screening for diabetes in children over 10 years of age (or at the onset of puberty if it occurs at a younger age) who are overweight or obese and have two or more additional risk factors such as family history of type 2 diabetes in a first- or second-degree relative, high-risk ethnicity, acanthosis nigricans, or PCOS [73]. The ADA recommends measurement of fasting plasma glucose (FPG) level in these patients.

In the author's clinic, children and adolescents who are noted to have multiple risk markers for dysglycemia (prediabetes or diabetes) undergo an oral glucose tolerance test with fasting and 2 hour blood samples for glucose and insulin. HbA1c level in the questionable zone for prediabetes (5.7-6.4% per ADA guidelines) is considered as a risk factor. A fasting glucose of 100 to 125 mg/dL is indicative of impaired fasting glucose, and a level of ≥126 mg per dL is consistent with the diagnosis of diabetes. Patients with intermediate or conflicting results for any of these tests should undergo repeat testing and be monitored for future development of diabetes. Definitive diagnosis of diabetes mellitus requires meeting diagnostic criteria on at least two separate occasions [70].

In 2011, an expert panel from the United States National Heart, Lung, and Blood Institute (NHLBI), issued integrated guidelines for cardiovascular risk reduction, endorsed by the American Academy of Pediatrics [74]. The panel recommended initial lipid screening with fasting lipid profile for children between ages two and eight years, with a BMI ≥95th percentile (or other risk factors for cardiovascular disease, such as family history of dyslipidemia/ early cardiovascular disease and or morbidity in first or second degree relatives, history of diabetes, hypertension or smoking in child). The panel recommended universal lipid screening with a nonfasting non HDL-C (HDL-C subtracted from the total cholesterol measurement) for children ages 9-11 years and 17-21 years. For children ages 9 and above with a BMI ≥85th percentile or other risk factors as listed above, lipid screening is recommended [74]. Cut-offs for normal are a fasting total cholesterol of <170 mg/dL, a LDL cholesterol of <110 mg/dL, non-HDL cholesterol of <120 mg/dl, triglycerides of <75 mg/dl for ages 0-9 years and <90 mg/dl for ages 10-19 years, and HDL cholesterol of >45 mg/dl. Abnormal values compatible with dyslipidemia are a fasting total cholesterol of ≥200 mg/dL, a LDL cholesterol of ≥130 mg/dL, non-HDL cholesterol of ≥ 145 mg/dl, triglycerides of ≥100 mg/dl for ages 0-9 and ≥130 mg/dl for ages 10-19 years, and HDL cholesterol of <40 mg/dl. Overweight/obese children with hyperlipidemia should be monitored and treated. Stepwise approach includes medical nutrition therapy (with lifestyle modification referring to increased physical activity) and medical therapy [74 - 76].

Liver function tests should be obtained because nonalcoholic fatty liver disease (NAFLD) is typically asymptomatic [19, 38]. Obese children with an elevation of ALT greater than two times the upper limit of normal, persisting for more than three months should be evaluated for the presence of NAFLD and other chronic liver problems. Assessment for other comorbidities, such as sleep apnea and polycystic ovary syndrome, depends on the detection of risk factors or symptoms, and should be done on a case by case format if indicated. Vitamin D deficiency has been noted commonly among obese children and adolescents either because of generalized vitamin and mineral deficiencies secondary to poor eating habits, and/or due to sequestration in excess adipose tissue. Studies from various geographical regions reported Vitamin D deficiency in about half of children and adults with severe obesity, and depicted association with higher BMI and features of the MetS [77 - 80]. No guidelines exist recommending routine screening of overweight children for Vitamin D status, therefore clinical judgment is recommended. If screening for vitamin D deficiency, serum 25(OH) vitamin D level should be measured. The reference range varies by region, but levels <20 ng/mL are generally considered deficient. If deficiency is found, vitamin D supplementation should be initiated to avoid long-term consequences.

Additional testing should be performed if there are findings consistent with hypothyroidism, PCOS, Cushing syndrome, and sleep apnea [5, 17, 44, 81]. Syndromic obesity should be evaluated in children with developmental delay or dysmorphic features (Table **2**). Endocrine causes of obesity are unlikely if the growth velocity is normal during childhood or early adolescence [44].

**Radiographic Evaluation** may be considered if indicated. For example, plain radiographs of the lower extremities should be obtained if there are clinical findings consistent with slipped capital femoral epiphysis (hip or knee pain, limited range of motion, abnormal gait) or Blount disease (bowed tibia). Abdominal ultrasonography may be indicated in children with findings consistent with gallstones (*e.g,* abdominal pain, abnormal transaminases) [5, 18]. Abdominal ultrasonography may be used to confirm the presence of fatty liver.

## TREATMENT

The pharmacotherapy options for the treatment of pediatric obesity are scanty. Lifestyle modification with components of medical nutrition therapy, physical activity and behavior modification is the key treatment approach for exogenous obesity in children and adolescents. Treatment should help reverse the disproportionately high ratio of energy intake to energy expenditure to reverse the positive energy balance. It is of utmost importance to involve the family/ caregivers.

Treatment should be targeted at primary and secondary prevention. Prevention efforts should start early, when an increasing BMI trend is noted. If the yearly increase in the BMI is more than three to four units (kg/m$^2$) and starting to cross percentile lines (even when the BMI is still below the 85th percentile, and particularly if the child is older than four years), this should prompt the clinician to discuss these observations with the family [5]. Providing simple tips for maintaining a healthy weight by nutrition modification and, increased physical activity and parenting strategies to support these goals will be a good start.

If the child is overweight or obese he or she should be screened for comorbidities of obesity. The clinician should provide counseling to optimize lifestyle habits with a goal of slowing the rate of weight gain. These families should receive nutrition and lifestyle counseling. These children require regular follow-up to monitor progress [5, 11]. Progression of linear growth, as applicable to certain children and adolescents, will also contribute to improvement in the BMI throughout the process of weight management interventions.

The 2011 NHLBI Expert Panel guidelines for cardiovascular health and risk reduction in children and adolescents [74] is a comprehensive reference prepared to assist pediatric health care providers in both the promotion of cardiovascular health and the identification and management of specific risk factors.

A stepwise approach is recommended in goal setting. Primordial prevention is the prevention of risk-factor development. Primary prevention refers to effective management of identified risk factors for ameliorating future problems such as cardiovascular disease, prediabetes, diabetes and other potential complications.

Children who have comorbidities of obesity should be consulted with appropriate subspecialty services. When available, children may be referred to pediatric obesity centers for dietary, pharmacologic, and/or surgical therapy, as applicable.

Treatment of obesity must help reach a negative energy balance [82]. Reduced-energy diets regardless of macronutrient composition result with clinically meaningful weight loss in adults. The association between pediatric obesity and the consumption of high calorie, high-fat, high-carbohydrate and low-fiber foods has been reported [83]. The specific approaches proven to result with improvement of obesity in children include elimination of sugar-containing beverages and a transition to low-glycemic index diet [10, 83, 84]. It is pivotal to increase awareness of the children and parents/ caregivers of the caloric content of beverages and limit consumption of caloric beverages. Physical activity intervention is the other essential component of the management. A recent systematic review and meta analysis reported that both diet-only and diet plus exercise approaches helped achieve weight loss and improve metabolic parameters [84]. Interventions combining exercise with diet resulted with better improvements in HDL-C, fasting glucose and fasting insulin [84].

Behavior modification involves motivation to limit screen time and increase physical activity, psychologic training to make a change in eating behaviors or exercise, family counseling to encourage for weight loss goals, and school-based changes to promote physical activity and healthy eating [5, 10]. Mobile and wireless health technologies and exergaming (video gaming that involves gross motor movement) may help develop effective intervention strategies [10]. Even though several medications are marketed to treat obesity, only a limited number of those are approved for children under 16 years of age. These medications resulted with limited improvement when used as an adjunct to exercise and nutrition modification. Due to serious adverse effects, majority of the medications proposed to treat obesity have been removed from use in children and adolescents. Phentermine and similar anorexiant medications which alter the release and reuptake of neurotransmitters are to be listed in this group. Pharmacologic treatment may be considered in selected patients, particularly those with severe comorbidities, when lifestyle intervention fails to result with weight loss [5, 10, 85]. Sibutramine (appetite suppressor: inhibits norepinephrine, serotonin and dopamine reuptake) is FDA-approved for treatment of obesity in adolescents above 16 years of age. Studies involving Sibutramine and behavioral therapy have shown decrease in BMI (2.9-3.6 kg/m2) [10]. Orlistat (gastrointestinal lipase inhibitor) is approved by the FDA for management of obesity in adolescents 12-16 years of age. Drug-related adverse effects, such as oily stools/spotting, have limited its use. Metformin is a biguanide approved by the FDA for treatment of type 2 diabetes mellitus in children aged 10 years and older. Metformin reduces hepatic glucose output and increases insulin sensitivity in peripheral tissues. Randomized controlled trials have been performed, evaluating metformin as an "obesity medication" in adolescents. The degree of long-term improvement in body weight or its complications is unknown. Metformin may be considered in the presence of clinically significant insulin resistance and or prediabetes. Leptin has been shown effective at reducing BMI in individuals with leptin deficiency, which is a rare condition [86]. Octreotide (a somatostatin analog) has been used in the treatment of hypothalamic obesity and shown to suppress insulin, and stabilize weight and BMI [10, 87]. Lack of coverage of medications by insurance, high out-of-pocket costs and adverse effects are among the restricting factors.

Bariatric surgery is the most definitive and longest lasting form of weight loss treatment. In adults, and to a smaller extent in adolescents, bariatric surgery has been shown to help accomplish significant weight loss and improvement or resolution of comorbidities, such as type 2 diabetes, hypertension and obstructive sleep apnea [10]. However significant acute and chronic complications ranging from wound infections to life-threatening problems such as bowel obstruction/perforation have been reported [4, 5, 10, 88]. Patients with severe pediatric obesity (BMI equal to or above the 99th percentile) may require consideration for this approach. Management of comorbid conditions with appropriate treatment strategies is essential. For example hormonal contraceptives are the first-line management for menstrual abnormalities and hirsutism/acne in

PCOS and metformin has also been used. Hypertension may necessitate medical treatment.

In some clinical centers for children and adolescents, specialty clinics have been developed for the management of obesity. If subspecialty center is not available, a well-organized and comprehensive evaluation strategy can be incorporated into the routine clinical practice. This should enable identification of the comorbidities and the required subspecialty referrals. Some clinic models, including our current practice, involve a nurse educator/nutritionist providing lifestyle counseling for children and families. This model was started during our participation in a collaborative effort to tackle pediatric obesity in our communities, entitled Healthy Green and Into the Outdoors. The collaboration was organized by the Community Foundation of North Louisiana, and supported by a grant from Blue Cross Blue Shield Foundation of Louisiana. The lifestyle counselor meets the child/family after the initial evaluation by the physician.

There is a crucial need for pediatric obesity advocacy. This clearly demands the clinician's involvement beyond the office, requires collaboration with the community and public policy makers. The 2005 Institute of Medicine Report recommends that clinicians, regardless of specialty, serve as role models and provide leadership in their communities for obesity prevention initiatives [89]. Pediatricians and pediatric subspecialists should routinely discuss obesity prevention and recommendations with patients and families [18]. Clinicians should consider advocating for and providing healthy food options in hospitals. In various areas of the United States, successful models have been established involving the medical/hospital staff in community advocacy programs, community/hospital partnerships, locally and at the state level. Physicians' participation may involve speaking at public forums and attending community/school board meetings to offer medical expertise on the issue of pediatric obesity. The American Board of Pediatrics maintenance of board certification (MOC) programs involve several projects focusing on pediatric obesity. These help with knowledge acquisition, self-efficacy, and physician compliance with recommended practice recommendations for the screening, prevention, and management of pediatric obesity [90].

## CONCLUSION

Pediatric care providers should universally assess children for obesity and risk of obesity to improve early identification and management. Calculation of the BMI and plotting on an appropriate reference curve should be part of the routine clinical assessment of all children with ages 2 years and above. The sequential follow up for the trends may provide invaluable and timely information to track overweight/obesity trends and may be instrumental to initiate primary and/or secondary prevention. Obesity prevention messages can be provided as applicable, weight control interventions initiated for those with excess weight [11, 91].

Clinical approach to pediatric overweight/obesity must be comprehensive and multi-faceted. The clinician's role should not be not restricted to the clinic but should expand to the community for advocacy efforts [11]. Collaborations among health-care systems, community and school systems may be instrumental [10]. A structured and comprehensive approach dealing with the pediatric obesity problem at the present will be expected to contribute to improvement in public health for the future generations.

## CONFLICT OF INTEREST

The authors declare no conflict of interest, financial or otherwise.

## ACKNOWLEDGEMENTS

Declared none.

## REFERENCES

[1] Han JC, Kimm SY. Childhood Obesity-2010: Progress and Challenges. Lancet 2010; 375(9727): 1737-48.
[http://dx.doi.org/10.1016/S0140-6736(10)60171-7]

[2] Ogden CL, Carroll MD, Kit BK, Flegal KM. Prevalence of and adult obesity in the United States, 2011-2012. JAMA Pediatr 2014; 311(8): 806-14.
[http://dx.doi.org/10.1001/jama.2014.732]

[3] Hubbard VS. Defining overweight and obesity: what are the issues? Am J Clin Nutr 2000; 72: 1067-8.

[4] Nicolai JP, Lupiani JH, Wolf AJ. An Integrative approach to obesity. In: Rakel D, Ed. Integrative Medicine. 3rd ed. Philadelphia, PA: W.B. Saunders (Elsevier) 2012; pp. 364-75.

[5] Klish WJ. Clinical evaluation of the obese child and adolescent. In: Motil KJ, Geffner M, Hoppin AG, Eds. Up to date. www.uptodate.com©2016 UpToDate. 2016.

[6] BMI curves. http://www.cdc.gov/growthcharts.

[7] Cole TJ, Bellizzi MC, Flegal KM, Dietz WH. Establishing a standard definition for child and obesity worldwide: International survey. BMJ 2000; 320: 1240-3.
[http://dx.doi.org/10.1136/bmj.320.7244.1240]

[8] De Onis M, Garza C, Victora CG, *et al.* The WHO Multicentre Growth Reference Study: planning, study design and methodology. Food Nutr Bull 2004; 25(1) (Suppl.): S15-26.
[http://dx.doi.org/10.1177/15648265040251S103]

[9] De Onis M, Onyanga AW, Borghi E, Siyam A, Nishida C, Siekmann J. Development of a WHO growth reference for school-aged children and adolescents. Bull World Health Organ 2007; 85(9): 660-7.
[http://dx.doi.org/10.2471/BLT.07.043497]

[10]    Katzmarzyk PT, Barlow S, Bouchard C, *et al.* An evolving scientific basis for the prevention and treatment of pediatric obesity. Int J Obes 2014; 38(7): 887-905.
[http://dx.doi.org/10.1038/ijo.2014.49]

[11]    Gungor NK. Overweight and obesity in children and adolescents. J Clin Res Pediatr Endocrinol 2014; 6(3): 129-43.
[http://dx.doi.org/10.4274/jcrpe.1471]

[12]    Ramachandrappa S, Farooqi IS. Genetic approaches to understanding human obesity. J Clin Invest 2011; 121: 2080-6.
[http://dx.doi.org/10.1172/JCI46044]

[13]    Karra E, Chandarana K, Batterham RL. The role of peptide YY in appetite regulation and obesity. J Physiol 2009; 587(1): 19-25.
[http://dx.doi.org/10.1113/jphysiol.2008.164269]

[14]    Cummings DE, Overduin J. Gastrointestinal regulation of food intake. J Clin Invest 2007; 117: 13-23.
[http://dx.doi.org/10.1172/JCI30227]

[15]    Farooqi S, O'Rahilly S. Genetics of obesity in humans. Endocr Rev 2006; 27: 710-8.
[http://dx.doi.org/10.1210/er.2006-0040]

[16]    Ogden CL, Carroll MD, Kit BK, Flegal KM. Prevalence of obesity and trends in body mass index among US children and adolescents, 1999-2010. JAMA 2012; 307(5): 483-90.
[http://dx.doi.org/10.1001/jama.2012.40]

[17]    Daniels SR. Complications of obesity in children and adolescents. Int J Obes 2009; 33 (Suppl. 1): S60-5.
[http://dx.doi.org/10.1038/ijo.2009.20]

[18]    Huang JS, Barlow SE, Quiros-Tejeira RE, *et al.* The NASPGHAN Obesity Task Force. Consensus Statement: Childhood Obesity for Pediatric Gastroenterologists. J Pediatr Gastroenterol Nutr 2013; 56: 99-109.
[http://dx.doi.org/10.1097/MPG.0b013e31826d3c62]

[19]    Gungor N, Libman I, Arslanian S. Type 2 Diabetes Mellitus in Children and Adolescents. In: Pescovitz , Eugster , Eds. Pediatric Endocrinology: Mechanisms, Manifestations, and Management. Lippincott, Williams and Wilkins 2004; pp. 450-66.

[20]    Kahn SE. The importance of beta cell failure in the development and progression of type 2 diabetes. J Clin Endocrinol Metab 2001; 86: 4047-58.

[21]    Gungor N, Bacha F, Saad R, Janosky J, Arslanian S. Youth Type 2 Diabetes Mellitus: Insulin resistance, beta-cell failure or both? Diabetes Care 2005; 28: 638-44.
[http://dx.doi.org/10.2337/diacare.28.3.638]

[22]    Sinha R, Fisch G, Teague B, *et al.* Prevalence of impaired glucose tolerance among children and adolescents with marked obesity. N Engl J Med 2002; 346(11): 802-10.
[http://dx.doi.org/10.1056/NEJMoa012578]

[23]    Goran MI, Bergman RN, Avila Q, *et al.* Impaired glucose tolerance and reduced beta-cell function in overweight Latino children with a positive family history for type 2 diabetes. J Clin Endocrinol Metab 2004; 89(1): 207-12.
[http://dx.doi.org/10.1210/jc.2003-031402]

[24]    Wiegand S, Maikowski U, Blankenstein O, Biebermann H, Tarnow P, Grüters A. Type 2 diabetes and impaired glucose tolerance in European children and adolescents with obesity - a problem that is no longer restricted to minority groups. Eur J Endocrinol 2004; 151(2): 199-206.
[http://dx.doi.org/10.1530/eje.0.1510199]

[25]    Aye T, Levitsky LL. Type 2 diabetes: an epidemic disease in childhood. Curr Opin Pediatr 2003; 15: 411-5.

[http://dx.doi.org/10.1097/00008480-200308000-00010]

[26]   SEARCH for Diabetes in Youth Study Group. Liese AD, D'Agostino RB Jr, Hamman RF, Kilgo PD, Lawrence JM, Liu LL, Loots B, Linder B, Marcovina S, Rodriguez B,Standiford D, Williams DE. The burden of diabetes mellitus among US youth: prevalence estimates from the SEARCH for Diabetes in Youth Study. Pediatrics 2006; 118: 1510-8.
       [http://dx.doi.org/10.1542/peds.2006-0690]

[27]   Lee L, Sanders RA. Metabolic syndrome. Pediatr Rev 2012; 33: 459-66.
       [http://dx.doi.org/10.1542/pir.33-10-459]

[28]   Calles-Escandon J, Cipolla M. Diabetes and endothelial dysfunction: a clinical perspective. Endocr Rev 2001; 22(1): 36-52.
       [http://dx.doi.org/10.1210/edrv.22.1.0417]

[29]   Meyer AA, Kundt G, Steiner M, Schuff-Werner P, Kienast W. Impaired flow-mediated vasodilation, carotid artery intima-media thickening, and elevated endothelial plasma markers in obese children: the impact of cardiovascular risk factors. Pediatrics 2006; 117(5): 1560-7.
       [http://dx.doi.org/10.1542/peds.2005-2140]

[30]   Berenson GS, Srinivasan SR, Bao W, Newman WP III, Tracy RE, Wattigney WA. Association between multiple cardiovascular risk factors and atherosclerosis in children and young adults. The Bogalusa Heart Study. N Engl J Med 1998; 338(23): 1650-6.
       [http://dx.doi.org/10.1056/NEJM199806043382302]

[31]   Li S, Chen W, Srinivasan SR, Xu J, Berenson GS. Relation of childhood obesity/cardiometabolic phenotypes to adult cardiometabolic profile: the Bogalusa Heart Study. Am J Epidemiol 2012; 176 (Suppl. 7): S142-9.
       [http://dx.doi.org/10.1093/aje/kws236]

[32]   Legro RS, Arslanian SA, Ehrmann DA, *et al.* Diagnosis and treatment of polycystic ovary syndrome: An Endocrine Society Clinical Practice Guideline. J Clin Endocrinol Metab 2013; 98(12): 4565-92.
       [http://dx.doi.org/10.1210/jc.2013-2350]

[33]   Witchel S. F, Oberfield S, Rosenfield R, L, Codner E, Bonny A, Ibáñez L, Pena A, Horikawa R, Gomez-Lobo V, Joel D, Tfayli H, Arslanian S, Dabadghao P, Garcia Rudaz C, Lee P, A, The Diagnosis of Polycystic Ovary Syndrome during Adolescence. Horm Res Paediatr 2015; 83: 376-89.
       [http://dx.doi.org/10.1159/000375530]

[34]   Kaplowitz PB, Slora EJ, Wasserman RC, Pedlow SE, Herman-Giddens ME. Earlier onset of puberty in girls: relation to increased body mass index and race. Pediatrics 2001; 108: 347-53.
       [http://dx.doi.org/10.1542/peds.108.2.347]

[35]   Kaplowitz P. Delayed puberty in obese boys: comparison with constitutional delayed puberty and response to testosterone therapy. J Pediatr 1998; 133(6): 745-9.
       [http://dx.doi.org/10.1016/S0022-3476(98)70144-1]

[36]   Pacifico L, Anania C, Ferraro F, Andreoli GM, Chiesa C. Thyroid function in childhood obesity and metabolic comorbidity. Clin Chim Acta 2012; 18(413): 396-405.
       [http://dx.doi.org/10.1016/j.cca.2011.11.013]

[37]   Srinivasan SR, Bao W, Wattigney WA, Berenson GS. Adolescent overweight is associated with adult overweight and related multiple cardiovascular risk factors: the Bogalusa Heart Study. Metabolism 1996; 45(2): 235-40.
       [http://dx.doi.org/10.1016/S0026-0495(96)90060-8]

[38]   Lavine JE, Schwimmer JB, Van Natta ML, *et al.* Nonalcoholic Steatohepatitis Clinical Research Network. Effect of vitamin E or metformin for treatment of nonalcoholic fatty liver disease in children and adolescents: the TONIC randomized controlled trial. JAMA 2011; 305(16): 1659-68.
       [http://dx.doi.org/10.1001/jama.2011.520]

[39] Schwimmer JB, Deutsch R, Rauch JB, Behling C, Newbury R, Lavine JE. Obesity, insulin resistance, and other clinicopathological correlates of pediatric nonalcoholic fatty liver disease. J Pediatr 2003; 143(4): 500-5.
[http://dx.doi.org/10.1067/S0022-3476(03)00325-1]

[40] de la Eva R, Baur LA, Donaghue KC, Waters KA. Metabolic correlates with obstructive sleep apnea in obese subjects. J Pediatr 2002; 140: 654-9.
[http://dx.doi.org/10.1067/mpd.2002.123765]

[41] Section on Pediatric Pulmonology, Subcommittee on Obstructive Sleep Apnea Syndrome. American Academy of Pediatrics. Clinical practice guideline: diagnosis and management of childhood obstructive sleep apnea syndrome. Pediatrics 2002; 109(4): 704-12.
[http://dx.doi.org/10.1542/peds.109.4.704]

[42] Gettys FK, Jackson JB, Frick SL. Obesity in pediatric orthopaedics. Orthop Clin North Am 2011; 42(1): 95-105.
[http://dx.doi.org/10.1016/j.ocl.2010.08.005]

[43] Ball AK, Clarke CE. Idiopathic intracranial hypertension. Lancet Neurol 2006; 5: 433-42.
[http://dx.doi.org/10.1016/S1474-4422(06)70442-2]

[44] August GP, Caprio S, Fennoy I, *et al.* Endocrine Society. Prevention and treatment of pediatric obesity: an endocrine society clinical practice guideline based on expert opinion. J Clin Endocrinol Metab 2008; 93(12): 4576-99.
[http://dx.doi.org/10.1210/jc.2007-2458]

[45] Lau K, Höger PH. Skin diseases associated with obesity in children. Bundesgesundheitsblatt Gesundheitsforschung Gesundheitsschutz 2013; 56(4): 539-42. [Article in German].
[http://dx.doi.org/10.1007/s00103-012-1641-x]

[46] Sinha S, Schwartz RA. Juvenile acanthosis nigricans. J Am Acad Dermatol 2007; 57(3): 502-8.
[http://dx.doi.org/10.1016/j.jaad.2006.08.016]

[47] Armstrong S, Lazorick S, Hampl S, *et al.* Physical examination findings among children and adolescents with obesity: An evidence-based review. Pediatrics 137(2): e20151766.
[http://dx.doi.org/10.1542/peds.2015-1766]

[48] Vander WJ, Mitchell ER. Psychological complications of pediatric obesity. Pediatr Clin North Am 2011; 58: 1393-401.
[http://dx.doi.org/10.1016/j.pcl.2011.09.008]

[49] Maloney AE. Pediatric obesity: a review for the child psychiatrist. Child Adolesc Psychiatr Clin N Am 2010; (19): 353-70.
[http://dx.doi.org/10.1016/j.chc.2010.01.005]

[50] Hebebrand J, Herpertz-Dahlmann B. Psychological and psychiatric aspects of pediatric obesity. Child Adolesc Psychiatr Clin N Am 2009; 18(1): 49-65.
[http://dx.doi.org/10.1016/j.chc.2008.08.002]

[51] Wardle J, Cooke L. The impact of obesity on psychological well-being. Clinical Endocrinology & Metabolism 2005; 19(3): 421-40.
[http://dx.doi.org/10.1016/j.beem.2005.04.006]

[52] Casazza K, Fontaine KR, Astrup A, *et al.* Myths, Presumptions, and Facts about Obesity. N Engl J Med 2013; 368: 446-54.
[http://dx.doi.org/10.1056/NEJMsa1208051]

[53] Leslie WS, Hankey CR, Lean ME. Weight gain as an adverse effect of some commonly prescribed drugs: a systematic review. Q J Med 2007; 100: 395-404.
[http://dx.doi.org/10.1093/qjmed/hcm044]

[54]    Cheskin LJ, Bartlett SJ, Zayas R, Twilley CH, Allison DB, Contoreggi C. Prescription medications: a modifiable contributor to obesity. South Med J 1999; 92(9): 898-904.
[http://dx.doi.org/10.1097/00007611-199909000-00009]

[55]    Bougnères P, Pantalone L, Linglart A, *et al.* Endocrine manifestations of the rapid-onset obesity with hypoventilation, hypothalamic, autonomic dysregulation, and neural tumor syndrome in childhood. J Clin Endocrinol Metab 2008; 93: 3971.
[http://dx.doi.org/10.1210/jc.2008-0238]

[56]    Whitaker RC, Wright JA, Pepe MS, *et al.* Predicting obesity in young adulthood from childhood and parental obesity. N Engl J Med 1997; 337: 869.
[http://dx.doi.org/10.1056/NEJM199709253371301]

[57]    Blair NJ, Thompson JM, Black PN, *et al.* Risk factors for obesity in 7-year-old European children: the Auckland Birthweight Collaborative Study. Arch Dis Child 2007; 92: 866.
[http://dx.doi.org/10.1136/adc.2007.116855]

[58]    Reilly JJ, Armstrong J, Dorosty AR, *et al.* Early life risk factors for obesity in childhood: cohort study. BMJ 2005; 330: 1357.
[http://dx.doi.org/10.1136/bmj.38470.670903.E0]

[59]    Rudolf M. Predicting babies' risk of obesity. Arch Dis Child 2011; 96: 995.
[http://dx.doi.org/10.1136/adc.2010.197251]

[60]    Puhl RM, Latner JD. Stigma, obesity and the health of the nation's children. Psychol Bull 2007; 133: 557-80.
[http://dx.doi.org/10.1037/0033-2909.133.4.557]

[61]    Edmunds LD. Parents' perceptions of health professionals' responses when seeking help for their overweight children. Fam Pract 2005; 22: 287-92.
[http://dx.doi.org/10.1093/fampra/cmh729]

[62]    Rodin RL, Alexander MH, Guillory J, *et al.* Physician counseling to prevent overweight in children and adolescents: American College of Preventive Medicine Position Statement. J Public Health Manag Pract 2007; 13: 655-61.
[http://dx.doi.org/10.1097/01.PHH.0000296144.25165.92]

[63]    Fernández JR, Redden DT, Pietrobelli A, Allison DB. Waist circumference percentiles in nationally representative samples of African-American, European-American, and Mexican-American children and adolescents. J Pediatr 2004; 145(4): 439-44.
[http://dx.doi.org/10.1016/j.jpeds.2004.06.044]

[64]    National High Blood Pressure Education Program Working Group on High Blood Pressure in Children and Adolescents. The fourth report on the diagnosis, evaluation, and treatment of high blood pressure in children and adolescents. Pediatrics 2004; 114(2 Suppl 4th Report): 555-76.

[65]    Krebs NF, Himes JH, Jacobson D, Nicklas TA, Guilday P, Styne D. Assessment of child and adolescent overweight and obesity. Pediatrics 2007; 120 (Suppl. 4): S193.
[http://dx.doi.org/10.1542/peds.2007-2329D]

[66]    Brara SM, Koebnick C, Porter AH, Langer-Gould A. Pediatric idiopathic intracranial hypertension and extreme childhood obesity. J Pediatr 2012; 161(4): 602-7.
[http://dx.doi.org/10.1016/j.jpeds.2012.03.047]

[67]    Green JS, Parfrey PS, Harnett JD, *et al.* The cardinal manifestations of Bardet-Biedl syndrome, a form of Laurence-Moon-Biedl syndrome. N Engl J Med 1989; 321(15): 1002.
[http://dx.doi.org/10.1056/NEJM198910123211503]

[68]    Dietz WH, Robinson TN. Clinical practice. Overweight children and adolescents. N Engl J Med 2005; 352: 2100.
[http://dx.doi.org/10.1056/NEJMcp043052]

[69]    Kroenke K, Spitzer RL, Williams JB. The PHQ-9: Validity of a brief depression severity measure. Gen Intern Med 2001; 16(9): 606-13.
[http://dx.doi.org/10.1046/j.1525-1497.2001.016009606.x]

[70]    American Diabetes Association Position Statement. Diagnosis and Classification of Diabetes Mellitus. Diabetes Care 2010; 33: S62-9.
[http://dx.doi.org/10.2337/dc10-S062]

[71]    Kapadia CR. Are the ADA Hemoglobin a1c criteria relevant for the diagnosis of type 2 diabetes in youth? Curr Diab Rep 2013; 13: 51-5.
[http://dx.doi.org/10.1007/s11892-012-0343-y]

[72]    Levy-Marchal C, Arslanian S, Cutfield W, et al. ESPE-LWPES-ISPAD-APPES-APEG-SLEP-JSPE; Insulin Resistance in Children Consensus Conference Group. Insulin resistance in children: consensus, perspective, and future directions. J Clin Endocrinol Metab 2010; 95(12): 5189-98.
[http://dx.doi.org/10.1210/jc.2010-1047]

[73]    American Diabetes Association. Type 2 diabetes in children and adolescents. Diabetes Care 2000; 23: 381-9.
[http://dx.doi.org/10.2337/diacare.23.3.381]

[74]    Expert Panel on Integrated Guidelines for Cardiovascular Health and Risk Reduction in Children and Adolescents, National Heart, Lung, and Blood Institute. Expert panel on integrated guidelines for cardiovascular health and risk reduction in children and adolescents: summary report. Pediatrics 2011; 128 (Suppl. 5): 213-56.
[http://dx.doi.org/10.1542/peds.2009-2107C]

[75]    Daniels SR. Management of hyperlipidemia in pediatrics. Curr Opin Cardiol 2012; 27: 92-7.
[http://dx.doi.org/10.1097/HCO.0b013e32834fea6c]

[76]    Bamba V. Update on screening, etiology and treatment of dyslipidemia in children. J Clin Endocrinol Metab 2014; 99(9): 3093-102.
[http://dx.doi.org/10.1210/jc.2013-3860]

[77]    Smotkin-Tangorra M, Purushothaman R, Gupta A, et al. Prevalence of vitamin D insufficiency in obese children and adolescents. J Pediatr Endocrinol Metab 2007; 20: 817.
[http://dx.doi.org/10.1515/JPEM.2007.20.7.817]

[78]    Botella-Carretero JI, Alvarez-Blasco F, Villafruela JJ, et al. Vitamin D deficiency is associated with the metabolic syndrome in morbid obesity. Clin Nutr 2007; 26: 573.
[http://dx.doi.org/10.1016/j.clnu.2007.05.009]

[79]    Kelly A, Brooks LJ, Dougherty S, et al. A cross-sectional study of vitamin D and insulin resistance in children. Arch Dis Child 2011; 96: 447.
[http://dx.doi.org/10.1136/adc.2010.187591]

[80]    Turer CB, Lin H, Flores G. Prevalence of vitamin D deficiency among overweight and obese US children. Pediatrics 2013; 131: e152.
[http://dx.doi.org/10.1542/peds.2012-1711]

[81]    Yanovski JA, Cutler GB Jr. Glucocorticoid action and the clinical features of Cushing's syndrome. Endocrinol Metab Clin North Am 1994; 23: 487.

[82]    Dubnov-Raz G, Berry EM. The dietary treatment of obesity. Med Clin North Am 2011; 95: 939-52.
[http://dx.doi.org/10.1016/j.mcna.2011.06.006]

[83]    Pediatric overweight: A review of the literature. The Center for Weight and Health College of Natural Resources University of California, Berkeley 2001 June; http://cwh.berkeley.edu/sites/default/files/primary_pdfs/Pediatric_Overweight_LitRev.pdf

[84]    Ho M, Garnett SP, Baur LA, et al. Impact of Dietary and Exercise Interventions on Weight Change and Metabolic Outcomes in Obese Children and Adolescents: A Systematic Review and Meta-analysis

of Randomized Trials. JAMA Pediatr 2013; 167(8): 759-68.
[http://dx.doi.org/10.1001/jamapediatrics.2013.1453]

[85]  Wald AB, Uli NK. Pharmacotherapy in pediatric obesity: current agents and future directions. Rev Endocr Metab Disord 2009; 10(3): 205-14.
[http://dx.doi.org/10.1007/s11154-009-9111-y]

[86]  Farooqi IS, Jebb SA, Langmack G, *et al*. Effects of recombinant leptin therapy in a child with congenital leptin deficiency. N Engl J Med 1999; 341(12): 879-84.
[http://dx.doi.org/10.1056/NEJM199909163411204]

[87]  Lustig RH, Hinds PS, Ringwald-Smith K, *et al*. Octreotide therapy of pediatric hypothalamic obesity: a double-blind, placebo-controlled trial. J Clin Endocrinol Metab 2003; 88(6): 2586-92.
[http://dx.doi.org/10.1210/jc.2002-030003]

[88]  Inge TH, Miyano G, Bean J, *et al*. Reversal of type 2 diabetes mellitus and improvements in cardiovascular risk factors after surgical weight loss in adolescents. Pediatrics 2009; 123(1): 214-22.
[http://dx.doi.org/10.1542/peds.2008-0522]

[89]  Perkin RM, Swift JD, Newton DA, *et al*. Pediatric Hospital Medicine: Textbook of Inpatient Management. 2nd ed. Philadelphia, PA: Lippincott Williams & Wilkins 2008; p. 692.

[90]  Huang JS, Chun S, Sandhu A, Terrones L. Quality Improvement in Childhood Obesity Management through the Maintenance of Certification Process. J Pediatr 2013 Jun 26; pii: S0022-3476(13)00560-.
[http://dx.doi.org/10.1016/j.jpeds.2013.05.011]

[91]  Barlow SE. Expert Committee. Expert committee recommendations regarding the prevention, assessment, and treatment of child and adolescent overweight and obesity: summary report. Pediatrics 2007; 120 (Suppl. 4): S164-92.
[http://dx.doi.org/10.1542/peds.2007-2329C]

# CHAPTER 10

# Current Concepts in the Management of Hyperthyroidism

## Abha Choudhary*

*Division of Pediatric Endocrinology, Department of Pediatrics, UT Southwestern Medical Center, Dallas, TX, USA*

**Abstract:** Graves' disease (GD) is the most common cause of hyperthyroidism in children and adolescents. It is an autoimmune disorder, caused by immunologic stimulation of the thyroid stimulating hormone receptor (TSHR). Thyrotropin stimulating immunoglobulin (TSI) binds to TSHR and leads to thyroid hormone overproduction. Clinical features include fatigue, tremors, palpitations, heat intolerance and poor school performance. The diagnosis is by findings of increased heart rate and goiter in the setting of suppressed thyrotropin stimulating hormone and elevated free thyroxine. Radioactive iodine uptake and serum antibody measurements help to determine the cause of hyperthyroidism. Treatment options for GD include antithyroid drugs, radioactive iodine or surgery. Lasting remission occurs in 15 to 30% of children with GD. Thus, a majority of children will require definitive therapy with radioactive iodine or thyroidectomy. A discussion of advantages and risks of each therapeutic option is essential to help the patient and family select a treatment option.

**Keywords:** Adolescents, Children, Graves' disease, Hashitoxicosis, Hepatotoxicity, Hyperthyroidism, Methimazole, Radioactive iodine, Radioactive iodine uptake, Thyroidectomy.

## INTRODUCTION
## Epidemiology

Graves' disease (GD) accounts for 10 to 15% of the childhood thyroid diseases. It is the most common cause of hyperthyroidism in children. The incidence of hyperthyroidism in adults worldwide has been reported to be 23-93/100,000 inhabitants per year [1]. The incidence in children is estimated to be 0.9 per 100,000 in national prospective surveillance study from the United Kingdom and Ireland. Autoimmune thyrotoxicosis accounted for 96% of the cases [2]. The incidence of GD is estimated to be 0.1 per 100,000 person-years in young

---

* **Corresponding author Abha Choudhary**: Division of Pediatric Endocrinology, Department of Pediatrics, UT Southwestern Medical Center, Dallas, TX, USA; Tel: 214 648 3501; Fax: 214 456 2940; Email: AChoudhary@uams.edu

Seckin Ulualp (Ed.)

children, while it is 3 per 100,000 person-years in adolescents. The prevalence in United States is 1 in 10,000 person-years. GD is rare in less than 5 years of age and has a peak incidence at 10 to 15 years of age, more common in females than males (5:1). GD is more common in children with other autoimmune conditions and in those with family history of autoimmune thyroid disease [3, 4].

**Pathogenesis**

The cause of GD is unclear, but it is thought to result from a complex interaction of genetic, immune and environmental factors. The immune system produces the thyroid stimulating hormone receptor antibody (TRAb), which is directed against the thyroid stimulating hormone receptor (TSHR). The TRAb can either stimulate or inhibit thyroid hormone secretion. GD occurs from formation of stimulating antibodies to the TSHR called the thyrotropin stimulating immunoglobulins (TSI). It is a functional assay which measures the production of cyclic adenosine monophosphate in cultured thyroid follicular cells. TSI binds to and also stimulates the TSHR on the thyroid follicular cells, leading to increased vascularity of the gland, follicular hypertrophy/ hyperplasia and increased production of the thyroid hormone. The thyroid gland displays lymphocytic infiltration with T-lymphocyte abnormalities and an absence of follicular destruction. T cells activate local inflammation and tissue remodeling by producing cytokines, leading to B-cell dysregulation and autoantibody formation. An imbalance between pathogenic and regulatory T cells is thought to be involved in both the development of GD and its severity [3].

Graves' ophthalmopathy, an immune mediated condition is caused by cross-reactivity of TSI with a TSHR like protein in retro-orbital tissue and extraocular muscle. This leads to local inflammation and infiltration of glycosaminoglycans resulting in edema, muscle swelling and increase in intraorbital pressure causing the characteristic eye findings [5, 7].

Transient hyperthyroidism may result from destruction of thyroid follicular cells by an autoimmune or infectious process, which leads to unregulated release of preformed hormone into the circulation. Subacute thyroiditis occurs from an infection or inflammation and usually resolves in a few months with normalization of thyroid functions. Hyperthyroidism is also seen in McCune-Albright syndrome (somatic-activating mutation of the GNAS gene). It results in increased stimulatory G protein signaling that causes hyperfunction of glycoprotein hormone receptors, autonomous cell proliferation and hormone hypersecretion. Thyrotropin stimulating hormone (TSH) secreting pituitary adenoma and pituitary resistance to thyroid hormone are caused by unregulated overproduction of TSH [6, 7].

## Etiology

The most common cause of hyperthyroidism in children is GD. Other causes include acute or sub-acute thyroiditis, T4 ingestion and thyrotoxic phase of chronic lymphocytic thyroiditis (Hashitoxicosis). Hyperthyroidism is also seen in autonomously functioning thyroid nodule, toxic adenoma, multinodular goiter, McCune Albright syndrome, struma ovarii and TSH producing pituitary adenomas [5, 7, 8]. Etiology is listed in Table **1**.

Table 1. Causes of Hyperthyroidism.

| Condition | Mechanism | Thyroid Exam | Antibody | RAIU |
|---|---|---|---|---|
| **Increased Secretion of Thyroid Hormone** | | | | |
| Graves' disease | Thyrotropin receptor-stimulating antibodies (TRAb) | Symmetric, non tender goiter | TSI+ Anti-thyroglobulin and thyroid peroxidase antibody +/- | Diffusely ↑ |
| Toxic multinodular goiter | Autonomous overproduction of thyroid hormone | Multiple nodules | Negative | ↑ multifocal uptake |
| Toxic adenoma | Autonomous overproduction of thyroid hormone | Single nodule | Negative | ↑ uptake in a single focus |
| TSH secreting pituitary adenoma | Autonomous production of TSH | Normal or symmetric goiter | Negative | ↑ |
| Pituitary resistance to thyroid hormone | Overproduction of TSH | Symmetric goiter | Negative | Diffusely ↑ |
| **Excess Secretion of Preformed Thyroid Hormone** | | | | |
| Chronic lymphocytic thyroiditis (Hashitoxicosis) | Autoimmune Release of preformed hormone | Firm goiter | Anti-thyroglobulin and thyroid peroxidase antibody + | ↓ |
| Subacute thyroiditis | Viral Release of preformed hormones | Painful goiter | Negative | ↓ |
| **Drug Induced Hyperthyroidism** | | | | |
| Factitious thyroiditis | Intake of thyroxine | No goiter | Negative, low TSH | ↓ |
| Iodine induced | Exposure to contrast agent | Often multinodular | Negative | ↑ |

TSH: Thyroid stimulating hormone; TSI: thyrotropin stimulating immunoglobulins; TRAb: thyroid stimulating hormone receptor antibody.

## CLINICAL PRESENTATION

The onset of symptoms is subtle and a high index of suspicion is needed in diagnosing children. Prompt treatment is important due to its unique effects on growth, pubertal development and neurodevelopmental outcomes in children.

GD can present insidiously with emotional lability, fatigue, sleep disturbances and increased appetite. School aged children are sometimes brought to medical attention for evaluation of attention deficit hyperactivity disorder because of their inability to concentrate and poor school performance. Prepubertal children most commonly present with poor weight gain and diarrhea, whereas adolescents present with irritability, fatigue, palpitations, heat intolerance, fine tremors and a goiter. Younger children typically have a delay in diagnosis and this leads to increased height, advanced bone age and poor weight. On physical examination, thyromegaly is present in 95% of the cases. The gland is symmetrically enlarged, smooth and non-tender. Other signs include tachycardia, fine tremors, warm skin, muscle weakness, increased pulse pressure and exaggerated deep tendon reflexes. Ophthalmic abnormalities such as staring eyes, proptosis, retraction of upper eye lid and wide palpebral fissure can occur in 40% of children and adolescents and is less severe than seen in adults. Pretibial myxedema and dermopathy are rare in children. Thyroid storm is also rare in children and is characterized by increased metabolism with excessive release of thyroid hormones leading to severe hyperthyroid symptoms [4, 5, 8, 9]. Signs and symptoms of GD are listed in Table **2**.

**Table 2. Signs and Symptoms of Graves' disease in children.**

| Signs | Symptoms |
|---|---|
| Smooth, symmetric, non- tender goiter | Hyperactivity |
| Tachycardia, rarely atrial fibrillation | Palpitations |
| Weight loss | Fatigue |
| Heat intolerance | Poor school performance, decreased attention span |
| Tremor | Emotional lability |
| Hypertension | Increased appetite |
| Hair loss | Increased frequency of bowel movements |
| Advanced bone age and height velocity | Excessive sweating |
| Eye findings- staring, lid lag, exophthalmos | Difficulty sleeping |
| Proximal muscle weakness and wasting | Amenorrhea or oligomenorrhea |

## DIAGNOSTIC EVALUATION

### Laboratory Evaluation

Laboratory evaluation includes serum thyroid stimulating hormone (TSH), free thyroxine (FT4), total triiodothyronine (TT3), TSI, thyroid peroxidase and anti-thyroglobulin antibody levels. Complete blood count and liver function tests are obtained at baseline.

Serum TSH level is suppressed and FT4 and TT3 values are elevated in hyperthyroidism. TSI is positive in 90% of the cases of GD. Thyroid peroxidase and thyroglobulin antibodies are positive in autoimmune thyroiditis and maybe positive in GD as well [9].

### Imaging Studies

#### *Thyroid Ultrasound*

It is performed if the thyroid gland is asymmetric or a palpable nodule is noted. If a nodule is confirmed, a fine needle aspiration biopsy should be performed as well as $^{123}$I or $^{99}$Tc scan. Differentiated thyroid cancer may be seen concurrently with GD or in an autonomous nodule.

#### *Thyroid Uptake Studies*

Thyroid uptake scan is performed in cases of unclear etiology of hyperthyroidism. The thyroid gland can actively concentrate iodine and radioactive iodine (RAI). $^{123}$I is the radionucleotide of choice for thyroid uptake since it has a short half-life and delivers a smaller radiation dose as compared with $^{131}$I. Radiolabelled technetium ($^{99}$Tc) can also be used since technetium is trapped by the thyroid gland but not organized. $^{99}$Tc scan is sometimes preferred because it is less expensive, quicker and involves less total body radiation.

The uptake scan shows increased uptake to 50 to 80% throughout the gland in GD. Conditions such as sub-acute thyroiditis or early phase of autoimmune thyroiditis are associated with decreased uptake as low as $\leq 2\%$ [8, 9].

## TREATMENT OPTIONS

Current treatment approaches for GD include antithyroid drugs (ATDs), surgery and radioactive iodine ablation ($^{131}$I). There is no specific cure for the disease and each treatment option is associated with complications. ATDs are the initial treatment options in GD. They palliate the hyperthyroid state until it sponta-neously resolves or definitive treatment is done. Refer to Fig. (**1**) and Table **3** for an overview on the management options.

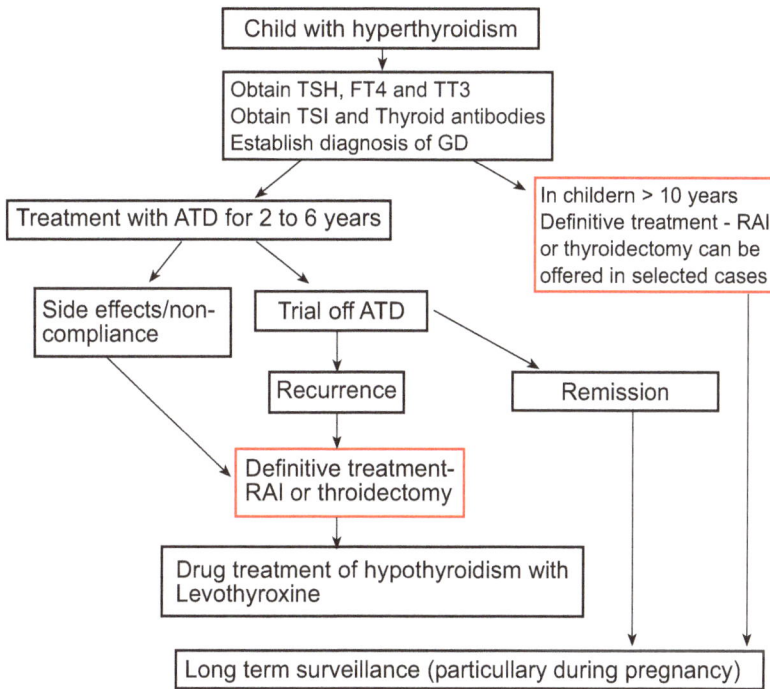

**Fig. (1).** Algorithm for diagnosis and management of Graves' disease in children.
TSH: Thyroid stimulating hormone; FT4: free thyroxine, TT3: Total triiodothyronine, TSI: thyrotropin stimulating immunoglobulins; GD: Graves' disease; ATD: anti-thyroid drugs; RAI: radioactive iodine ablation

**Table 3. Treatment options.**

|  | Indications | Contraindications | Advantages |
|---|---|---|---|
| **Antithyroid drugs** | First line of treatment in children<br>If greater chances of remission (mild disease, small goiter, low titers of TRAb) | Major adverse drug reaction | Non invasive<br>No hospital stay needed<br>Less initial cost<br>Low risk of permanent hypothyroidism<br>Possible remission |
| **Radioactive iodine** | >10 years of age<br>If child not in remission after 1 to 2 years of MMI<br>Major adverse drug reaction to ATD | Pregnancy<br>Breastfeeding<br>Coexisting thyroid cancer<br>Unable to follow radiation safety precautions | Definitive cure of hyperthyroidism<br>No surgical/ anesthesia risk<br>No effect on infertility, birth defects, cancer<br>Reduction in goiter size |

*(Table 3) contd.....*

|  | Indications | Contraindications | Advantages |
|---|---|---|---|
| **Surgery** | Large goiter (>80gm) Suspicion of thyroid malignancy If planning a pregnancy in 4 to 6 months | Coexisting conditions which increase the anesthesia and surgery risk | Rapid control of hyperthyroidism |

TRAb: thyroid stimulating hormone receptor antibody; MMI: methimazole; ATD: antithyroid drugs
Adapted from Management Guidelines of the American Thyroid Association and American Association of Clinical Endocrinologists (2011) [11].

## Antithyroid Drugs

ATDs are Thionamide derivatives which were introduced in early 1940s by Astwood. Thiouracil, the first compound used clinically was associated with toxic side effects and was replaced by Propylthiouracil (PTU) in 1947. Methimazole (MMI) has been the treatment option for GD since 1950. MMI is 10 to 20 times more potent than PTU and has a longer half- life. In 2008, a number of cases describing PTU- induced liver failure requiring transplant emerged. The risk was estimated to be 1 in 2000 children. In April 2010, the United States Food and Drug Administration issued a black box warning stating that PTU should not be used in children, except in special circumstances. PTU can sometimes be used short term with extreme caution in patients who have had a toxic reaction to MMI while waiting for definitive therapy. If started on PTU, patient and families should be informed of the risk of liver failure. If they note signs and symptoms of liver toxicity like itching, jaundice, abdominal pain, light colored stools, dark urine or anorexia, the medication should be stopped and medical attention should be sought promptly [10].

### Mechanism of Action

ATDs act by inhibiting oxidation and organic binding of thyroid iodine thus impairing thyroid hormone synthesis [8, 10].

### MMI and Monitoring Therapy

MMI is the drug of choice for GD. The typical dose is 0.2 to 0.5 mg/kg/day once a day or in divided doses. The dose can range from 0.1 to 1 mg/kg/day. It is available in 5, 10 and 20 mg tablets. The following doses can be used in guiding therapy. In infants: 1.25 mg/day; 1 to 5 years: 2.5 to 5 mg/day; 5 to 10 years: 5 to 10 mg/day and 10 to 18 years: 10 to 20 mg/day. The doses can be doubled in severe hyperthyroidism. Complete blood counts, liver function tests, pregnancy test (for girls in the reproductive age group), should be performed prior to starting therapy [11]. Thyroid function tests should be obtained 1 month after starting therapy. After FT4 levels normalize, the MMI dose is reduced by 50% to maintain a euthyroid state. TSH takes months to normalize and hence should not be used in guiding the change in dose.

Two approaches have been discussed. Some use the "block and replace" approach and add levothyroxine while not changing the MMI dose to achieve euthyroidism. With this approach, there is a greater risk of side effects since there is a dose response relationship for some MMI related complications. The other approach is the dose titration which involves adjusting the doses of the MMI to achieve euthyroidism. Compliance may also be an issue in some children, who may find it easier to take one drug rather than two drugs. The American Thyroid Association guidelines suggest using the dose titration method by using the lowest dose of MMI rather than the block and replace approach [3, 10 - 12].

### Adverse Drug Reaction

Minor side effects can occur in 17% of the children on MMI which includes rash, hives, arthralgia and nausea. Major side effects include Stevens- Johnson syndrome, agranulocytosis, neutropenia, thrombocytopenia, cholestatic jaundice, hepatitis and vasculitis. These typically occur in the first 6 months of starting therapy but can occur anytime during the course of therapy [13]. Agranulocytosis is dose dependent and typically develops in the first 100 days of therapy. Pediatric patients and their families should be informed of the side effects, the necessity of stopping the medications and informing their physician if they develop pruritic rash, jaundice, acolic stools or dark urine, arthralgias, abdominal pain, nausea, fatigue, fever or pharyngitis [11]. In the pediatric population, anti-neutrophilic cytoplasmic antibody (ANCA) - mediated disease has been described with PTU or MMI. These antibodies can cause serious vasculitis event, hence it is reasonable to check ANCAs on children who have been on ATDs for greater than 2 years. ATDs can cross the placenta and has an increased risk of birth defects. MMI embryopathy causes choanal atresia, esophageal atresia, growth retardation and developmental delay. PTU is the drug of choice during the first trimester of pregnancy because of the potential teratogenic effects of MMI [9].

### Remission

Remission of GD is defined as biochemical euthyroidism or hypothyroidism for one year or more after discontinuation of ATDs. The remission rates in children are reported to be 20 to 30% after many years of ATDs [14, 15]. A French study showed that prolonged ATDs were associated with 50% remission rates. 154 children with GD diagnosed between 1997 and 2002 were examined following treatment with carbimazole. The estimated remission rates were 20%, 37%, 45% and 49% after 4, 6, 8 and 10 years of therapy respectively [16]. The chance of remission after 2 years of ATDs is low if the thyroid gland is large (more than 2.5 times normal size for age), young child (<12 years), not Caucasian, serum TRAb levels are above normal on therapy and elevated FT4 at diagnosis (>4 ng/dl) [11, 15, 17, 18]. The 2011 American Thyroid Association (ATA) and American Association of Clinical Endocrinologist (AACE) management guidelines recommend continuing ATD in children for two years if there are no major side effects. If children develop serious allergic reaction to MMI, radioactive iodine or surgery should be considered [11].

## Beta Adrenergic Antagonists

Beta adrenergic antagonists are useful in the management of GD because it helps to decrease sympathetic symptoms like sweating, tremor, palpitations and anxiety. Propranolol, atenolol or metaprolol can be used to control GD symptoms. Atenolol is preferred for its cardioselective nature. When the thyroid hormone levels normalize, they can be stopped [8, 9].

## Radioactive Iodine

Radioactive iodine (RAI; $^{131}$I) use for thyroid ablation was introduced in 1940s by Saul Hertz and co-workers at the Massachusetts Institute of Technology and Massachusetts General Hospital. RAI uptake by the thyroid is not distinguishable from ordinary iodine, thus RAI is trapped in the thyroid cell. After being taken up by the thyroid cells, beta- emission causes destruction of the iodine trapping cells. It results in fibrosis and glandular atrophy. If $^{131}$I therapy is chosen, it should be administered as a single dose to render the patient hypothyroid [7, 11, 12]. It should not be used to cause euthyroidism in children as this leads to partially irradiated residual thyroid tissue which can be associated with a risk of thyroid cancer. Typically administered thyroid doses of 150μCi/gm generate radiation doses of 12,000 cGy to the thyroid. Larger doses (>150 μCi of $^{131}$I per gram of thyroid tissue) are preferred over smaller doses of radioactive iodine. Hypothyroidism is achieved in approximately 60 to 95% of patients with a dose of $^{131}$I 150 – 200 μCi per gram of thyroid tissue [11, 19, 20].

Dosages of radioiodine administered are based on iodine uptake and gland size using the Quimby-Marinelli equation: dosage (radiation; in Gy) = 90 × oral $^{131}$Idose (μCi) × oral 24-hr uptake (%) / gland mass (gm) × 100%). This calculation assumes an effective half life of 6 days for $^{131}$I. Thyroid size is estimated by palpation or ultrasound (ultrasound volume = 0.48 × length × depth × width) [10]. An advantage of calculated dose is that it may be possible to administer lower doses if the iodine uptake is high.

## Preparation

The ATDs are discontinued 3–5 days before [131]I is administered. The circulating levels of thyroid hormones may increase 4 to 10 days after the ablation when the thyroid hormones are released from degenerating follicular cells. Following the ablation, TSH and FT4 levels should be obtained every month. Biochemical euthyroidism or hypothyroidism is achieved in 6 to 12 weeks after [131]I treatment. Until then, the symptoms of hyperthyroidism can be controlled using beta adrenergic antagonists. MMI or Lugol's solution can be used one week after [131]I to decrease biochemical hyperthyroidism without affecting the outcome of RAI [8]. Children with FT4 >5ng/dl should be pretreated with MMI and beta adrenergic antagonists until FT4 normalizes before proceeding with [131]I therapy [11].

## Side Effects

Side effects of [131]I therapy include mild tenderness over the thyroid in the first week after ablation. This can be treated with acetaminophen or non-steroidal anti-inflammatory drugs for 24 to 48 hrs. There are rare reports of thyroid storm in children with severe hyperthyroidism receiving [131]I.

## RAI Precautions

RAI is excreted in saliva urine and stool. Significant radioactivity is retained within the thyroid for several days. Hence radiation precautions are recommended which include absence from school, not sharing utensils and not kissing or sitting next to pregnant women and babies for 1 week [11].

## Follow Up

If hyperthyroidism persists 6 months after [131]I, a second dose can be given. Patients with very large thyroid gland (>80 gm) and high TRAb levels have lower responses to [131]I therapy.

## Indications

[131]I is an effective therapy for GD and may be considered for children who are not in remission after 1 - 2 years of MMI therapy or in those who have major adverse side effects to the ATDs [19]. It can also be offered as the initial therapy in adolescents [19].

## Outcome

The benefits of RAI is the ease of administration, reduced need for long term follow up and absence of long term side effects [9, 21]. The most extensive study in children involved 36 year outcomes of 116 patients who were < 20 year old when treated with [131]I therapy for GD. There was no evidence of increased cancer risk in this population. There has been no evidence of adverse effects to offspring of children treated with [131]I, increase in rate of infertility, spontaneous abortion or congenital anomalies in offspring of patients treated with [131]I [22].

The risk of thyroid cancer after external radiation is highest in children < 5 years of age and decline with advancing age. The American Thyroid Association recommends to avoid RAI in children <5 years of age and limit the dose to 10 mCi in children who are 5 to 10 years of age [11]. [131]I therapy in patients older than 10 years of age is acceptable if the activity is > 150 µCi/g of thyroid tissue. The need for [131]I in a young child may occur when the child develops a toxic reaction to an ATD, proper surgical expertise is not accessible, or the child is not a suitable surgical candidate.

## Surgery

The oldest form of definitive GD therapy is thyroidectomy. The Nobel Prize in Physiology and Medicine was awarded to Koker in 1909 for development in this field. When surgery is chosen as therapy, near total or total-thyroidectomy is recommended and should be performed by a high volume thyroid surgeon. Surgery leads to hypothyroidism in children who undergo total thyroidectomy, whereas after subtotal thyroidectomy, hyperthyroidism recurs in 10-15% of the patients.

### *Indications*

Surgery is preferred in children < 5 years when definitive therapy is needed, in individuals with large thyroid glands (>80 gm) where the response to [131]I is poor and in a late adolescent who is considering pregnancy. It should be performed by an experienced and high volume thyroid surgeon [11, 23].

### *Preparation for Surgery*

The patient should be rendered euthyroid with ATDs or inorganic iodine. Iodine drops (5 to 10 drops three times a day) are given 7 to 10 days prior to surgery. This stops the thyroid hormone production and causes the gland to become firm and less vascular, facilitating surgery.

### *Complications*

Postoperatively, children are at a high risk for acute complications such as hypocalcemia, hemorrhage and recurrent laryngeal nerve paresis. In children, rates from 0–6 years were 22%, from 7–12 years, 11%; and from 13 to 17 years,

11% [24, 25]. Long term complications include hypoparathyroidism and recurrent laryngeal nerve injury.

## *Follow Up*

Follow up is essential for all patients treated for GD. It should include regular examination of the thyroid gland and thyroid function tests once to twice a year.

## OTHER CAUSES OF HYPERTHYROIDISM AND MANAGEMENT

**Chronic Lymphocytic Thyroiditis**- 5 to 10% of children present with a thyrotoxic phase called Hashitoxicosis. The hyperthyroidism is due to inflammation and autonomous release of preformed and stored thyroid hormones. It typically lasts for a few months. The hyperthyroidism is mild and transient. The thyroid peroxidase and anti-thyroglobulin antibodies are positive and TSI is negative. RAI uptake is low or absent. Symptomatic treatment with beta adrenergic antagonists is recommended in children with palpitations, tremors, tachycardia and hypertension.

**Sub-acute Thyroiditis**- It is also known as De Quervain's disease and is due to a viral infection of the thyroid. The inflammation results in autonomous release of preformed and stored hormones which leads to hyperthyroidism. Fever, thyroid tenderness and hyperthyroidism may last for several weeks. The erythrocyte sedimentation rate is elevated. The TSH is suppressed and the FT4 and TT3 are high. Thyroid antibodies are negative and RAI uptake is low or absent. Non-steroidal anti-inflammatory drugs and beta adrenergic antagonists are used for symptomatic treatment. This disease is self-limited, running its course over a period of 2 to 5 months.

**Acute Thyroiditis-** It is characterized by fever, sore throat, painful thyroid swelling and erythema of the overlying skin. Surgical incision and drainage with appropriate antibiotics are required.

**Toxic Adenoma or Solitary Thyroid Nodule-** These are uncommon and are suspected in the setting of hyperthyroidism and presence of a thyroid nodule. Warm or hot nodules can lead to excessive production of thyroid hormone. Activating mutations of TSHR and stimulatory G protein have been described in hyperfunctioning nodules. Thyroid antibodies are negative. RAI uptake will show uptake only in the functioning nodule. The treatment is ATDs but ultimately surgical excision is required.

**Toxic Multinodular Goiter-** These are also uncommon cause of hyperthyroidism in children. They are suspected in the setting of hyperthyroidism and multiple nodules. Thyroid antibodies are negative and RAI shows uptake in multiple nodules. It can be treated with ATDs and eventually thyroidectomy or [131]I should be considered.

**TSH-secreting Pituitary Adenoma**- Hypersecretion of TSH from a pituitary adenoma is a rare cause of hyperthyroidism in children. Laboratory evaluation shows an elevated FT4 and TT3 with inappropriately normal or slightly elevated TSH with a high serum TSH alpha subunit concentration. This diagnosis is confirmed on magnetic resonance imaging and treatment is resection of the pituitary tumor.

**Iodine-induced Hyperthyroidism**- Contrast agents can induce thyrotoxicosis.

**Radiation Induced Hyperthyroidism-** Childhood cancer survivors can have thyrotoxicosis associated with radiation.

**Resistance to Thyroid Hormone-** It is an autosomal dominant disorder due to mutation in the thyroid hormone beta receptor gene (TRβ). Children present with a goiter, elevated FT4 and normal to slightly elevated TSH. Children with generalized resistance to thyroid hormone are usually euthyroid, while those with pituitary resistance can have thyrotoxic clinical features. Most patients with generalized resistance require no treatment.

**Mutation in the TSH Receptor Gene-** It is an autosomal disorder caused by mutations in the thyrotropin receptor gene on the long arm of chromosome 14. It is also called non autoimmune hereditary hyperthyroidism. FT4 and TT3 are increased with a suppressed TSH. The TSI is negative. Diffuse goiter is present with a negative maternal history of thyroid disease. Treatment is with ATD's.

**McCune- Albright Syndrome-** It is a sporadic disease characterized by the triad of polyostotic fibrous dysplasia, cutaneous pigmentation (Café- au-lait macule) and precocious puberty. It is caused by an activating mutation of the alpha subunit of the stimulatory G protein. Diffuse enlargement of the thyroid occurs early which then evolves into a multinodular goiter. The TSH is suppressed with increased RAI uptake. Surgical excision is indicated.

**Factitious Thyrotoxicosis-** can be seen in adolescents who ingest thyroxine to lose weight. RAI uptake will be low or absent.

**Thyroid Storm-** It is an endocrine emergency and is a life-threatening condition. It is characterized by multisystem organ failure and clinical features including nausea, vomiting, diarrhea, tachycardia, hepatic dysfunction, hyperthermia, hypotension, arrhythmias and congestive heart failure. Neuropsychiatric manifestations are agitation, delirium, psychosis, stupor and coma. Factors that precipitate thyroid storm include acute cessation of ATDs, surgery in inadequately treated hyperthyroidism and acute illnesses. The recommendations for treatment are monitoring in intensive care unit, treatment with beta adrenergic antagonists, ATDs, inorganic iodine and glucocorticoids [11].

**Neonatal Thyrotoxicosis-** Neonatal GD is due to transplacental passage of maternal TSI antibodies. The incidence is estimated to be 1 in 25,000 neonates. It occurs in infants of mothers with active GD or in those previously treated with RAI or surgery due to persistant TSI. It is most likely if maternal TSI exceeds 500%. Clinical features include tachycardia, irritability, hyperactivity, restlessness, diarrhea and poor weight gain. Severe neonatal thyrotoxicosis can be complicated by congestive heart failure. Management includes use of inorganic iodine which inhibits organification of iodine and thyroid hormone release, ATDs and beta adrenergic antagonists. Neonatal GD resolves 3 to 12 weeks after birth [3, 4, 7, 8].

## CONCLUSIONS

GD is the most common cause of hyperthyroidism in children. ATDs are the first line of treatment, although ultimately definitive treatment is needed. Selecting a treatment approach for childhood GD can be challenging. It is important to discuss the risks and benefits of each therapeutic option to help the patient and family select a treatment plan.

For children less than 5 years of age, MMI should be considered as the first-line therapy. Young children are less likely to have remission on drug treatment and prolonged drug therapy may be necessary. If there are no adverse side effects with MMI, it is reasonable to continue MMI until the child is old enough for $^{131}$I. If adverse drug reaction occurs, or there is the desire to avoid prolonged drug use, thyroidectomy or $^{131}$I can be considered. 15% of children with GD present between 6 years and 10 years of age. MMI is the first line drug therapy for this age group. Children who are 10 years of age and older constitute 80% of GD. For this age group, either MMI therapy can be considered if prognostic factors suggest likelihood of remission or radioactive iodine can be considered as an initial therapy if the chances of remission appear poor [8, 11, 19, 23].

## CONFLICT OF INTEREST

The author declares no conflict of interest, financial or otherwise.

## ACKNOWLEDGMENTS

Declared none.

## REFERENCES

[1]      Abraham-Nordling M, Byström K, Törring O, *et al.* Incidence of hyperthyroidism in Sweden. Eur J Endocrinol 2011; 165(6): 899-905.
[http://dx.doi.org/10.1530/EJE-11-0548]

[2]      Williamson S, Greene SA. Incidence of thyrotoxicosis in childhood: a national population based study in the UK and Ireland. Clin Endocrinol (Oxf) 2010; 72(3): 358-63.
[http://dx.doi.org/10.1111/j.1365-2265.2009.03717.x]

[3]      Léger J, Kaguelidou F, Alberti C, Carel JC. Graves' disease in children. Best Pract Res Clin Endocrinol Metab 2014; 28(2): 233-43.
[http://dx.doi.org/10.1016/j.beem.2013.08.008]

[4]      Zimmerman D, Lteif AN. Thyrotoxicosis in children. Endocrinol Metab Clin North Am 1998; 27(1): 109-26.
[http://dx.doi.org/10.1016/S0889-8529(05)70302-9]

[5]      Cooper DS. Hyperthyroidism. Lancet 2003; 362(9382): 459-68.
[http://dx.doi.org/10.1016/S0140-6736(03)14073-1]

[6]      Brent GA. Clinical practice. Graves' disease. N Engl J Med 2008; 358(24): 2594-605.
[http://dx.doi.org/10.1056/NEJMcp0801880]

[7]      Srinivasan S, Misra M. Hyperthyroidism in children. Pediatr Rev 2015; 36(6): 239-48.
[http://dx.doi.org/10.1542/pir.36-6-239]

[8]      Rivkees SA. Thyroid Disorders in Children and Adolescents. In: Ma S, Ed. Pediatric Endocrinology. Philadelphia: Elsevier 2014; pp. 444-70.

[9]      Bansal S, Umpaichitra V, Desai N. Perez- Colon S. Pediatric graves' disease. Int J Endocrinol 2015; 1(1)
[http://dx.doi.org/10.16966/ ijemd.104]

[10]     Rivkees SA. Pediatric Graves' disease: management in the post-propylthiouracil Era. Int J Pediatr Endocrinol 2014; 2014(1): 10.
[http://dx.doi.org/10.1186/1687-9856-2014-10]

[11]     Bahn RS, Burch HB, Cooper DS, *et al.* American Thyroid Association. American Association of Clinical Endocrinologists. Hyperthyroidism and other causes of thyrotoxicosis: management guidelines of the American Thyroid Association and American Association of Clinical Endocrinologists. Endocr Pract 2011; 17(3): 456-520.
[http://dx.doi.org/10.4158/EP.17.3.456]

[12]     Hegedüs L. Treatment of Graves' hyperthyroidism: evidence-based and emerging modalities. Endocrinol Metab Clin North Am 2009 Jun; 38(2): 355-71, ix.
[http://dx.doi.org/10.1016/j.ecl.2009.01.009]

[13]     Kaguelidou F, Carel JC, Léger J. Graves' disease in childhood: advances in management with antithyroid drug therapy. Horm Res 2009; 71(6): 310-7.
[http://dx.doi.org/10.1159/000223414]

[14]     Glaser NS, Styne DM. Predicting the likelihood of remission in children with Graves' disease: a prospective, multicenter study. Pediatrics 2008; 121(3): e481-8.
[http://dx.doi.org/10.1542/peds.2007-1535]

[15]     Kaguelidou F1. Alberti C, Castanet M, Guitteny MA, Czernichow P, Léger J; French Childhood Graves' Disease Study Group. Predictors of autoimmune hyperthyroidism relapse in children after

discontinuation of antithyroid drug treatment. J Clin Endocrinol Metab 2008; 93(10): 3817-26.
[http://dx.doi.org/10.1210/jc.2008-0842]

[16]     Léger J, Gelwane G, Kaguelidou F, Benmerad M, Alberti C. French Childhood Graves' Disease Study Group. Positive impact of long-term antithyroid drug treatment on the outcome of children with Graves' disease: national long-term cohort study. J Clin Endocrinol Metab 2012; 97(1): 110-9.
[http://dx.doi.org/10.1210/jc.2011-1944]

[17]     Vitti P, Rago T, Chiovato L, *et al.* Clinical features of patients with Graves' disease undergoing remission after antithyroid drug treatment. Thyroid 1997; 7(3): 369-75.
[http://dx.doi.org/10.1089/thy.1997.7.369]

[18]     Bauer AJ. Approach to the pediatric patient with Graves' disease: when is definitive therapy warranted? J Clin Endocrinol Metab 2011; 96(3): 580-8.
[http://dx.doi.org/10.1210/jc.2010-0898]

[19]     Rivkees SA, Sklar C, Freemark M. Clinical review 99: The management of Graves' disease in children, with special emphasis on radioiodine treatment. J Clin Endocrinol Metab 1998; 83(11): 3767-76.

[20]     Lee HS, Hwang JS. The treatment of Graves' disease in children and adolescents. Ann Pediatr Endocrinol Metab 2014; 19(3): 122-6.
[http://dx.doi.org/10.6065/apem.2014.19.3.122]

[21]     Okawa ER, Grant FD, Smith JR. Pediatric Graves' disease: decisions regarding therapy. Curr Opin Pediatr 2015; 27(4): 442-7.
[http://dx.doi.org/10.1097/MOP.0000000000000241]

[22]     Read CH Jr, Tansey MJ, Menda Y. A 36-year retrospective analysis of the efficacy and safety of radioactive iodine in treating young Graves' patients. J Clin Endocrinol Metab 2004; 89(9): 4229-33.
[http://dx.doi.org/10.1210/jc.2003-031223]

[23]     Rivkees SA. Pediatric Graves' disease: controversies in management. Horm Res Paediatr 2010; 74(5): 305-11.
[http://dx.doi.org/10.1159/000320028]

[24]     Sosa JA, Tuggle CT, Wang TS, *et al.* Clinical and economic outcomes of thyroid and parathyroid surgery in children. J Clin Endocrinol Metab 2008; 93(8): 3058-65.
[http://dx.doi.org/10.1210/jc.2008-0660]

[25]     Burch HB, Burman KD, Cooper DS. 2011 survey of clinical practice patterns in the management of Graves' disease. J Clin Endocrinol Metab 2012; 97(12): 4549-58.
[http://dx.doi.org/10.1210/jc.2012-2802]

# CHAPTER 11

# Recent Advances in Pediatric Asthma

Amine   Daher,   Tanya   M.   Martínez   Fernández   and   Yadira   M.
Rivera-Sánchez*

*University of Texas Southwestern (UTSW) Medical Center, Dallas Children's Health, Dallas, Texas, USA*

**Abstract:** In the past decade, there have been great advances in the approach to and management of pediatric asthma. Recent progress includes improved definitions, established guidelines, and novel therapeutic modalities. There is growing recognition that asthma is a heterogeneous entity and as such, individualized therapy is now standard when creating intervention plans. Asthma severity is classically categorized based on the concepts of impairment and risk. As more specific data is gathered on asthma subgroups, molecular pathways and cluster analysis, there has been a movement for categorizing patients into asthma phenotypes, which could serve to tailor therapies and optimize clinical response. This chapter will review the pathophysiologic processes involved in asthma; expose the latest definitions of asthma and management guidelines; discuss the implications of the "phenotypic" approach in pediatric asthma and present an overview of pertinent recent therapeutic advances.

**Keywords:** Asthma guidelines, Asthma pathophysiology, Asthma phenotypes, Inhaled corticosteroids, Macrolides, Mepolizumab, Omalizumab, Pediatric asthma, Type 2 Hi asthma, Type 2 Lo asthma, Vitamin D.

## INTRODUCTION

Asthma is the most common chronic disease in children and affects over 6 million children in the US [1]. It has been increasingly recognized as a heterogeneous disorder in terms of its phenotypic presentation, pathophysiology and response to therapy. Asthma patients experience recurrent symptoms of airflow obstruction due to airway inflammation, bronchial hyper-responsiveness and in some cases progressive permanent changes [1]. The essence of asthma therapy is control of symptoms and inflammation coupled with treatment of bronchospasms and exacerbations while giving proper consideration to potential contribution from comorbidities. We will briefly review common established therapies as well as

* **Corresponding author Yadira M. Rivera-Sánchez**: University of Texas Southwestern (UTSW) Medical Center, Dallas Children's Health, Dallas, Texas, USA; Tel: (214) 456-4630/(214) 456-5406; Email: Yadira.Rivera-Sanchez@utsouthwestern.edu

**Seckin Ulualp (Ed.)**

novel and developing therapies in the care of pediatric patients with asthma.

## DEFINITION OF ASTHMA AND CURRENT STANDARD OF CARE

Asthma is a global health concern with prevalence estimated at 1-18% of the world's population. The Global Initiative For Asthma (GINA) established in 2002, defines asthma as a heterogeneous disease, usually characterized by chronic airway inflammation in which patients have a history of wheezing, shortness of breath, chest tightness and cough that vary over time and in intensity, together with variable expiratory airflow limitation [2]. A definition for severe asthma was recently developed by both the European Respiratory Society and the American Thoracic Society [3]. It includes patients greater than six years of age who require at least high dose inhaled corticosteroids (ICS) augmented by a second controller to achieve adequate control [3].

Current guidelines offer a standardized approach to asthma therapy. The overall strategy includes assessment of severity and control of symptoms as well as contributing co-morbidities such as obesity, gastroesophageal reflux, psychiatric disorders and rhinosinusitis. Long-term therapeutic goals focus on use of controller medications, relievers and add-on therapies in order to achieve good symptom control as well as a reduction in exacerbations, lung function limitation and side effects of treatment. We refer the reader to a published standardized stepwise approach for the use of inhaled corticosteroids, short acting beta agonists, long acting beta agonists and leukotriene antagonists in the management of asthma [1]. More novel and developing therapies are discussed in later sections of this chapter.

## ASTHMA PATHOPHYSIOLOGY

Asthma symptoms stem from airflow limitation due to bronchoconstriction, airway hyper-responsiveness and edema. These, in the setting of chronic inflammation, can progressively lead to airway remodeling. In this section, we will define those processes as well as discuss the various chemical and cellular participants in the pathophysiology of asthma.

Acute bronchoconstriction is the rapid narrowing of airways resulting from airway smooth muscle constriction. Airway hyper-responsiveness is the unbalanced bronchoconstriction response of airways to various stimuli. Airway edema participates in airflow obstruction through mucosal swelling, increased mucus secretions and plug formation. In some asthma patients, permanent histologic changes such as smooth muscle and mucus glands hyperplasia as well as angiogenesis can occur. These histologic changes are collectively referred to as airway remodeling and account for the lack of complete reversibility often seen in chronic asthma [1, 4].

Neonates have a predominant Th2 phenotype. With time, various exposures tend to shift the immune system towards the Th1 system. In children with asthma, there is an imbalance between the Th1 and Th2 immune pathways manifested by high prevalence of atopic conditions. The hygiene hypothesis proposes for example, that among other exposures, having older siblings and or attending day care can lead to beneficial effects by decreasing the risk of developing atopic diseases. This decrease in atopy is the direct result of infectious exposures balancing in turn the Th1 and Th2 components of the immune system [4].

Inhalation of allergens leads to an inflammatory cascade in asthma patients that is, in most cases, eosinophilic and IgE mediated. Allergens cross-link IgE bound to mucosal mast cells and trigger the release of preformed histamines and leukotrienes. This is known as the "early phase reaction" leading to acute bronchoconstriction [4]. The inflammation seen in asthma requires the interaction of many cell lines, each with characteristic contributions. Upon activation, mucosal mast cells release pre-formed histamines and other mediators leading to bronchoconstriction. Airway eosinophils also release several pro-inflammatory cytokines. In atopic asthma patients, the degree of eosinophilia often correlates with the severity of asthma and decreases with the use of steroid therapy. Some patients with asthma have a predominance of airway neutrophils. Neutrophils contribution to inflammation in asthma is not well understood. Data suggests, however, that in asthma patients, the presence of neutrophils as the predominant cell line correlates with steroid resistance [1, 4].

In addition, asthma inflammation strongly depends on the interplay of a multitude of signaling molecules such as IgE, cytokines and leukotrienes. These molecules are the target of many research and established therapies. IgE is an allergen specific antibody essential to the allergic inflammation of asthma. It binds mast cells as well as other inflammatory cells and promotes bronchoconstriction as well as the release of other inflammatory cytokines [1]. Key Th2 cytokines include: IL-5 promotes bone marrow proliferation of eosinophils and survival in the periphery; IL-4 and IL-13 promote a Th2 response and IgE production [1]. Leukotrienes are released upon activation of mast cells and lead to bronchoconstriction [1].

In summary, in asthma there is an imbalance between the Th1 (protective) and Th2 (allergic) immune systems. The inflammatory cascade is the product of the interaction of many Th2 cell lines and signaling molecules. Clinical symptoms of asthma result from airflow limitation due to acute bronchoconstriction in the early phase followed by inflammation, increased mucus secretion and airway hyper-responsiveness. In some patients, airway remodeling with permanent histologic changes and decreased lung function ensues.

## A PHENOTYPIC APPROACH TO ASTHMA

Categorizing asthma patients into various phenotypes follows from our expanding understanding of asthma pathophysiologic processes. A number of phenotypes have now been proposed based on criteria including these processes as well as various patient related clinical characteristics and differential response to therapies. In this section, we will review literature that supports a "phenotypic approach" to asthma management.

In 2001, Roorda *et al* attempted to determine a sub-population of preschool children with asthma symptoms that would have the best response to inhaled corticosteroids. In this study, the authors pooled the populations of two previous studies comparing fluticasone to placebo in 305 preschool children and evaluated the relationship between response to ICS treatment and various patient characteristics. They found that among asthmatic preschool children, those with frequent symptoms and a family history of asthma were most likely to respond to treatment with ICS [5]. The authors also went on to suggest that the variable response to ICS based on family history of asthma suggests that more than a single pathophysiologic process is involved. In 2009, a post hoc subgroup analysis of the Prevention of Early Asthma in Kids (PEAK) study; a multicenter, placebo-controlled trial of inhaled fluticasone *versus* placebo in preschool children, also found that preschool children with asthma symptoms do not uniformly respond to ICS. The authors evaluated the relationship between atopic and demographic characteristics of 285 preschool children with a positive asthma predictive index and positive response to ICS. In the study population, best response to ICS was found in Caucasian male subjects who had frequent symptoms, were sensitized to aeroallergens and had an emergency department visit or hospitalization in the past year [6]. A post hoc analysis of 163 children included in the Best Add-on Therapy Giving Effective Response (BADGER) trial looking into the relationship between treatment response and patient characteristics found that response to step up therapies was differential with respect to eczema and race [7]. The authors noted that step up therapy to long acting beta agonists (LABA) was best in children without eczema, regardless of race. In those with eczema, race seemed to predict response to step up therapy. Their findings suggested that African Americans benefitted most from high dose ICS, Hispanics from leukotrienes antagonists (LTRA), whereas Caucasians had an equal response to addition of either LABA or LTRA [7].

Severe pediatric asthma may be defined by high impairment and frequent exacerbations despite high dose ICS in those with a high prevalence of atopy. The strong association to atopy differentiates pediatric from adult severe asthma. From a histological standpoint, it may be inferred that severe pediatric asthma is a phenotype in and of itself, which may be associated to airway remodeling as well as altered antioxidant and inflammation regulation resulting in a primarily steroid responsive disease. It is important to note, however, that within the severe pediatric asthma phenotype, there is variation to steroid responsiveness [8]. Statistical cluster analyses of pediatric patients included in the Severe Asthma Research Program study identified four phenotypic clusters of pediatric patients with asthma based on lung function, duration of asthma symptoms and controller use. Patients with severe pediatric asthma were present in all four clusters further supporting the notion that pediatric severe asthma is a heterogeneous disorder [8].

Cluster analysis of large clinical trials has been a powerful tool assisting researchers in the identification of asthma phenotypes. Howrylak *et al* described five clinical clusters when analyzing the 1041 children included in the Childhood Asthma Management Program. The clusters were based on 3 characteristics: atopy, airway obstruction and burden of exacerbations. Cluster grouping was reflective of disease severity and was predictive of time to first systemic steroids course. Perhaps the most important finding was that patients remained within their clusters over time and that ICS use did not alter which cluster subjects were classified into. The latter finding suggests that while ICS use improves symptoms, they may not have a significant effect on disease progression [9].

In addition to clinical and inflammatory phenotyping, asthma patients can be characterized by molecular phenotyping. As identification of new biomarkers and therapeutic targets arise, phenotypic classification based on cytokine activity such as Type 2 Hi and Type 2 Lo may have practical applications. Type 2 Hi asthma is associated to a prevalent TH2 eosinophilic and inflammatory cytokine response and has been noted to exhibit a good response to steroids treatment. Type 2 Lo asthma, on the other hand, is associated to a more prominent neutrophilic (or non-eosinophilic) inflammation, obesity related asthma and compared to Type 2 Hi phenotype, a reduced responsiveness to treatment with steroids [10].

**Intermittent Inhaled Corticosteroids**

The use of daily inhaled corticosteroids (ICS) is the current gold standard maintenance therapy for persistent asthma. However, there are two pediatric populations for which the benefits of daily ICS remain to be conclusively established: 1- children with intermittent wheezing and symptom -free intervals; and 2- preschool aged children with viral-induced wheezing. The practical allure of limiting ICS administration to an "as needed" basis, as well as concerns over the adverse effects of potentially unnecessary steroids exposure in children led to several studies looking into intermittent ICS use in pediatric patients with wheezing.

As early as two decades ago, clinical trials of intermittent ICS use in patients with episodes of wheezing suggested potential improvement in symptoms but were not conclusive. In 2006, the PEAK trial showed an increase in symptom-free days with daily administration of ICS compared to placebo in preschool age children at high risk for asthma [11]. However, a small decrease in height gain in the treatment group was noted. Furthermore, subsequent analyses showed that response to daily ICS was not uniform within the study population of toddlers at high risk for asthma. Those findings reiterated the need to identify, among toddlers with wheezing, a sub-population that could benefit from intermittent ICS.

In 2009, Ducharme *et al* compared the efficacy of high dose fluticasone (750 µg twice daily for up to 10 days *vs.* placebo) in reducing oral corticosteroid (OCS) use when administered early in viral illnesses. They studied 129 children aged 1 to 6 years presenting with recurrent viral-induced wheezing. This study did show a decrease in OCS need but raised concerns of decreased weight and height gain in the treatment group [12]. Despite promising results, the authors did not recommend this regimen of intermittent high dose fluticasone with viral-induced wheezing before a better understanding of potential adverse effects. Subsequently, Zeiger *et al* compared daily low-dose (0.5 mg nightly) and intermittent high-dose (1 mg twice daily for 7 days) nebulized budesonide in 278 patients aged 12 to 53 months. They found that, in the select population of young children with frequent wheezing and at least one exacerbation requiring oral steroids in the past year, yet with low impairment and few severe exacerbations (less than 7 courses of oral steroids and 2 admissions in the previous year), daily nebulized budesonide was not superior to intermittent high dose with regards to frequency of exacerbations [13]. Furthermore, they found that the cumulative exposure to budesonide was less in the intermittent group. An interesting remark by the authors and based on the findings of the study is that intermittent ICS should be initiated at the beginning of symptoms that previously preceded wheezing in each child rather than systematically at the start of an upper respiratory illness [13].

Finally, a Cochrane review meta-analysis published in 2015 comparing intermittent ICS with placebo in the management of persistent asthma found that in children, intermittent ICS seems to lead to a decreased use of oral steroids. However, the overall evidence was not strong [14].

## Omalizumab: The First "Biologic" Used Commercially for the Treatment of Asthma

Omalizumab is a humanized murine monoclonal IgG antibody specific for the mast and basophil binding sites on human IgE. Omalizumab's immediate effect is to dramatically decrease circulating levels of free IgE. The first benefit of its use in the management of asthma comes from this substantial reduction in available free IgE which when present, directly interferes with the allergic inflammatory cascade described earlier in this chapter. In addition, as a consequence of decreased circulating free IgE; mast cells, basophils and dendritic cells down regulate their IgE specific cell surface receptors, further dampening the allergic inflammatory cascade upon exposure to allergens [15].

Humbert *et al* demonstrated that patients with persistent severe allergic asthma which was poorly controlled despite high-dose ICS and a LABA had a significant decrease in both asthma exacerbations and emergency department visits with the addition of Omalizumab to their regimen [16]. Of relevance for the pediatric practitioner, is to note, that the population in this study consisted of patients with uncontrolled persistent severe allergic asthma whose age ranged from 12 to 75 years and had serum IgE levels which ranged from 30 to 700 IU/mL. The safety and efficacy of Omalizumab in pediatric patients age 6 to 12 years was later demonstrated by Lanier *et al* in 2009. In their study, they chose a population of pediatric patients who despite optimal available therapy had poorly controlled persistent severe allergic asthma and whose serum IgE levels ranged from 30 to 1300 IU/mL (mean 469.7 IU/mL). They concluded that Omalizumab was both safe and beneficial in this population [17].

Since then, many studies in both the United States and other countries have corroborated the safety and efficacy of Omalizumab in the pediatric population of severe allergic asthma patients who are $\geq 6$ years of age [18, 19]. A recent systematic review of placebo controlled studies of Omalizumab in children confirms the benefits and acceptable safety profile of Omalizumab as add-on therapy for moderate to severe allergic pediatric asthma [20].

As the use of Omalizumab in the severe allergic pediatric asthma population becomes increasingly widespread, there is upcoming research into its potential use in non-atopic asthma through its effect on local inflammation [15]. If and how this will play a role in the management of the pediatric patients with non-atopic asthma, is not yet clear. The substantial cost of treatment may also impede expanding its use until further research demonstrates clear benefits outside the scope of allergic asthma.

## Mepolizumab

As previously described, IL-5 plays a major role in the eosinophilic inflammatory cascade seen in asthma. It is necessary for production, maturation and survival of eosinophils. As such, IL-5 has been the target of many recent asthma therapies. Mepolizumab is a humanized monoclonal antibody with high affinity to IL-5 that inhibits its binding to the IL-5 receptor on the surface of eosinophils. Initial clinical trials of Mepolizumab in asthmatics failed to show significant clinical benefit despite a clear decrease in blood and sputum eosinophils [21]. Therefore, further clinical research was developed to evaluate if specific asthma populations would be likely to benefit from Mepolizumab.

Nair *et al* compared Mepolizumab with placebo in adults with persistent sputum eosinophilia despite high dose ICS and oral steroids. They found that in this population, Mepolizumab helped decrease steroid use without clinical deterioration [22]. The authors concluded that in order to further study the potential benefits of Mepolizumab it is paramount to focus on asthma patients with significant airway eosinophilia: a conclusion well in line with Mepolizumab's mechanism of action. In the same year, a larger study of adults with refractory eosinophilic asthma showed that Mepolizumab led to significantly fewer severe exacerbations compared to placebo despite no improvement in day to day symptoms [23]. These studies shaped the path for Mepolizumab to be used as a steroid sparing agent and as preventative treatment for severe asthma exacerbations in patients with airway eosinophilia.

Two large clinical trials were published defining the benefits of Mepolizumab add on therapy in severe asthma. In the MENSA clinical trial, Ortega et al demonstrated that, use of either intravenous or subcutaneous formulations of Mepolizumab resulted in a reduction of asthma exacerbations in a group of 576 severe eosinophilic asthma patients over 12 years of age. In addition, improvement in quality of life and questionnaire defined asthma control were noted when compared with placebo [24]. The SIRIUS clinical trial by Bel et al found that addition of Mepolizumab therapy to a group of 135 patients over 16 years of age with severe steroids dependent eosinophilic asthma led to successful decrease in systemic steroids doses compared to placebo [25]. In addition, a recent Cochrane review published in 2015 concluded that although there is evidence favoring the use of Mepolizumab in reducing exacerbations of severe eosinophilic asthmatics, further research is necessary to more discretely identify the populations most likely to benefit from it [26].

In summary, the availability of Mepolizumab further expands the arsenal of treatment options available for severe asthma., Although there is growing evidence that Mepolizumab therapy decreases frequency of severe exacerbations and steroids requirements in severe eosinophilic asthmatics, there is no clear benefit on daily symptoms. Further research is needed to shed light on a number of yet unanswered questions regarding this newly FDA approved therapy. These include the identification of biomarkers that may best predict response to therapy, optimal dose and formulation for different ages and subgroups, appropriate end

points to be used for therapy as well as effective and safe age range in pediatric patients [27].

## The Developing Role of Vitamin D Deficiency and Supplementation in Pediatric Asthma

In the past decade, a number of studies aimed to define the relationship between vitamin D deficiency and asthma. There is increasing evidence that Vitamin D has a role in the adaptive and innate immune response, which may result in modulation of both asthma severity and the response to respiratory infections. Increased maternal vitamin D intake during pregnancy has been shown to offer some degree of protection against the development of wheezing in infants. Epidemiologic studies suggest that lower vitamin D levels are present in pediatric patients with asthma. In addition, there is evidence that the response to steroids in steroid-resistant asthmatic patients may be enhanced by vitamin D.

Vitamin D receptors are found on a number of cells involved in the immune response [28]. These receptors form part of the steroid hormone nuclear receptor family and may thus potentiate the response to glucocorticosteroid therapy [29]. Vitamin D appears to act on T regulatory lymphocytes involved in cytokine regulation [29 - 31] including the promotion of IL-10, an anti-inflammatory cytokine. The exact role of vitamin D in asthma pathophysiology, however, is complex and remains unclear.

Brehm *et al* published a landmark study of 616 children with asthma in Costa Rica in which they found that Vitamin D levels considered insufficient or deficient were prevalent (3.4% and 24.6%, respectively) among children with asthma. Furthermore, lower levels were associated with elevated IgE and eosinophils as well as an increased frequency of hospitalizations [32]. The following year, they again published an association between lower vitamin levels and the frequency of severe asthma exacerbations in 1024 mild to moderate asthmatic children enrolled in the long standing multicenter Childhood Asthma Management Program study [33]. They did not, however, find in this larger and more ethnically diverse cohort, the previously described association of low vitamin D levels with markers of atopy. Published evidence also suggests lower vitamin D levels in children with severe therapy resistant asthma. In this group, lower levels were associated with reduced asthma control and increased airway smooth muscle mass suggesting a potential relationship with airway remodeling [34].

It remains unclear which patients would benefit from vitamin D supplementation, how much to supplement and whether timing of supplements (*i.e.* treatment in younger patients) may lead to specific long term benefits in asthma control. A recent meta-analysis found that there is low quality evidence confirming a reduction of asthma exacerbations in children treated with vitamin D [35]. However, there is lack of consensus as to the vitamin D level required for optimal immune function. Experts consider levels of 25-hydroxy vitamin D, the major circulating form of vitamin D, below 30 ng/mL as insufficient making this a reasonable target goal for supplementation [36].

## Macrolides as Anti-Inflammatory and the Differential Response to Azithromycin

Macrolides have both antimicrobial and anti-inflammatory effects, which have made them treatment options for several chronic inflammatory respiratory illnesses. There is evidence for the benefit of azithromycin therapy as a long-term adjunct to therapy in cystic fibrosis and bronchiectasis. However, the potential benefit in asthma therapy is not clear [37].

Limited animal and human data suggests that there may be some benefit in macrolide therapy in asthma. In a murine model of chronic asthma, azithromycin reduced smooth airway remodeling, likely through a neutrophil-related anti-inflammatory effect [38]. A randomized placebo controlled trial of 109 patients with severe asthma looked at the effects of azithromycin as an adjunct to standard therapy [39]. Although the study did not find benefit in the use of azithromycin add-on therapy for the study population as a whole, a reduction in exacerbations and respiratory infections was noted in a subgroup analysis of patients treated with azithromycin who had non-eosinophilic severe asthma. These results further support a phenotypic approach to asthma therapy [39]. Macrolides with no antimicrobial effects are being studied as anti-inflammatory adjuncts, but this research is still in its early phases [40].

## CONCLUSION

In summary, asthma is a heterogeneous disease. It is the most common chronic disease in children. Clinical symptoms of asthma result from airflow limitation due to acute bronchoconstriction in the early phase followed by inflammation, increased mucus secretion and airway hyper-responsiveness. In some patients, the result is airway remodeling with permanent histologic changes and decreased lung function. New insights into the variable phenotypes of this disease have led to a more targeted approach to the diagnosis and management of asthma. A new generation of therapeutics is emerging with biological agents such as omalizumab being incorporated as part of the standard of care in pediatric asthma. However, further research is still required as we explore newer biological agents and utilize baseline phenotypic characteristics to guide their use.

## CONFLICT OF INTEREST

The authors declares no conflict of interest, financial or otherwise.

## ACKNOWLEDGEMENTS

Declared none.

## REFERENCES

[1]   National Asthma Education and Prevention Program. Expert Panel Report 3 (EPR-3): Guidelines for the Diagnosis and Management of Asthma-Summary Report 2007. J Allergy Clin Immunol 2007; 120(5) (Suppl.): S94-S138.
      [http://dx.doi.org/10.1016/j.jaci.2007.09.029] [PMID: 17983880]

[2]   Global Initiative for Asthma. Global Strategy for Asthma Management and Prevention 2015.

[3]   Chung KF, Wenzel SE, Brozek JL, *et al.* International ERS/ATS guidelines on definition, evaluation and treatment of severe asthma. Eur Respir J 2014; 43(2): 343-73.
      [http://dx.doi.org/10.1183/09031936.00202013] [PMID: 24337046]

[4]   Busse WW, Lemanske RF Jr. Asthma. N Engl J Med 2001; 344(5): 350-62.
      [http://dx.doi.org/10.1056/NEJM200102013440507] [PMID: 11172168]

[5]   Roorda RJ, Mezei G, Bisgaard H, Maden C. Response of preschool children with asthma symptoms to fluticasone propionate. J Allergy Clin Immunol 2001; 108(4): 540-6.
      [http://dx.doi.org/10.1067/mai.2001.118789] [PMID: 11590379]

[6]   Bacharier LB, Guilber TW, Zeiger RS, *et al.* Patient characteristics associated with improved outcomes with use of an inhaled corticosteroid in preschool children at risk for asthma. J Allergy Clin Immunol 2009; 123(5): 1077-82. 1082 e1-5

[7]   Malka J, Mauger DT, Covar R, *et al.* Eczema and race as combined determinants for differential response to step-up asthma therapy. J Allergy Clin Immunol 2014; 134(2): 483-5.
      [http://dx.doi.org/10.1016/j.jaci.2014.03.039] [PMID: 24835502]

[8]   Fitzpatrick AM, Baena-Cagnani CE, Bacharier LB. Severe asthma in childhood: recent advances in phenotyping and pathogenesis. Curr Opin Allergy Clin Immunol 2012; 12(2): 193-201.
      [http://dx.doi.org/10.1097/ACI.0b013e32835090ac] [PMID: 22249197]

[9]   Howrylak JA, Fuhlbrigge AL, Strunk RC, *et al.* Classification of childhood asthma phenotypes and long-term clinical responses to inhaled anti-inflammatory medications. J Allergy Clin Immunol 2014; 133(5): 1289-300. 1300 e1-12

[10]  Gauthier M, Ray A, Wenzel SE. Evolving Concepts of Asthma. Am J Respir Crit Care Med 2015; 192(6): 660-8.
      [http://dx.doi.org/10.1164/rccm.201504-0763PP] [PMID: 26161792]

[11]  Horner CC, Bacharier LB. Management approaches to intermittent wheezing in young children. Curr Opin Allergy Clin Immunol 2007; 7(2): 180-4.

[http://dx.doi.org/10.1097/ACI.0b013e32807fafd2] [PMID: 17351473]

[12]   Ducharme FM, Lemire C, Noya FJ, *et al.* Preemptive use of high-dose fluticasone for virus-induced wheezing in young children. N Engl J Med 2009; 360(4): 339-53.
[http://dx.doi.org/10.1056/NEJMoa0808907] [PMID: 19164187]

[13]   Zeiger RS, Mauger D, Bacharier LB, *et al.* CARE Network of the National Heart, Lung, and Blood Institute. Daily or intermittent budesonide in preschool children with recurrent wheezing. N Engl J Med 2011; 365(21): 1990-2001.
[http://dx.doi.org/10.1056/NEJMoa1104647] [PMID: 22111718]

[14]   Chong J, Haran C, Chauhan BF, Asher I. Intermittent inhaled corticosteroid therapy versus placebo for persistent asthma in children and adults. Cochrane Database Syst Rev 2015; 7(7): CD011032.
[PMID: 26197430]

[15]   Domingo C. Omalizumab for severe asthma: efficacy beyond the atopic patient? Drugs 2014; 74(5): 521-33.
[http://dx.doi.org/10.1007/s40265-014-0203-y] [PMID: 24691707]

[16]   Humbert M, Beasley R, Ayres J, *et al.* Benefits of omalizumab as add-on therapy in patients with severe persistent asthma who are inadequately controlled despite best available therapy (GINA 2002 step 4 treatment): INNOVATE. Allergy 2005; 60(3): 309-16.
[http://dx.doi.org/10.1111/j.1398-9995.2004.00772.x] [PMID: 15679715]

[17]   Lanier B, Bridges T, Kulus M, Taylor AF, Berhane I, Vidaurre CF. Omalizumab for the treatment of exacerbations in children with inadequately controlled allergic (IgE-mediated) asthma. J Allergy Clin Immunol 2009; 124(6): 1210-6.
[http://dx.doi.org/10.1016/j.jaci.2009.09.021] [PMID: 19910033]

[18]   Odajima H, Ebisawa M, Nagakura T, *et al.* Omalizumab in Japanese children with severe allergic asthma uncontrolled with standard therapy. Allergol Int 2015; 64(4): 364-70.
[http://dx.doi.org/10.1016/j.alit.2015.05.006] [PMID: 26433533]

[19]   Deschildre A, Marguet C, Salleron J, *et al.* Add-on omalizumab in children with severe allergic asthma: a 1-year real life survey. Eur Respir J 2013; 42(5): 1224-33.
[http://dx.doi.org/10.1183/09031936.00149812] [PMID: 23520319]

[20]   Rodrigo GJ, Neffen H. Systematic review on the use of omalizumab for the treatment of asthmatic children and adolescents. Pediatr Allergy Immunol 2015; 26(6): 551-6.
[http://dx.doi.org/10.1111/pai.12405] [PMID: 25963882]

[21]   Menzella F, Lusuardi M, Galeone C, Taddei S, Zucchi L. Profile of anti-IL-5 mAb mepolizumab in the treatment of severe refractory asthma and hypereosinophilic diseases. J Asthma Allergy 2015; 8: 105-14.
[http://dx.doi.org/10.2147/JAA.S40244] [PMID: 26504401]

[22]   Nair P, Pizzichini MM, Kjarsgaard M, *et al.* Mepolizumab for prednisone-dependent asthma with sputum eosinophilia. N Engl J Med 2009; 360(10): 985-93.
[http://dx.doi.org/10.1056/NEJMoa0805435] [PMID: 19264687]

[23]   Haldar P, Brightling CE, Hargadon B, *et al.* Mepolizumab and exacerbations of refractory eosinophilic asthma. N Engl J Med 2009; 360(10): 973-84.
[http://dx.doi.org/10.1056/NEJMoa0808991] [PMID: 19264686]

[24]   Ortega HG, Liu MC, Pavord ID, *et al.* MENSA Investigators. Mepolizumab treatment in patients with severe eosinophilic asthma. N Engl J Med 2014; 371(13): 1198-207.
[http://dx.doi.org/10.1056/NEJMoa1403290] [PMID: 25199059]

[25]   Bel EH, Wenzel SE, Thompson PJ, *et al.* SIRIUS Investigators. Oral glucocorticoid-sparing effect of mepolizumab in eosinophilic asthma. N Engl J Med 2014; 371(13): 1189-97.
[http://dx.doi.org/10.1056/NEJMoa1403291] [PMID: 25199060]

[26]   Powell C, Milan SJ, Dwan K, Bax L, Walters N. Mepolizumab versus placebo for asthma. Cochrane

Database Syst Rev 2015; 7(7): CD010834.
[PMID: 26214266]

[27]   Patterson MF, Borish L, Kennedy JL. The past, present, and future of monoclonal antibodies to IL-5 and eosinophilic asthma: a review. J Asthma Allergy 2015; 8: 125-34.
[PMID: 26604804]

[28]   Provvedini DM, Tsoukas CD, Deftos LJ, Manolagas SC. 1,25-dihydroxyvitamin D3 receptors in human leukocytes. Science 1983; 221(4616): 1181-3.
[http://dx.doi.org/10.1126/science.6310748] [PMID: 6310748]

[29]   Xystrakis E, Kusumakar S, Boswell S, *et al.* Reversing the defective induction of IL-10-secreting regulatory T cells in glucocorticoid-resistant asthma patients. J Clin Invest 2006; 116(1): 146-55.
[http://dx.doi.org/10.1172/JCI21759] [PMID: 16341266]

[30]   Gregori S, Casorati M, Amuchastegui S, Smiroldo S, Davalli AM, Adorini L. Regulatory T cells induced by 1 alpha,25-dihydroxyvitamin D3 and mycophenolate mofetil treatment mediate transplantation tolerance. J Immunol 2001; 167(4): 1945-53.
[http://dx.doi.org/10.4049/jimmunol.167.4.1945] [PMID: 11489974]

[31]   Gregori S, Giarratana N, Smiroldo S, Uskokovic M, Adorini L. A 1alpha,25-dihydroxyvitamin D(3) analog enhances regulatory T-cells and arrests autoimmune diabetes in NOD mice. Diabetes 2002; 51(5): 1367-74.
[http://dx.doi.org/10.2337/diabetes.51.5.1367] [PMID: 11978632]

[32]   Brehm JM, Celedón JC, Soto-Quiros ME, *et al.* Serum vitamin D levels and markers of severity of childhood asthma in Costa Rica. Am J Respir Crit Care Med 2009; 179(9): 765-71.
[http://dx.doi.org/10.1164/rccm.200808-1361OC] [PMID: 19179486]

[33]   Brehm JM, Schuemann B, Fuhlbrigge AL, *et al.* Serum vitamin D levels and severe asthma exacerbations in the Childhood Asthma Management Program study. J Allergy Clin Immunol 2010; 126(1): 52-8 e5.

[34]   Gupta A, Sjoukes A, Richards D, *et al.* Relationship between serum vitamin D, disease severity, and airway remodeling in children with asthma. Am J Respir Crit Care Med 2011; 184(12): 1342-9.
[http://dx.doi.org/10.1164/rccm.201107-1239OC] [PMID: 21908411]

[35]   Riverin BD, Maguire JL, Li P, Vitamin D. Vitamin D Supplementation for Childhood Asthma: A Systematic Review and Meta-Analysis. PLoS One 2015; 10(8): e0136841.
[http://dx.doi.org/10.1371/journal.pone.0136841] [PMID: 26322509]

[36]   Rance K. The emerging role of Vitamin D in asthma management. J Am Assoc Nurse Pract 2014; 26(5): 263-7.
[PMID: 24170480]

[37]   Crosbie PA, Woodhead MA. Long-term macrolide therapy in chronic inflammatory airway diseases. Eur Respir J 2009; 33(1): 171-81.
[http://dx.doi.org/10.1183/09031936.00042208] [PMID: 19118228]

[38]   Kang JY, Jo MR, Kang HH, *et al.* Long-term azithromycin ameliorates not only airway inflammation but also remodeling in a murine model of chronic asthma. Pulm Pharmacol Ther 2016; 36: 37-45.
[http://dx.doi.org/10.1016/j.pupt.2015.12.002] [PMID: 26778828]

[39]   Brusselle GG, Vanderstichele C, Jordens P, *et al.* Azithromycin for prevention of exacerbations in severe asthma (AZISAST): a multicentre randomised double-blind placebo-controlled trial. Thorax 2013; 68(4): 322-9.
[http://dx.doi.org/10.1136/thoraxjnl-2012-202698] [PMID: 23291349]

[40]   Cameron EJ, McSharry C, Chaudhuri R, Farrow S, Thomson NC. Long-term macrolide treatment of chronic inflammatory airway diseases: risks, benefits and future developments. Clin Exp Allergy 2012; 42(9): 1302-12.
[http://dx.doi.org/10.1111/j.1365-2222.2012.03979.x] [PMID: 22925316]

# CHAPTER 12

# Evaluation and Treatment of Bronchiolitis

## Derek L. Pepiak[*]

*Department of Pediatrics, Ochsner for Children and The University of Queensland School of Medicine, Ochsner Clinical School, New Orleans, Louisiana, USA*

**Abstract:** Bronchiolitis is the most common cause of hospitalization in infants and children less than 2 years of age. Patients typically present with signs of an upper respiratory tract infection that then progress to symptoms consistent with a lower respiratory tract infection. The key to diagnosis is the history and physical examination; labs and chest radiography are not routinely necessary or recommended. Treatment is largely supportive as many of the therapies that are effective in other respiratory diseases are ineffective in the treatment of bronchiolitis. Emphasis should therefore be on prevention and reducing transmission of the disease. Areas of focus for the prevention of bronchiolitis include administration of palivizumab prophylaxis in selected infants and children, hand hygiene, elimination of tobacco smoke exposure, encouragement of breastfeeding, and family education.

**Keywords:** Breastfeeding, Bronchiolitis, Bronchodilators, Children, Corticosteroids, Hand hygiene, Hypertonic saline, Infants, Oxygen, Palivizumab, RSV, Respiratory distress, Respiratory syncytial virus, Smoking.

## INTRODUCTION

Bronchiolitis is a clinically diagnosed condition in patients less than 2 years of age that usually begins with symptoms of an upper respiratory tract infection. Initial presentation with coryza and low-grade fever is common. Typically this progresses to a lower respiratory tract infection manifesting as cough, tachypnea, retractions, nasal flaring, wheezes, and/or crackles. The pathogenesis of bronchiolitis includes acute inflammation, edema, sloughing and necrosis of epithelial cells of the small bronchi and bronchioles, increased mucus production, bronchospasm, obstruction of small airways, and atelectasis [1]. Multiple viruses have been isolated as the cause of bronchiolitis. Respiratory syncytial virus (RSV) is by far the most common cause of bronchiolitis, accounting for 50%-80% of cases [2]. Ninety percent of children are infected with RSV within the first 2 years

---

[*] **Corresponding author Derek L. Pepiak**: Department of Pediatrics, Ochsner for Children and The University of Queensland School of Medicine, Ochsner Clinical School, New Orleans, Louisiana, USA; Tel: 504-390-0245; Email: dpepia@lsuhsc.edu

of life [3]. The highest incidence of RSV bronchiolitis occurs in North America between December and April [4]. Other viral etiologies of bronchiolitis include rhinovirus, parainfluenza virus type 3, human metapneumovirus, influenza, adenovirus, coronavirus, and enterovirus [5]. In North America, bronchiolitis is the most common cause of hospitalization in infants less than 12 months of age, accounting for approximately 100,000 admissions per year at an estimated cost of $1.73 billion [6 - 8].

## CLINICAL FEATURES

### Clinical Presentation and Course

During the first few days of illness, most infants present with a 1- to 3-day history of mild upper respiratory tract infection symptoms such as conjunctivitis, otitis media, nasal congestion, rhinitis, pharyngitis, and fever [9]. Decreased oral intake may also be present. Up to 40% of patients then progress to a lower respiratory tract infection with tachypnea, retractions, wheezing, and/or crackles on days 2-3 of illness [10]. Symptoms usually peak on days 5-7 and then gradually resolve. The mean duration of illness is 15 days with resolution of symptoms within 3-4 weeks [11, 12].

### Criteria for Admission

No clear criteria exist for determining which infants should be admitted to the hospital. Generally, hospitalization is considered for infants who present with lethargy, dehydration, apnea, or moderate to severe respiratory distress, manifested as nasal flaring, retractions, or a respiratory rate greater than 60-70 breaths per minute [13, 14]. Risk factors for more severe disease presentation requiring admission include prematurity, age less than 12 weeks, chronic lung disease, congenital and anatomical defects of the airway, congenital heart disease, immunodeficiency, and neuromuscular disorders [5]. The average length of stay in the hospital is 3-4 days [15, 16].

### Short-term Complications

While bronchiolitis has a high degree of morbidity, it is associated with a low degree of mortality. Mortality rates are estimated to be around 1% [17 - 19]. However, mortality rates can increase to 3.5% in patients with bronchiolitis when additional cardiac or chronic lung conditions are present [20]. The risk of apnea is increased in infants with RSV bronchiolitis, with rates ranging from 1.2% to as high as 23.8% [21, 22]. The risk for intubation in bronchiolitis, either secondary to disease progression or due to apnea, is approximately 5% [18]. Acute otitis media may be present in 50%-60% of patients with bronchiolitis [23, 24].

Secondary bacterial infection, with the exception of acute otitis media, is uncommon in infants with bronchiolitis [25]. Children with bronchiolitis have been reported to have inappropriate secretion of antidiuretic hormone, and close monitoring of fluid status is recommended [26, 27].

## Long-term Complications

Most infants with bronchiolitis recover with no long-term sequelae. However, long-term complications may include development of bronchiolitis obliterans, allergic sensitization, and recurrent wheezing [28]. Some studies have shown an association between bronchiolitis in infancy and subsequent development of atopic illnesses such as asthma later in life [29]. However, the connection between bronchiolitis and asthma is controversial as other studies have not supported a relationship between the two [30, 31].

## EVALUATION AND DIAGNOSIS

The diagnosis of bronchiolitis is essentially a clinical one. The typical history has been discussed earlier. Physical examination findings can vary between patients and can also fluctuate over time in the same patient; serial assessment of an infant with bronchiolitis is often necessary to monitor the progression and resolution of the disease. Patients often present with excessive nasal secretions leading to upper airway obstruction, manifesting as transmitted inspiratory and expiratory wheezing. Nasal obstruction from secretions may limit the ability of the infant to take adequate nutrition, ultimately leading to dehydration. Work of breathing is usually increased as shown by nasal flaring, intercostal retractions, subcostal retractions, and use of accessory muscles. Auscultation of the chest often reveals diffuse bilateral crackles and wheezes, as well as a prolonged expiratory phase of respiration. Hyperinflation of the lungs from air trapping may allow the liver and spleen to be palpable in the abdomen on examination.

The main goal for the history and physical examination is to determine which infants who present with wheezing and other respiratory symptoms likely have viral bronchiolitis versus another disorder [32]. In addition to bronchiolitis, the differential diagnosis of infants less than 2 years of age who present with wheezing and/or other lower respiratory tract symptoms includes adenoidal hypertrophy, retropharyngeal abscess, croup, asthma, recurrent viral-induced wheezing, bacterial pneumonia, cystic fibrosis, malacia of the airways, foreign body aspiration, aspiration pneumonia, congenital heart disease, congestive heart failure, and vascular rings [33, 34].

In 2014, the American Academy of Pediatrics (AAP) updated their guidelines for diagnosis, management, and prevention of bronchiolitis [32]. The guidelines advise clinicians to diagnose bronchiolitis and assess disease severity on the basis of history and physical examination alone. Numerous scoring systems have been developed to attempt to classify respiratory distress and disease severity. No system has been routinely adopted due to lack of predictive validity [35].

Once a clinician has diagnosed bronchiolitis based on history and physical examination, chest radiographs and laboratory studies should not be routinely obtained. A review of the current evidence did not support the use of chest radiographs in children with bronchiolitis as they do not correlate with disease severity [32]. Chest imaging in bronchiolitis often reveals hyperinflation with flattened diaphragms, airway wall thickening, peribronchial infiltrates, and patchy atelectasis. It is can be difficult to distinguish bronchiolitis-related atelectasis from consolidation, resulting in increased use of antibiotics and increased length of stay [36]. The current AAP guidelines advise clinicians to limit chest radiography to patients who may need admission to the intensive care unit or who present with signs and symptoms of other airway compromise or complication such as the presence or development of a pneumothorax [32].

Sensitive polymerase chain reaction assays are now readily available for a variety of viral agents. Some studies have shown that identification of the causative viral agent during emergency room evaluation or in hospitalized patients can decrease the use of antibiotic therapy and assist in the utilization of antiinfluenza therapy [37 - 42]. However, the current AAP guidelines recommend routine virologic testing only in infants hospitalized for bronchiolitis who have been receiving monthly prophylaxis with palivizumab. In this case, testing should be performed to see if RSV is the etiologic agent. If testing for RSV is positive, it is recommended that monthly palivizumab prophylaxis be discontinued based on the very low likelihood of a second RSV infection in the same year [32].

## TREATMENT

Both the AAP and the Scottish Intercollegiate Guidelines Network (SIGN) have issued comprehensive evidence based guidelines for the diagnosis, treatment, and prevention of bronchiolitis [13, 32]. The SIGN guidelines were last updated in 2006; the AAP guidelines were updated in 2014. The hallmark of treatment for bronchiolitis remains supportive care. Many infants with only mild symptoms can be treated at home. Infants with more severe disease, approximately 2%-3% of infants, are often hospitalized. A variety of treatment modalities for bronchiolitis have been proposed and attempted over the years. The following sections discuss the most recent recommendations based on the available evidence.

## Nutrition and Hydration

Approximately 30% of infants admitted for bronchiolitis will require fluid replacement therapy [43]. Infants with feeding difficulty secondary to respiratory distress may receive replacement *via* intravenous access or a nasogastric tube; there is no clear evidence that one route is advantageous over the other. Infants may be at risk for fluid retention secondary to increased production of antidiuretic hormone in bronchiolitis [26, 27, 44]. If hypotonic fluids are used for fluid replacement or maintenance needs, infants may be at risk for hyponatremia; therefore isotonic fluids may be safer. In infants with milder symptoms who are able to breastfeed, breastfeeding should be encouraged as breast milk has been shown to have neutralizing activity against RSV and contains RSV immunoglobulins A and G and interferon-α [45, 46].

## Albuterol

Bronchodilators have often been used in the management of bronchiolitis. The 2006 AAP guidelines recommended a trial of albuterol for patients with bronchiolitis. However, as of the 2014 update, the AAP now advises against the use of albuterol in infants and children with bronchiolitis. Bronchodilators may improve clinical symptom scores but have not been shown to affect disease resolution, need for hospitalization, or length of stay. The adverse effects, such as tachycardia and tremors, as well as the cost of the medication, outweigh the potential benefits. In most reviewed studies, children with severe disease and respiratory failure were excluded in analyzing the effect of bronchodilators and as such the recommendation against the use of albuterol may not apply to these patients [32].

## Epinephrine

Another bronchodilator, nebulized epinephrine, is commonly used in the treatment of bronchiolitis. In two studies comparing nebulized epinephrine to placebo or albuterol in hospitalized patients, there was no improvement in length of stay or other inpatient outcomes [47, 48]. Therefore, the AAP guidelines do not recommend the use of epinephrine in the hospital setting. The Canadian Bronchiolitis Epinephrine Steroid Trial involved 800 patients with bronchiolitis seen in the emergency department and compared hospitalization rates over a 7-day period. Patients received one of the following: nebulized epinephrine plus oral dexamethasone, nebulized epinephrine plus oral placebo, nebulized placebo plus oral dexamethasone, or nebulized placebo plus oral placebo. Patients who received nebulized epinephrine and oral dexamethasone had a lower likelihood of admission by day 7 compared to those who received the double placebo; however, this effect was not statistically significant after adjusting for multiple comparisons

[49]. The current evidence therefore does not support the use of nebulized epinephrine in the outpatient setting, although further studies are needed [32].

## Mucolytics

Given the role of mucus plugging in bronchiolitis, treatments aimed at thinning the airway secretions have been attempted in bronchiolitis. Hypertonic saline is one such intervention. Evidence suggests that nebulized hypertonic saline improves mucociliary clearance in both normal and diseased lungs by causing osmotic movement of water into the airways, thinning airway mucus [50 - 52]. Current evidence indicates that the use of nebulized 3% saline is effective in improving symptoms of mild and moderate bronchiolitis after 24 hours of use. It has also been shown to reduce hospital length of stay when the duration of stay exceeds 3 days. It does not appear to be effective in reducing hospitalizations when used in the emergency department. The AAP does not recommend the use of nebulized hypertonic saline in the emergency department but gives a weak recommendation for its use in infants and children admitted for bronchiolitis [32].

## Nasal Suctioning

Nasal suctioning is a common therapy in bronchiolitis given the copious thick secretions and the impact of nasal obstruction on feeding. There is little evidence to support frequent deep suctioning with a nasopharyngeal catheter. Deep suctioning *via* a catheter can be traumatic, produce edema, and result in further nasal obstruction [32]. Mechanical aspiration *via* nasal bulb suction or nasal aspirator, often in combination with saline nose drops, is commonly used.

## Corticosteroids

Corticosteroids can significantly improve symptoms in respiratory diseases such as asthma and croup. However, evidence shows that steroid use in patients with bronchiolitis does not significantly reduce admissions or reduce length of stay for inpatients [53]. As previously discussed, the Canadian Epinephrine Steroid Trial showed a reduction in hospitalization, but this reduction in length of stay did not reach statistical significance once adjusted for multiple comparisons. Further studies are needed before a recommendation for routine use of dexamethasone and nebulized epinephrine can be provided. Corticosteroid therapy may also prolong viral shedding in patients with bronchiolitis [54]. As of their most recent update, the AAP advises clinicians not to administer systemic corticosteroids to infants with bronchiolitis. There is currently no evidence to recommend the use of inhaled steroids for the treatment of acute bronchiolitis.

## Supplemental Oxygen and Continuous Pulse Oximetry

The need for supplemental oxygen based on pulse oximetry is one of the major determinants in the hospitalization of infant with bronchiolitis; unfortunately, the accuracy of pulse oximetry, especially in the range of 76%-90%, is poor [55]. Transient desaturations can be a normal finding in healthy infants. Oxygen saturation is often a primary measure that determines length of stay in bronchiolitis [56, 57]. Twenty-five percent of patients have an unnecessarily prolonged hospitalization due to the perceived need for oxygen supplementation [58]. The AAP guidelines state that clinicians may choose not to use supplemental oxygen for saturations exceeding 90% and may choose not to use continuous pulse oximetry. For patients requiring supplemental oxygen, delivery *via* heated, humidified, high-flow nasal cannula (HFNC) is becoming more widespread. However, the absence of trials evaluating the efficacy of HFNC precluded any specific recommendation from the AAP in the 2014 guidelines. Continuous positive airway pressure (CPAP) can be used as a means to avoid intubation in infants with respiratory failure. Systematic reviews of CPAP use in bronchiolitis have been inconclusive, and there are no specific recommendations on its use. Heliox therapy has been used in the treatment of asthma exacerbations and has also been attempted in bronchiolitis; currently there is not enough evidence to support its use in infants with bronchiolitis.

## Chest Physiotherapy

While chest physiotherapy can be a useful tool to aid in the clearance of secretions in a variety of pulmonary and neuromuscular disorders, current literature has shown no benefit of its use in patients hospitalized for bronchiolitis, and thus, the AAP does not recommend it. However, in patients admitted for bronchiolitis who also have comorbidities that impair clearance of secretions, chest physiotherapy may be warranted [59].

## Leukotriene Modifiers

Leukotrienes have been thought to play a role in airway inflammation in bronchiolitis, and the use of leukotriene modifiers has been studied in this condition. A 2015 meta-analysis found no effect on duration of hospitalization or clinical status in children with bronchiolitis [60]. There is currently insufficient evidence to recommend leukotriene modifiers in the treatment of bronchiolitis.

## Antibiotics and Antivirals

Given the young age at which patients present with bronchiolitis, antibiotics are often prescribed due to concern for undetected bacterial infection. Febrile infants without a known source for their fever may have a risk of bacteremia as high as 7%; patients with a distinct viral syndrome such as bronchiolitis have a less than 1% risk of bacterial infection of the cerebrospinal fluid or blood [61]. In addition, it is unusual for infants with bronchiolitis to have a bacterial pneumonia [62]. Current AAP guidelines advise that clinicians should not administer antibacterial medications to infants and children with a diagnosis of bronchiolitis unless there is a concomitant bacterial infection or a strong suspicion of one [32].

Ribavirin is an antiviral medication licensed for use for RSV bronchiolitis. Its use may decrease the number of days of hospitalization and mechanical ventilation, but it did not reduce the progression of respiratory disease or mortality [63]. Ribavirin is not recommended for routine use in children with bronchiolitis.

## PREVENTION

Multiple strategies exist to reduce the risk and severity of bronchiolitis. These include administration of palivizumab prophylaxis to appropriate infants and children, proper hand hygiene, elimination of tobacco smoke exposure, encouragement of breastfeeding of infants, and family education.

### Palivizumab

Palivizumab is a humanized monoclonal antibody against the RSV F glycoprotein. It has been shown to decrease the risk of hospitalization due to severe RSV infection in certain infants at increased risk of RSV bronchiolitis. Due to the high cost of the medication, the AAP guidelines for administration have become increasingly restrictive. Palivizumab is not recommended for otherwise healthy infants born after 29 weeks' gestational age. It is recommended during the first year of life in infants with hemodynamically significant heart disease or chronic lung disease of prematurity, defined as preterm infants born at less than 32 weeks' gestational age who require greater than 21% oxygen for at least the first 28 days of life. Palivizumab is given at a dose of 15 mg/kg once per month for a maximum of 5 doses during RSV season to infants who qualify during their first year of life. Palivizumab is only given in the second year of life to children who meet the criteria of chronic lung disease of infancy who continue to require supplemental oxygen, diuretic therapy, or chronic corticosteroid therapy within 6 months of the onset of the second RSV season. Prophylactic palivizumab is not routinely recommended for patients with Down syndrome, cystic fibrosis, neuromuscular disease, pulmonary abnormalities, or immune compromise. There are exceptions when a patient with one of these conditions may be considered for prophylaxis. These exceptions include patients with Down syndrome who qualify based on cardiac disease or prematurity during the first year of life; patients with cystic fibrosis with clinical evidence of lung disease during the first year of life;

infants in their first year of life with neuromuscular disease or a congenital anomaly that impacts their efforts to clear secretions due to ineffective cough; and patients undergoing hematopoietic stem cell transplant during RSV season who are severely immunosuppressed [32, 64, 65]. If a patient who is receiving monthly prophylaxis for RSV is hospitalized for RSV bronchiolitis, monthly prophylaxis should be discontinued for the remainder of the season.

## Hand Hygiene

No other intervention can do more to prevent the spread of RSV than thorough and consistent hand hygiene. RSV can remain infectious on countertops for greater than 6 hours, on gowns or paper tissues for 20-30 minutes, and on skin for up to 20 minutes [66]. It is recommended that all people disinfect their hands before and after direct contact with a patient, after contact with inanimate objects in the direct vicinity of the patient, and after removing gloves. Alcohol-based rubs should be used for hand decontamination; if alcohol-based rubs are not available or hands are visibly dirty, individuals should use soap and water to wash their hands [32].

## Tobacco Smoke Exposure

Exposure to tobacco smoke increases the risk and severity of bronchiolitis. Clinicians should inquire about the exposure of infants and children to tobacco smoke when assessing them for bronchiolitis [32]. Parents should be fully educated about the importance of not allowing smoking in the home. Smoke lingers on clothes and in the environment for prolonged periods of time [67]. As such, it should be made clear to the family that smoking outdoors poses risks to infants and children as well.

## Breastfeeding

Respiratory infections have been shown to be significantly less common in infants who are breastfed for at least 6 months. There is an overall 72% reduction in the risk of hospitalization due to respiratory disease in infants exclusively breastfed for 4 or more months compared to those who were formula fed [68]. In addition, evidence has shown that the duration of exclusive breastfeeding was inversely proportional to the length of oxygen use and the length of hospitalization in previously healthy infants with acute bronchiolitis [69]. As such, clinicians should encourage exclusive breastfeeding for at least 6 months to decrease the morbidity of respiratory infections [32].

## Family Education

The AAP's final recommendation on the prevention of bronchiolitis deals with family education and advises clinicians and nurses to educate personnel and family members on evidence-based diagnosis, treatment, and prevention of bronchiolitis. Families should be made aware that their child may continue to have symptoms for 2-3 weeks and that this is the normal course of bronchiolitis. Children with RSV continue to shed virus for 1-2 weeks, and family members should be educated about prevention of disease transmission [32].

## CONCLUSION

Bronchiolitis, especially secondary to RSV, continues to remain one of the most common respiratory infections in infants worldwide. The associated healthcare cost in the United States alone is more than $1.5 billion per year. Despite a number of therapies that are beneficial in the treatment of other respiratory illnesses, supportive care continues to be the mainstay of treatment for bronchiolitis. The key to reducing the associated costs, hospitalizations, morbidity, and mortality of bronchiolitis is to continue to increase the focus on prevention.

## CONFLICT OF INTEREST

The author declares no conflict of interest, financial or otherwise.

## ACKNOWLEDGEMENTS

None declared.

## REFERENCES

[1]    American academy of pediatrics subcommittee on diagnosis and management of bronchiolitis. Diagnosis and management of bronchiolitis. Pediatrics 2006; 118: 1774-93.
       [http://dx.doi.org/10.1542/peds.2006-2223]

[2]    Wright AL, Taussig LM, Ray CG, Harrison HR, Holberg CJ. The Tucson Children's Respiratory Study II. Lower respiratory tract illness in the first year of life. Am J Epidemiol 1989; 129: 1232-46.
       [http://dx.doi.org/10.1093/oxfordjournals.aje.a115243]

[3]    Greenough A, Cox S, Alexander J. Health care utilisation of infants with chronic lung disease, related to hospitalisation for RSV infection. Arch Dis Child 2001; 85: 463-8.
       [http://dx.doi.org/10.1136/adc.85.6.463]

[4]    Centers for disease control and prevention (CDC). Respiratory syncytial virus activity - United States, July 2008-December 2009. MMWR Morb Mortal Wkly Rep 2010; 59: 230-3.

[5]    Zorc JJ, Hall CB. Bronchiolitis: recent evidence on diagnosis and management. Pediatrics 2010; 125: 342-9.
       [http://dx.doi.org/10.1542/peds.2009-2092]

[6]　Hall CB, Weinberg GA, Iwane MK. The burden of respiratory syncytial virus infection in young children.N Engl J Med 2009; 360: 588-98.
[http://dx.doi.org/10.1056/NEJMoa0804877]

[7]　Pelletier AJ, Mansbach JM, Camargo CA Jr. Direct medical costs of bronchiolitis hospitalizations in the United States. Pediatrics 2006; 118: 2418-23.
[http://dx.doi.org/10.1542/peds.2006-1193]

[8]　Hasegawa K, Tsugawa Y, Brown DF, Mansbach JM, Camargo CA Jr. Trends in bronchiolitis hospitalizations in the United States, 2000-2009. Pediatrics 2013; 132: 28-36.
[http://dx.doi.org/10.1542/peds.2012-3877]

[9]　Turcios NL. Gauging the severity of bronchiolitis. J Respir Dis 1994; 15: 875.

[10]　Checchia P. Identification and management of severe respiratory syncytial virus. Am J Health Syst Pharm 2008; 65: S7-S12.
[http://dx.doi.org/10.2146/ajhp080439]

[11]　Plint AC, Johnson DW, Wiebe N. Practice Variation among Pediatric Emergency Departments in the Treatment of Bronchiolitis.Acad Emerg Med 2004; 11: 353-60.
[http://dx.doi.org/10.1197/j.aem.2003.12.003]

[12]　Petruzella FD, Gorelick MH. Duration of illness in infants with bronchiolitis evaluated in the emergency department. Pediatrics 2010; 126: 285-90.
[http://dx.doi.org/10.1542/peds.2009-2189]

[13]　Scottish Intercollegiate Guidelines Network. Bronchiolitis in children. A national clinical guideline 2006. Available from: http://www.sign.ac.uk/pdf/sign91.pdf

[14]　Tapiainen T, Aittoniemi J, Immonen J. Finnish guidelines for the treatment of laryngitis, wheezing bronchitis and bronchiolitis in children.Acta Paediatr 2016; 105: 44-9.
[http://dx.doi.org/10.1111/apa.13162]

[15]　Mansbach JM, McAdam AJ, Clark S. Prospective multicenter study of the viral etiology of bronchiolitis in the emergency department. Acad Emerg Med 2008; 15: 111-8.
[http://dx.doi.org/10.1111/j.1553-2712.2007.00034.x]

[16]　Shay DK, Holman RC, Newman RD, Liu LL, Stout JW, Anderson LJ. Bronchiolitis-associated hospitalizations among US children, 1980-1996. JAMA 1999; 282: 1440-6.
[http://dx.doi.org/10.1001/jama.282.15.1440]

[17]　Yanney M, Vyas H. The treatment of bronchiolitis. Arch Dis Child 2008; 93: 793-8.
[http://dx.doi.org/10.1136/adc.2007.128736]

[18]　Jorgensen J, Wei JL, Sykes KJ. Incidence of and Risk Factors for Airway Complications Following Endotracheal Intubation for Bronchiolitis.Otolaryngol Head Neck Surg 2007; 137: 394-9.
[http://dx.doi.org/10.1016/j.otohns.2007.03.041]

[19]　Johnston C, de Carvalho WB, Piva J, Garcia PC, Fonseca MC. Risk factors for extubation failure in infants with severe acute bronchiolitis. Respir Care 2010; 55: 328-33.

[20]　Navas L, Wang E, de Carvalho V, Robinson J. Pediatric Investigators Collaborative Network on Infections in Canada. Improved outcome of respiratory syncytial virus infection in a high-risk hospitalized population of Canadian children. J Pediatr 1992; 121: 348-54.
[http://dx.doi.org/10.1016/S0022-3476(05)90000-0]

[21]　Kneyber MC, Brandenburg AH, de Groot R. Risk factors for respiratory syncytial virus associated apnoea.Eur J Pediatr 1998; 157: 331-5.
[http://dx.doi.org/10.1007/s004310050822]

[22]　Wahab AA, Dawod ST, Raman HA. Clinical characteristics of respiratory syncytial virus infection in hospitalized healthy infants and young children in Qatar. J Trop Pediatr 2001; 47: 363-6.
[http://dx.doi.org/10.1093/tropej/47.6.363]

[23]   Shazberg G, Revel-Vilk S, Shoseyov D, Ben-Ami A, Klar A, Hurvitz H. The clinical course of bronchiolitis associated with acute otitis media. Arch Dis Child 2000; 83: 317-9.
[http://dx.doi.org/10.1136/adc.83.4.317]

[24]   Andrade MA, Hoberman A, Glustein J, Paradise JL, Wald ER. Acute otitis media in children with bronchiolitis. Pediatrics 1998; 101: 617-9.
[http://dx.doi.org/10.1542/peds.101.4.617]

[25]   Hall CB, Powell KR, Schnabel KC, Gala CL, Pincus PH. Risk of secondary bacterial infection in infants hospitalized with respiratory syncytial viral infection. J Pediatr 1988; 113: 266-71.
[http://dx.doi.org/10.1016/S0022-3476(88)80263-4]

[26]   van Steensel-Moll HA, Hazelzet JA, van der Voort E, Neijens HJ, Hackeng WH. Excessive secretion of antidiuretic hormone in infections with respiratory syncytial virus. Arch Dis Child 1990; 65: 1237-9.
[http://dx.doi.org/10.1136/adc.65.11.1237]

[27]   Gozal D, Colin AA, Jaffe M, Hochberg Z. Water, electrolyte, and endocrine homeostasis in infants with bronchiolitis. Pediatr Res 1990; 27: 204-9.
[http://dx.doi.org/10.1203/00006450-199002000-00023]

[28]   Bont L. Current concepts of the pathogenesis of RSV bronchiolitis. Adv Exp Med Biol 2009; 634: 31-40.
[http://dx.doi.org/10.1007/978-0-387-79838-7_3]

[29]   Sigurs N, Gustafsson PM, Bjarnason R. Severe Respiratory Syncytial Virus Bronchiolitis in Infancy and Asthma and Allergy at Age 13.Am J Respir Crit Care Med 2005; 171: 137-41.
[http://dx.doi.org/10.1164/rccm.200406-730OC]

[30]   Stein RT, Sherrill D, Morgan WJ. Respiratory syncytial virus in early life and risk of wheeze and allergy by age 13 years.Lancet 1999; 354: 541-5.
[http://dx.doi.org/10.1016/S0140-6736(98)10321-5]

[31]   Henderson J, Hilliard TN, Sherriff A, Stalker D, Al Shammari N, Thomas HM. Hospitalization for RSV bronchiolitis before 12 months of age and subsequent asthma, atopy and wheeze: a longitudinal birth cohort study. Pediatr Allergy Immunol 2005; 16: 386-92.
[http://dx.doi.org/10.1111/j.1399-3038.2005.00298.x]

[32]   Ralston SL, Lieberthal AS, Meissner HC. Clinical Practice Guideline: The Diagnosis, Management, and Prevention of Bronchiolitis.Pediatrics 2014; 134: e1474-502.
[http://dx.doi.org/10.1542/peds.2014-2742]

[33]   Mansbach JM, Piedra PA, Teach SJ, *et al.* MARC-30 Investigators. Prospective multicenter study of viral etiology and hospital length of stay in children with severe bronchiolitis. Arch Pediatr Adolesc Med 2012; 166: 700-6.
[http://dx.doi.org/10.1001/archpediatrics.2011.1669]

[34]   Welliver RC. Bronchiolitis and Infectious Asthma. In: Cherry JD, Demmler-Harrison GJ, Kaplan SL, Steinbach WJ, Hotez P, Eds. Feigin and Cherry's Textbook of Pediatric Infectious Diseases. 7th ed. Philadelphia: Elsevier Saunders 2014; p. 271.

[35]   Destino L, Weisgerber MC, Soung P. Validity of Respiratory Scores in Bronchiolitis.Hosp Pediatr 2012; 2: 202-9.
[http://dx.doi.org/10.1542/hpeds.2012-0013]

[36]   Abbott GF, Rosado-de-Christenson ML, Rossi SE, Suster S. Imaging of small airways disease. J Thorac Imaging 2009; 24: 285-98.
[http://dx.doi.org/10.1097/RTI.0b013e3181c1ab83]

[37]   Harris JA, Huskins WC, Langley JM, Siegel JD. Pediatric Special Interest Group of the Society for Healthcare Epidemiology of America. Health care epidemiology perspective on the October 2006 recommendations of the Subcommittee on Diagnosis and Management of Bronchiolitis. Pediatrics

2007; 120: 890-2.
[http://dx.doi.org/10.1542/peds.2007-1305]

[38]   Smyth RL, Openshaw PJ. Bronchiolitis. Lancet 2006; 368: 312-22.
[http://dx.doi.org/10.1016/S0140-6736(06)69077-6]

[39]   Vogel AM, Lennon DR, Harding JE. Variations in bronchiolitis management between five New Zealand hospitals: Can we do better?J Paediatr Child Health 2003; 39: 40-5.
[http://dx.doi.org/10.1046/j.1440-1754.2003.00069.x]

[40]   Adcock PM, Stout GG, Hauck MA, Marshall GS. Effect of rapid viral diagnosis on the management of children hospitalized with lower respiratory tract infection. Pediatr Infect Dis J 1997; 16: 842-6.
[http://dx.doi.org/10.1097/00006454-199709000-00005]

[41]   Doan QH, Kissoon N, Dobson S. A randomized, controlled trial of the impact of early and rapid diagnosis of viral infections in children brought to an emergency department with febrile respiratory tract illnesses.J Pediatr 2009; 154: 91-5.
[http://dx.doi.org/10.1016/j.jpeds.2008.07.043]

[42]   Doan Q, Enarson P, Kissoon N. Rapid viral diagnosis for acute febrile respiratory illness in children in the Emergency Department.Cochrane Database Syst Rev 2014; 9: CD006452.

[43]   Johnson DW, Adair C, Brant R, Holmwood J, Mitchell I. Differences in admission rates of children with bronchiolitis by pediatric and general emergency departments. Pediatrics 2002; 110: e49.
[http://dx.doi.org/10.1542/peds.110.4.e49]

[44]   Rivers RP, Forsling ML, Olver RP. Inappropriate secretion of antidiuretic hormone in infants with respiratory infections. Arch Dis Child 1981; 56: 358-63.
[http://dx.doi.org/10.1136/adc.56.5.358]

[45]   Laegreid A, Kolstø Otnaess AB, Orstavik I, Carlsen KH. Neutralizing activity in human milk fractions against respiratory syncytial virus. Acta Paediatr Scand 1986; 75: 696-701.
[http://dx.doi.org/10.1111/j.1651-2227.1986.tb10276.x]

[46]   Chiba Y, Minagawa T, Mito K, *et al.* Effect of breast feeding on responses of systemic interferon and virus specific lymphocyte transformation in infants with respiratory syncytial virus infectionJ Med Virol 1987; 21: 7 14.
[http://dx.doi.org/10.1002/jmv.1890210103]

[47]   Wainwright C, Altamirano L, Cheney M, *et al.* A multicenter, randomized, double-blind, controlled trial of nebulized epinephrine in infants with acute bronchiolitis.N Engl J Med 2003; 349: 27-35.
[http://dx.doi.org/10.1056/NEJMoa022226]

[48]   Patel H, Gouin S, Platt RW. Randomized, double-blind, placebo-controlled trial of oral albuterol in infants with mild-to-moderate acute viral bronchiolitis. J Pediatr 2003; 142: 509-14.
[http://dx.doi.org/10.1067/mpd.2003.196]

[49]   Plint AC, Johnson DW, Patel H, *et al.* Pediatric Emergency Research Canada (PERC). Epinephrine and dexamethasone in children with bronchiolitis. N Engl J Med 2009; 360: 2079-89.
[http://dx.doi.org/10.1056/NEJMoa0900544]

[50]   Wark PA, McDonald V, Jones AP. Nebulised hypertonic saline for cystic fibrosis. Cochrane Database Syst Rev 2005; 3: CD001506.

[51]   Daviskas E, Anderson SD, Gonda I, *et al.* Inhalation of hypertonic saline aerosol enhances mucociliary clearance in asthmatic and healthy subjects.Eur Respir J 1996; 9: 725-32.
[http://dx.doi.org/10.1183/09031936.96.09040725]

[52]   Sood N, Bennett WD, Zeman K, *et al.* Increasing concentration of inhaled saline with or without amiloride: effect on mucociliary clearance in normal subjects.Am J Respir Crit Care Med 2003; 167: 158-63.
[http://dx.doi.org/10.1164/rccm.200204-293OC]

[53]   Fernandes RM, Bialy LM, Vandermeer B, *et al.* Glucocorticoids for acute viral bronchiolitis in infants and young children.Cochrane Database Syst Rev 2013; 6: CD004878.

[54]   Hall CB, Powell KR, MacDonald NE, *et al.* Respiratory syncytial viral infection in children with compromised immune functionN Engl J Med 1986; 315: 77-81.
[http://dx.doi.org/10.1056/NEJM198607103150201]

[55]   Ross PA, Newth CJ, Khemani RG. Accuracy of pulse oximetry in children. Pediatrics 2014; 133: 22-9.
[http://dx.doi.org/10.1542/peds.2013-1760]

[56]   Unger S, Cunningham S. Effect of oxygen supplementation on length of stay for infants hospitalized with acute viral bronchiolitis. Pediatrics 2008; 121: 470-5.
[http://dx.doi.org/10.1542/peds.2007-1135]

[57]   Cunningham S, McMurray A. Observational study of two oxygen saturation targets for discharge in bronchiolitis. Arch Dis Child 2012; 97: 361-3.
[http://dx.doi.org/10.1136/adc.2010.205211]

[58]   Schroeder AR, Marmor AK, Pantell RH, Newman TB. Impact of pulse oximetry and oxygen therapy on length of stay in bronchiolitis hospitalizations. Arch Pediatr Adolesc Med 2004; 158: 527-30.
[http://dx.doi.org/10.1001/archpedi.158.6.527]

[59]   National Institute for Health and Care Excellence. Bronchiolitis: diagnosis and management of bronchiolitis in children. Clinical Guideline NG 9 2015 June; Available from: https://www.nice.org.uk/guidance/ng9

[60]   Liu F, Ouyang J, Sharma AN, *et al.* Leukotriene inhibitors for bronchiolitis in infants and young children.Cochrane Database Syst Rev 2015; 3: CD010636.

[61]   Spurling GK, Doust J, Del Mar CB, Eriksson L. Antibiotics for bronchiolitis in children. Cochrane Database Syst Rev 2011; 6: CD005189.

[62]   Pinto LA, Pitrez PM, Luisi F, *et al.* Azithromycin therapy in hospitalized infants with acute bronchiolitis is not associated with better clinical outcomes: a randomized, double-blinded, and placebo-controlled clinical trial.J Pediatr 2012; 161: 1104-8.
[http://dx.doi.org/10.1016/j.jpeds.2012.05.053]

[63]   Ventre K, Randolph AG. Ribavirin for respiratory syncytial virus infection of the lower respiratory tract in infants and young children. Cochrane Database Syst Rev 2007; 1: CD000181.

[64]   Megged O, Schlesinger Y. Down syndrome and respiratory syncytial virus infection. Pediatr Infect Dis J 2010; 29: 672-3.
[http://dx.doi.org/10.1097/INF.0b013e3181d7ffa5]

[65]   El Saleeby CM, Somes GW, DeVincenzo JP, Gaur AH. Risk factors for severe respiratory syncytial virus disease in children with cancer: the importance of lymphopenia and young age. Pediatrics 2008; 121: 235-43.
[http://dx.doi.org/10.1542/peds.2007-1102]

[66]   Hall CB, Douglas RG Jr, Geiman JM. Possible transmission by fomites of respiratory syncytial virus. J Infect Dis 1980; 141: 98-102.
[http://dx.doi.org/10.1093/infdis/141.1.98]

[67]   Matt GE, Quintana PJ, Destaillats H, *et al.* Thirdhand tobacco smoke: emerging evidence and arguments for a multidisciplinary research agendaEnviron Health Perspect 2011; 119: 1218-26.
[http://dx.doi.org/10.1289/ehp.1103500]

[68]   Ip S, Chung M, Raman G, *et al.* Breastfeeding and maternal and infant health outcomes in developed countries.Evid Rep Technol Assess (Full Rep) 2007; 153: 1-186.

[69]   Dornelles CT, Piva JP, Marostica PJ. Nutritional status, breastfeeding, and evolution of infants with acute viral bronchiolitis. J Health Popul Nutr 2007; 25: 336-43.

# CHAPTER 13

# What is New with Management of Pediatric Central Sleep Apnea?

## S. Kamal Naqvi[*]

*Division of Respiratory and Sleep Medicine, Department of Pediatrics, UT Southwestern Medical Center, Dallas, Texas, USA*

**Abstract:** Central Sleep Apnea (CSA) in children is a far less studied and understood abnormality compared to Obstructive Sleep Apnea (OSA). It is seen more often in younger patient population mostly with co-morbidity. There are structural abnormalities in the brain, spinal cord, airway and chest wall or functional disorders in respiratory control, hemoglobin concentration, swallowing or cardiovascular system, resulting in CSA. Clinical observation of central apneic events prompts further evaluation ideally done by performing Polysomnography testing (sleep study) to confirm the presence and estimate the severity.

Various medical and surgical treatment options result in improvement or resolution of the central apneic events. Majority of the patients show a gradual resolution of the disorder with age. However a minority of patients continue to manifest the disorder and require longer term treatment mostly by using respiratory support in the form of invasive or non-invasive ventilation. More research is needed to explore treatment options for children.

**Keywords:** Central sleep apnea, Pediatrics, Polysomnographic study, Sleep disordered breathing.

## INTRODUCTION

Sleep disordered breathing encompasses conditions from the more common obstructive sleep apnea (OSA) to obstructive hypoventilation, sleep related hypoxemia and central sleep apnea.

Central sleep apnea results from absent respiratory drive from breathing centers in the brainstem during sleep. There is a difference in the definition of CA for children and adults. The American Academy of Sleep Medicine (AASM) defines CA in children as cessation of breathing during sleep without any breathing effort

---

[*] **Corresponding author S. Kamal Naqvi**: Division of Respiratory and Sleep Medicine, Department of Pediatrics, UT Southwestern Medical Center, Dallas, Texas, USA; Tel: 214-456-8348; Fax: 214-456-5406; Email: kamal.naqvi@utsouthwestern.edu

for duration of 20 seconds or longer, or lasting at least 2 breaths' duration with 3% oxygen desaturation or arousal [1].

## Definitions

In children including infants, the CA is at least 2 breaths in duration and is associated with a decrease in heart rate to less than 50 beats per minute for at least 5 seconds, or less than 60 beats per minute for 15 seconds. Periodic breathing has been described as greater than 3 episodes of CA lasting 3 seconds separated by no more than 20 seconds of normal breathing.

Apnea following a sigh is not considered pathologic unless it is associated with arousal or desaturation. Isolated central apnea (Fig. **1A**), CA following post-arousal sigh breathing (see Fig. **1B**), and periodic breathing patterns (see Fig. **1C**) can be seen in healthy infants and children [2].

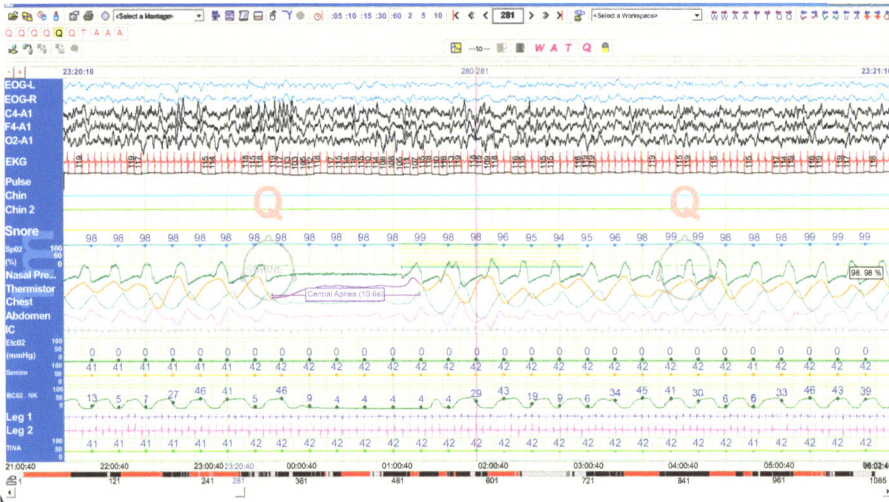

**Fig. (1A).** Sixty-second-long epoch showing central sleep apnea.

[1A,1B] Sixty-second-long [1C] 120 seconds-long epoch of the polysomnography of a 4-month-old child born at full term, referred for evaluation of sleep apnea because of observation by parent of apneic episodes. [1*A*] Central sleep apnea without arousal. [*B*] Central sleep apnea after arousal during Quiet sleep. [*C*] Periodic breathing during Active sleep. abdm, abdominal plethysmography; C4, central electroencephalogram leads; CHIN, chin electromyogram; EOG, L&R eye electromyogram; EKG, electrocardiogram; ETCO, end-tidal carbon dioxide tracing; F4, frontal electroencephalogram leads; O2, Occipital electro-encephalogram, FLOW, tracing of oral thermistor; Nasal Pressure for measurement of nasal air pressure; SNOR, snore micrograph; SpO2, continuous pulse oximetry; thor, thoracic plethysmography.

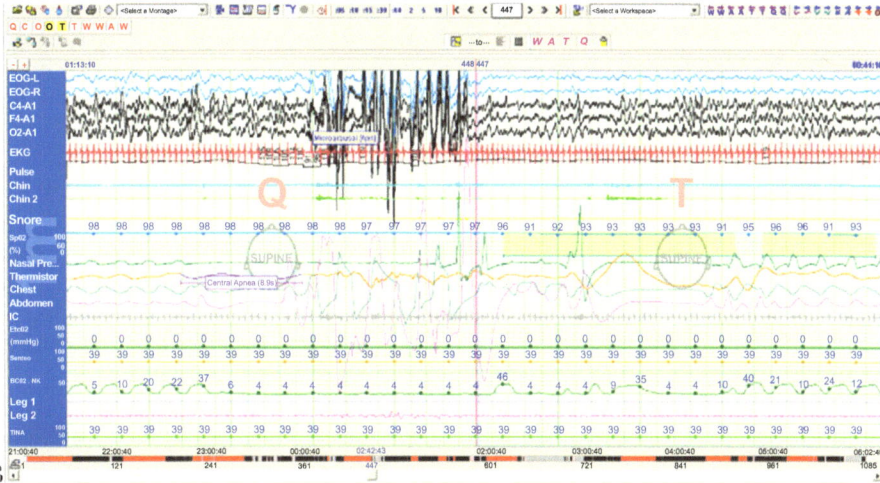

**Fig. (1B).** Sixty-seconds-long epoch showing central sleep apnea after arousal during Quiet sleep.

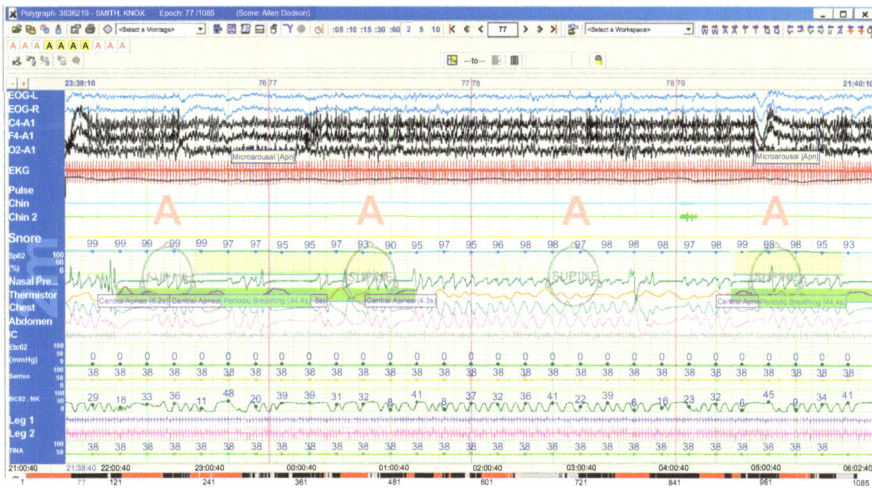

**Fig. (1C).** 120 seconds-long epoch showing periodic breathing during Active sleep.

Generally, it is common to see CA in healthy infants and children, but on rare occasions it can be a sign of significant pathologic consequences, such as congenital central hypoventilation syndrome or Arnold-Chiari malformation [3].

The severity of CA can be characterized using the central apnea index (CAI) while apnea-hypopnea index (AHI) usually refers to the obstructive type of the disorder and is the total number of events overnight divided by hours of sleep. There is no clear description in the literature of pathologic central apnea index but studies have considered a CAI from >1 to 5 per hour as abnormal [4 - 6].

Duration of these apneic events may be more indicative of an underlying pathology than just the index. The adverse consequences of moderate and severe CA are well known, but those of CA of milder degree are still debated[7].

The mild CA seen in otherwise healthy infants and young children tends to improve with age [5, 7]. With maturation of respiratory control and chest-wall mechanics, the apnea frequency is improved in almost all patients.

**Apnea in Normal Children and Infants**

Brief CA in full-term infants is seen commonly, especially in the early months of life. Both the duration and frequency of CA improves with age [8, 9].

There has been an effort in defining the prevalence of CA in healthy infants. Each study has used different criteria to define CA, different monitoring techniques, and different testing environments such as home *versus* in-laboratory polysomnography, which makes it difficult to make comparisons between the studies.

With the development of standardization of the definition of CA future studies are likely to be comparable leading to better understanding.

The Collaborative Home Infant Monitoring Evaluation (CHIME) study seems to be the largest and the most comprehensive study allowing comparison of breathing patterns during sleep in healthy term infants, siblings of infants with a family history of sudden infant death syndrome (SIDS), healthy preterm infants, and infants with apparent life-threatening events (ALTE) in both term and preterm subjects [10].

The study was conducted in over 1000 infants over 6 months' duration in their home environment. The investigators concluded that conventional events, described as apnea of 20 seconds' duration not associated with bradycardia, are common in otherwise healthy term infants. The study also reported that extreme events, described as apneas longer than 30 seconds associated with bradycardia, are more common in premature infants and tend to reduce in frequency after 43 weeks gestational age (GA).

Normative data on pediatric breathing patterns during sleep was presented by Uliel and colleagues who studied 70 subjects between the ages of 1 and 15 years who underwent a single-night sleep study in the laboratory. CA was defined as of at least 10 seconds' duration or any duration associated with desaturation of greater than 4% compared with baseline [5]. The investigators confirmed that CA is rare in children, and stated that CA with desaturation is even rarer. The study was conducted with a modern computer-based recording system and was manually scored by visual inspection.

The literature suggests that CA is common in early infancy and improves with age [11]. It is also noted that most central apnea events follow a sigh breath in older healthy children beyond infancy. In premature infants, the breathing pattern is not fully developed at the time of birth [12]. This situation may be complicated with the development of bronchopulmonary dysplasia with limited respiratory reserves, and/or cerebral palsy with associated poor neuromuscular control of upper airway [4] Thus, prematurity predisposes to both central and obstructive sleep apnea. Most studies performed in premature infants to assess the maturation of breathing are retrospective in nature.

Periodic breathing is also common in premature and young term infants [13]. Glotzbach and colleagues described the prevalence of periodic breathing in relatively mature preterm infants (30–35 weeks GA) in comparison with full-term infants.

The investigators reported a higher mean percentage value of periodic breathing and the longest episode of periodic breathing was higher in preterm infants than in full-term controls. Moreover, percentage and episodes of periodic breathing during sleep decreased as infants reached 39 to 41 weeks postconceptional age.

## Clinical Presentation of Central Apnea in Children

### *ALTE: Apparent Life-Threatening Event*

ALTE has been described as an episode that is frightening to the observer and characterized by some combination of apnea, color change, marked change in muscle tone, choking, and/or gagging. The pathophysiology of ALTE is multifactorial; occasionally it is a single event, and no significant pathologic features may be discovered despite extensive investigation [14].

In the past, it was proposed that some infants who die of SIDS had recurrent ALTE, but most patients with ALTE do not die [15].

There are several causes for ALTE, and it is difficult to focus on a single system function [16].

Apnea may not necessarily be part of the presentation in infants who present with ALTE. The AASM recommends performing polysomnography in infants with clinical suspicion of sleep-disordered breathing [17].

The relationship between gastroesophageal reflux (GER) and central and/or obstructive apnea has been debated frequently. Khan and colleagues studied both central and obstructive apnea in 50 infants with ALTE and 50 control subjects [18]. It was concluded that there is no temporal association between GER in the middle esophagus and apnea/bradycardia in both populations.

## Pathophysiology of Central Apnea in the Pediatric Population

The exact timing of the start of breathing movements in the human fetus is unclear. The fetal breathing movement in most mammals starts in the second trimester [19]. The fetal breathing movement is discontinuous, rhythmic, and nonsynchronized [20].

Perhaps an important aspect of breathing rhythm in the fetus is that it is vital for lung development during fetal life [21].

The control of breathing in fetal life is complex, and involves several inhibitory and excitatory stimuli. Some of the important modulators of breathing include central rhythm generators, central and peripheral chemoreceptors, sleep and wake states, and various neurotransmitters [22, 23].

Based on the animal model of respiratory control, there are 2 distinct groups of respiratory centers that function in harmony. The first, the parafacial nucleus, is located at the ventral surface of the hindbrain while the second, the pre-Bötzinger complex, is on the dorsal aspect. Both groups of neurons develop independently from each other in the hindbrain [24].

The parafacial nucleus predominantly controls expiration and functions by phasic inhibition of tonic background inspiratory activity via glutamatergic neurons [25].

The pre-Bötzinger complex predominately works as the inspiratory control. The development of these respiratory centers and the interaction between them is beyond the scope of this review.

Fetal breathing is stimulated with elevated carbon dioxide during low-voltage high-frequency electrocorticography, suggestive of wake state, and during both high-voltage and low-voltage electrocorticography with exposure to cold and carbon dioxide [26, 27]. Responses to hypoxia and hypercapnia in fetal life suggest that carotid chemoreceptors are already active in fetal life [28].

The other inhibitory stimuli for breathing in fetal life include adenosine and the placenta [29, 30]. Removal of placenta after birth may be a stimulus for continuous breathing [31]. Fetal breathing is also under behavioral control. It is stimulated during high-frequency, low-voltage electrocorticographic activity, which is characteristic of awake and REM sleep, and is inhibited during low-frequency, high-voltage electrocorticographic activity, with apnea being present.

Transition from fetal to neonatal life is probably the most complex transition in human life [32].

The irregular breathing pattern in preterm and term infants is also exacerbated by immature lung mechanics at the time of birth. Infants have low functional residual capacity, which results in hypoxemia even with brief CA and periodic breathing.

In full-term infants, breathing irregularities persist during 60% to 70% of the sleep time and decrease by 3 months of age [33]. Warm temperature induces apnea in term infants, and loss of body heat stimulates breathing [34].

Periodic breathing in premature infants is related to the carbon dioxide level and its relationship to the apnea threshold. Reduction in serum carbon dioxide below a certain point causes apnea during sleep, and this level is termed the apneic threshold. In premature infants, the apnea threshold is much closer to the eucapnia level in comparison with adults [35]. The apnea threshold is therefore frequently reached with common maneuvers such as an augmented breath, resulting in recurrent apnea that is seen in periodic breathing.

Another concept in understanding periodic breathing may be related to loop gain. Loop gain is described as a negative feedback system in which a disturbance (u) increases alveolar ventilation from a steady state. This increase in ventilation in turn reduces carbon dioxide, which evokes a negative corrective action (e) to suppress the disturbance. The ratio of e/u will define the loop gain of the system. In the high loop-gain system, the response is greater or equal to the disturbance, which results in an unstable system. For example, a sigh produces a sudden reduction of carbon dioxide levels, which evokes an exaggerated response from the central respiratory center and induces apnea, which in turn results in elevated levels of carbon dioxide. This process causes resumption of breathing but in an exaggerated fashion, leading to washout of carbon dioxide, bringing it below the apneic threshold; the cycle will thus repeat itself, resulting in the characteristic breathing pattern seen in periodic breathing.

## Evaluation

Polysomnography is considered the test of choice to diagnose sleep-disordered breathing in infants and children. This is done as in-laboratory testing, reported to be well tolerated by patients and family members [36]. A recent study has shown that a shorter 4-hour evening study is comparable with an overnight sleep study in the diagnosis of sleep-disordered breathing in children younger than 2 years [37].

A nap study, even shorter than a 4-hour study, is not considered to be equivalent to a full-night study and may miss sleep-disordered breathing [38]. The in-laboratory polysomnography testing assures accurate diagnosis of the nature of sleep-disordered breathing with additional assessment of non-breathing disorders such as parasomnia and has ability to intervene during the study as indicated. The disadvantages include prolonged test duration for young children and need for a parent to stay for the whole duration of data collection, expensive testing, and long waiting time for the study because of the shortage of child-friendly sleep laboratories.

Home monitoring has been used in several research studies to document sleep-disordered breathing in infants, but has not been widely accepted as a tool for clinical use. There are various portable testing modalities available for the assessment of sleep-disordered breathing in infants, including home pulse oximetry, pulse transit time, and multichannel unattended sleep studies [39, 40]. Portable monitoring provides the advantage to collect data in a patient's familiar surroundings and for an extended period of time. It is also inexpensive and readily available. The disadvantages include difficulty in accurate differentiation of sleep and wake stages, and multiple artifacts during the data collection.

While routine evaluation of children with elevated central apnea index by MRI is not indicated, providers should consider neuroimaging in children with CSA and abnormal neurologic examination findings or gastroesophageal reflux disease. Further research is necessary to identify other tests with improved diagnostic yield for evaluation of pediatric CSA [41].

## Medical Disorders Associated With Central Sleep Apnea

### Brain Tumors

Among the pediatric population referred to a sleep clinic who are affected by brain tumors, up to 90% involve tumors located within brainstem, thalamus, or hypothalamus [42]. In addition to daytime sleepiness, tumors in these locations can often cause respiratory irregularities during sleep when wakefulness-determined behavioral compensatory mechanisms are lost. Of the few reported cases of CSA involving tumors in this population, tumors have been located in the brainstem, fourth ventricle, posterior fossa, and spinal region. Thus, dysfunction or interruption of respiratory neural output at multiple sites within the central nervous system may cause CSA. Unlike patients with tumors and obstructive sleep apnea who are often also obese, CSA patients tend to be nonobese [43].

## Chiari Type I Malformation

Chiari type I malformation is associated with both obstructive apnea and CSA, affecting pediatric and adult populations. CSA and hypoventilation can be present in both rapid eye movement (REM) and non-REM (NREM) sleep. The extent of the malformation present and the downstream effects on control of breathing centers vary However, polysomnography changes correlate well with magnetic resonance imaging (MRI) findings [44, 45]. CSA tends to be more severe in children who present with syrinx and general crowding at the foramen magnum [46, 47].

## Endocrine and Hormonal Disturbances

Prader-Willi syndrome is known to be associated with sleep disordered breathing in children including obstructive sleep apnea, hypoventilation, central sleep apnea and even death with more frequent respiratory complications seen during upper respiratory infections.

Sleep disordered breathing is also significant because of potential growth of soft tissue in the airway in response to growth hormone treatment frequently used [48].

## Neuromuscular Disease

Congenital muscular dystrophies are inherited diseases affecting muscles. In addition to poor-quality sleep and seizures, sleep-disordered breathing is present in approximately 65% of cases [49, 50]. CSA is the most common form of sleep-related breathing instability in patients with congenital muscular dystrophies. The severity of CSA is related to the age of onset of symptoms and the rate of progression of muscle weakness. The primary mechanism by which CSA occurs in these patients is via an inability to translate respiratory neural drive from the respiratory centers (which may be perfectly normal) into functional motion of the respiratory muscles, because of muscle weakness. Whereas in some of these patients a degree of hypoventilation can occur during wakefulness leading to $CO_2$ retention, others remain normocapnic, with hypoventilation only occurring during sleep when wakefulness neurocompensatory mechanisms are lost. Thus, unlike other forms of CSA that typically worsen in NREM sleep, CSA in patients with congenital muscular dystrophies may be most pronounced during REM sleep against the background of already low drive to the intercostal muscles and accessory respiratory muscles [51 - 53].

Healthy infants ($\leq$ 18 months old) born and residing at high altitude show preserved sleep architecture but higher apnea-hypopnea indexes and more prominent desaturation with respiratory events than do those living at low altitude [54].

## Management of Central Apnea in Children

### *Treat The Underlying Cause*

The target in managing CA in infants and young children is aimed at normalization of breathing and stabilization of fluctuation in oxygen saturation. The available therapies for the treatment of apnea in infant serve as temporary therapies while awaiting maturity of the breathing apparatus of premature and full-term infants.

Supplemental oxygen therapy has been widely prescribed for CA and periodic breathing in both premature and full-term infants. In a small study of 15 preterm infants, supplemental oxygen improved apnea and periodic breathing.

Oxygen therapy prevents desaturation and improves breathing stability in infants. However, there is no clear guideline for its use in the treatment of CA in infants.

Stimulant medications such as theophylline and caffeine have been frequently prescribed and widely accepted therapy for CA and periodic breathing in preterm and term. In premature infants, the use of caffeine to stimulate breathing is targeted toward adenosine-induced breathing suppression that is normally seen in fetal life.

A meta-analysis of 6 clinical trials looking at the efficacy of methylxanthine in the treatment of apnea of prematurity reported a reduction in apnea severity and utilization of intermittent positive pressure therapy in the first 2 to 7 days [47].

In a randomized placebo-controlled trial of 2000 infants born at preterm and with apnea of prematurity, caffeine reduced the need for positive pressure ventilation and reduced the use of supplemental oxygen [55].

Some other nonconventional therapies for the treatment of CA have been researched in preterm infants. A small study of 24 premature infants born at 27 weeks GA with apnea of prematurity compared supine *versus* prone positioning, and concluded that more CA and less arousal was noted during prone sleeping position, whereas infants had more awakening and arousals per hour in a supine sleeping position, hence supine sleep position was suggested [56].

In a prospective, randomized controlled study of 27 preterm infants of similar GA, the short-term inhalation of 0.8% carbon dioxide had efficacy similar to that of theophylline in reducing the apnea [57].

Both of these trials were based on the fact that inhaled carbon dioxide will increase the carbon dioxide levels and prevent the apnea threshold being reaching in preterm infants, thus stabilizing breathing.

Positive pressure ventilation has been widely used in the treatment of CA and periodic breathing in preterm and term infants. Continuous positive airway pressure (CPAP) is one such modality. The underlying mechanism of improvement of CA was recently studied by Edwards and colleagues in a lamb model of periodic breathing [58]. CPAP reduced CA and mixed apnea in a dose-dependent manner, most likely by reducing the loop gain via an increase in the lung volume.

Other therapies that have been studied in preterm infants for treatment of CA and periodic breathing but not yet available for clinical use include stochastic mechanosensory stimulation (vibrotactile stimulation to stimulate breathing). In a small study of 10 relatively mature preterm infants (33 weeks), a low level of exogenous stochastic stimulation stabilized breathing during sleep and helped to reduce the incidence of apnea and periodic breathing [59].

Acetazolamide, a carbonic anhydrase inhibitor, has been used in the treatment of CA and periodic breathing. In a small study of 12 infants with recurrent hypoxemia, acetazolamide reduced the CA index and improved oxygen saturation [60].

Acetazolamide diminishes the ventilatory response of the peripheral chemoreceptors to hypoxia, decreases loop gain, and reduces the ventilatory response to arousals [64, 65]. In animal models, it has been shown to lower the PETCO2 apnea threshold and widen the difference between the eupneic and PETCO2 thresholds. Treatment of anemia of prematurity with blood transfusion has also been shown to reduce central apnea in preterm infants [61].

In adults, the use of supplemental $CO_2$ for hypocapnic central sleep apnea syndromes is old news. That $CO_2$ can stabilize respiration has been known for decades, but high concentrations fragment sleep by inducing arousals secondary to respiratory stimulation and sympathoexcitation [62, 63]. The key challenge has been delivery of $CO_2$ in a clinically adequate, tolerated, and precise manner.

Sleep stabilization has been advocated to be effective in adults showing stable respiration. Some additional therapies have been tried in adults with mixed success with scant data available on pediatric population. These include medications such as Clonidine, Nasal Expiratory Positive Pressure (Provent) and Hypoglossal Nerve Stimulation.

## *Treatment Options with Positive Pressure Ventilation*

In children with clinically significant central sleep apnea that persists while addressing the underlying cause require supporting the ventilation for some duration of time. This can be achieved with either invasive mechanical ventilation via tracheostomy or non-invasive positive pressure ventilation (NIPPV) by applying a nasal or full face interface.

There are valid concerns about efficacy and tolerance of NIPPV in young children when used at home. This includes appropriate size mask, constant supervision by a caregiver in assuring adequate seal and positioning of the mask and likely accidental removal of the mask by the child with acute consequences.

## CONCLUSION

Sleep disordered breathing especially central sleep apnea is a frequently seen clinical entity. There are treatable underlying conditions resulting in effective resolution of central apneas. However, a significant patient population continues to suffer from the disorder and require medication or equipment support for the ventilation for varying length of time. There are limitations in applying these devices to younger patients indicating a need for more pediatric specific studies.

## CONFLICT OF INTEREST

The author declares no conflict of interest, financial or otherwise.

## ACKNOWLEDGEMENTS

Declared none.

## REFERENCES

[1]     Berry RB, Budhiraja R, Gottlieb DJ, *et al.* Rules for scoring respiratory events in sleep: update of the 2007 AASM Manual for the Scoring of Sleep and Associated Events. Deliberations of the Sleep Apnea Definitions Task Force of the American Academy of Sleep Medicine. J Clin Sleep Med 2007; 15;8(5): 597-619.

[2]     Fukumizu M, Kohyama J. Central respiratory pauses, sighs, and gross body movements during sleep in children. Physiol Behav 2004; 82: 721-6.
        [http://dx.doi.org/10.1016/j.physbeh.2004.06.011]

[3]     Weese-Mayer DE, Berry-Kravis EM, Ceccherini I, *et al.* An official ATS clinical policy statement: congenital central hypoventilation syndrome: genetic basis, diagnosis, and management. Am J Respir Crit Care Med 2010; 181: 626-44.
        [http://dx.doi.org/10.1164/rccm.200807-1069ST]

[4]     Ng DK, Chan CH. A review of normal values of infant sleep polysomnography. Pediatr Neonatol 2013; 54: 82-7.
        [http://dx.doi.org/10.1016/j.pedneo.2012.11.011]

[5]     Uliel S, Tauman R, Greenfeld M, *et al.* Normal polysomnographic respiratory values in children and adolescents. Chest 2004; 125: 872-8.
[http://dx.doi.org/10.1378/chest.125.3.872]

[6]     Kritzinger FE, Al-Saleh S, Narang I. Descriptive analysis of central sleep apnea in childhood at a single center. Pediatr Pulmonol 2011; 46: 1023-30.
[http://dx.doi.org/10.1002/ppul.21469]

[7]     Marcus CL, Omlin KJ, Basinki DJ, *et al.* Normal polysomnographic values for children and adolescents. Am Rev Respir Dis 1992; 146: 1235-9.
[http://dx.doi.org/10.1164/ajrccm/146.5_Pt_1.1235]

[8]     Richards JM, Alexander JR, Shinebourne EA, *et al.* Sequential 22-hour profiles of breathing patterns and heart rate in 110 full-term infants during their first 6 months of life. Pediatrics 1984; 74: 763-77.

[9]     Hoppenbrouwers T, Hodgman JE, Harper RM, *et al.* Polygraphic studies of normal infants during the first six months of life: III. Incidence of apnea and periodic breathing. Pediatrics 1977; 60: 418-25.

[10]    Ramanathan R, Corwin MJ, Hunt CE, *et al.* Cardiorespiratory events recorded on home monitors: comparison of healthy infants with those at increased risk for SIDS. JAMA 2001; 285: 2199-207.
[http://dx.doi.org/10.1001/jama.285.17.2199]

[11]    Weese-Mayer DE, Corwin MJ, Peucker MR, *et al.* Comparison of apnea identified by respiratory inductance plethysmography with that detected by end-tidal CO(2) or thermistor. The CHIME Study Group. Am J Respir Crit Care Med 2000; 162: 471-80.
[http://dx.doi.org/10.1164/ajrccm.162.2.9904029]

[12]    Robertson CM, Watt MJ, Dinu IA. Outcomes for the extremely premature infant: what is new? And where are we going? Pediatr Neurol 2009; 40: 189-96.
[http://dx.doi.org/10.1016/j.pediatrneurol.2008.09.017]

[13]    Baraldi E, Filippone M. Chronic lung disease after premature birth. N Engl J Med 2007; 357: 1946-55.
[http://dx.doi.org/10.1056/NEJMra067279]

[14]    Samuels MP, Poets CF, Noyes JP, *et al.* Diagnosis and management after life threatening events in infants and young children who received cardiopulmonary resuscitation. BMJ 1993; 306: 489-92.
[http://dx.doi.org/10.1136/bmj.306.6876.489]

[15]    Infantile Apnea and Home Monitoring. NIH Consensus Statement Online 1986 Sep 29-Oct; 1;6(6): 1-10. Available at: http://consensus.nih.gov/1986/1986InfantApneaMonitoring058html.htm.

[16]    McGovern MC, Smith MB. Causes of apparent life threatening events in infants: a systematic review. Arch Dis Child 2004; 89: 1043-8.
[http://dx.doi.org/10.1136/adc.2003.031740]

[17]    Aurora RN, Zak RS, Karippot A, *et al.* Practice parameters for the respiratory indications for polysomnography in children. Sleep 2011; 34: 379-88.
[http://dx.doi.org/10.1093/sleep/34.3.379]

[18]    Kahn A, Rebuffat E, Sottiaux M, *et al.* Lack of temporal relation between acid reflux in the proximal oesophagus and cardiorespiratory events in sleeping infants. Eur J Pediatr 1992; 151: 208-12.
[http://dx.doi.org/10.1007/BF01954386]

[19]    Jansen AH, Chernick V. Development of respiratory control. Physiol Rev 1983; 63: 437-83.

[20]    Johnston BM, Gunn TR, Gluckman PD. Surface cooling rapidly induces coordinated activity in the upper and lower airway muscles of the fetal lamb in utero. Pediatr Res 1988; 23: 257-61.
[http://dx.doi.org/10.1203/00006450-198803000-00005]

[21]    Wallen-Mackenzie A, Gezelius H, Thoby-Brisson M, *et al.* Vesicular glutamate transporter 2 is required for central respiratory rhythm generation but not for locomotor central pattern generation. J Neurosci 2006; 26: 12294-307.
[http://dx.doi.org/10.1523/JNEUROSCI.3855-06.2006]

[22] Corcoran AE, Hodges MR, Wu Y, *et al.* Medullary serotonin neurons and central CO2 chemoreception. Respir Physiol Neurobiol 2009; 168: 49-58.
[http://dx.doi.org/10.1016/j.resp.2009.04.014]

[23] Wong-Riley MT, Liu Q. Neurochemical development of brain stem nuclei involved in the control of respiration. Respir Physiol Neurobiol 2005; 149: 83-98.
[http://dx.doi.org/10.1016/j.resp.2005.01.011]

[24] Bouvier J, Thoby-Brisson M, Renier N, *et al.* Hindbrain interneurons and axon guidance signaling critical for breathing. Nat Neurosci 2010; 13: 1066-74.
[http://dx.doi.org/10.1038/nn.2622]

[25] Janczewski WA, Feldman JL. Distinct rhythm generators for inspiration and expiration in the juvenile rat. J Physiol 2006; 570: 407-20.
[http://dx.doi.org/10.1113/jphysiol.2005.098848]

[26] Rigatto H, Lee D, Davi M, *et al.* Effect of increased arterial CO2 on fetal breathing and behavior in sheep. J Appl Physiol 1988; 64: 982-7.

[27] Kuipers IM, Maertzdorf WJ, De Jong DS, *et al.* The effect of hypercapnia and hypercapnia associated with central cooling on breathing in unanesthetized fetal lambs. Pediatr Res 1997; 41: 90-5.
[http://dx.doi.org/10.1203/00006450-199701000-00014]

[28] Blanco CE, Dawes GS, Hanson MA, *et al.* The response to hypoxia of arterial chemoreceptors in fetal sheep and new-born lambs. J Physiol 1984; 351: 25-37.
[http://dx.doi.org/10.1113/jphysiol.1984.sp015229]

[29] Adamson SL, Kuipers IM, Olson DM. Umbilical cord occlusion stimulates breathing independent of blood gases and pH. J Appl Physiol 1991; 70: 1796-809.

[30] Koos BJ, Maeda T, Jan C. Adenosine A(1) and A(2A) receptors modulate sleep state and breathing in fetal sheep. J Appl Physiol 2001; 91: 343-50.

[31] lvaro R, de Almeida V, al-Alaiyan S, *et al.* A placental extract inhibits breathing induced by umbilical cord occlusion in fetal sheep. J Dev Physiol 1993; 19: 23-8.

[32] Hillman NH, Kallapur SG, Jobe AH. Physiology of transition from intrauterine to extrauterine life. Clin Perinatol 2012; 39: 769-83.
[http://dx.doi.org/10.1016/j.clp.2012.09.009]

[33] Parmelee AH, Stern E, Harris MA. Maturation of respiration in prematures and young infants. Neuropadiatrie 1972; 3: 294-304.
[http://dx.doi.org/10.1055/s-0028-1091768]

[34] Tourneux P, Cardot V, Museux N, *et al.* Influence of thermal drive on central sleep apnea in the preterm neonate. Sleep 2008; 31: 549-56.
[http://dx.doi.org/10.1093/sleep/31.4.549]

[35] Khan A, Qurashi M, Kwiatkowski K, *et al.* Measurement of the CO2 apneic threshold in newborn infants: possible relevance for periodic breathing and apnea. J Appl Physiol 2005; 98: 1171-6.
[http://dx.doi.org/10.1152/japplphysiol.00574.2003]

[36] Das S, Mindell J, Millet GC, *et al.* Pediatric polysomnography: the patient and family perspective. J Clin Sleep Med 2011; 7: 81-7.

[37] Kahlke PE, Witmans MB, Alabdoulsalam T, *et al.* Full-night *versus* 4h evening polysomnography in children less than 2 years of age. Sleep Med 2013; 14: 177-82.
[http://dx.doi.org/10.1016/j.sleep.2012.10.016]

[38] Marcus CL, Keens TG, Ward SL. Comparison of nap and overnight polysomnography in children. Pediatr Pulmonol 1992; 13: 16-21.
[http://dx.doi.org/10.1002/ppul.1950130106]

[39]    Kirk VG, Bohn SG, Flemons WW, *et al.* Comparison of home oximetry monitoring with laboratory polysomnography in children. Chest 2003; 124: 1702-8.
[http://dx.doi.org/10.1378/chest.124.5.1702]

[40]    Foo JY, Parsley CL, Wilson SJ, *et al.* Detection of central respiratory events using pulse transit time in infants. Conf Proc IEEE Eng Med Biol Soc 2005; 3: 2579-82.

[41]    Woughter M1. Perkins AM2, Baldassari CM. Is MRI Necessary in the Evaluation of Pediatric Central Sleep Apnea? Otolaryngol Head Neck Surg 2015; 153(6): 1031-5.
[http://dx.doi.org/10.1177/0194599815597215]

[42]    Rosen GM, Shor AC, Geller TJ. Sleep in children with cancer. Curr Opin Pediatr 2008; 20: 676-68172.
[http://dx.doi.org/10.1097/MOP.0b013e328312c7ad]

[43]    Weintraub Z, Alvaro R, Kwiatkowski K, *et al.* Effects of inhaled oxygen (up to 40%) on periodic breathing and apnea in preterm infants. J Appl Physiol 1992; 72: 116-20.

[44]    Dhamija R, Wetjen NM, Slocumb NL, *et al.* The role of nocturnal polysomnography in assessing children with Chiari type I malformation. Clin Neurol Neurosurg 2013; 115: 1837-41.
[http://dx.doi.org/10.1016/j.clineuro.2013.05.025]

[45]    Khatwa U, Ramgopal S, Mylavarapu A, *et al.* MRI findings and sleep apnea in children with Chiari I malformation. Pediatr Neurol 2013; 48: 299-307.
[http://dx.doi.org/10.1016/j.pediatrneurol.2012.12.009]

[46]    Addo NK, Javadpour S, Kandasamy J, *et al.* Central sleep apnea and associated Chiari malformation in children with syndromic craniosynostosis: treatment and outcome data from a supraregional national craniofacial center. J Neurosurg Pediatr 2013; 11: 296-30173.
[http://dx.doi.org/10.3171/2012.11.PEDS12297]

[47]    Henderson-Smart DJ, Steer PA. Caffeine versus theophylline for apnea in preterm infants. Cochrane Database Syst Rev 2010. (CD000273)

[48]    Jennifer L. Miller, M.D. Sleep Disordered Breathing in Infants with Prader-Willi Syndrome During the First 6 Weeks of Growth Hormone Therapy: A Pilot Study. J Clin Sleep Med 2009; 5(5): 448-53.

[49]    Quijano-Roy S, Galan L, Ferreiro A, *et al.* Severe progressive form of congenital muscular dystrophy with calf pseudohypertrophy, macroglossia and respiratory insufficiency. Neuromuscul Disord 2002; 12: 466-75.
[http://dx.doi.org/10.1016/S0960-8966(01)00331-5]

[50]    Pinard JM, Azabou E, Essid N, *et al.* Sleep-disordered breathing in children with congenital muscular dystrophies. Eur J Paediatr Neurol 2012; 16: 619-24.
[http://dx.doi.org/10.1016/j.ejpn.2012.02.009]

[51]    Suresh S, Wales P, Dakin C, *et al.* Sleep-related breathing disorder in Duchenne muscular dystrophy: disease spectrum in the paediatric population. J Paediatr Child Health 2005; 41: 500-3.
[http://dx.doi.org/10.1111/j.1440-1754.2005.00691.x]

[52]    Labanowski M, Schmidt-Nowara W, Guilleminault C. Sleep and neuromuscular disease: frequency of sleep-disordered breathing in a neuromuscular disease clinic population. Neurology 1996; 47: 1173-80.
[http://dx.doi.org/10.1212/WNL.47.5.1173]

[53]    Kryger MH, Steljes DG, Yee WC, *et al.* Central sleep apnoea in congenital muscular dystrophy. J Neurol Neurosurg Psychiatry 1991; 54: 710-2.
[http://dx.doi.org/10.1136/jnnp.54.8.710]

[54]    Duenas-Meza E, Bazurto-Zapata MA, Gozal D, González-García M, Durán-Cantolla J, Torres-Duque CA. Overnight Polysomnographic Characteristics and Oxygen Saturation of Healthy Infants, 1 to 18 Months of Age, Born and Residing At High Altitude (2,640 Meters). Chest 2015; 148(1): 120-7.

[http://dx.doi.org/10.1378/chest.14-3207]

[55]    Schmidt B, Roberts RS, Davis P, *et al.* Caffeine therapy for apnea of prematurity. N Engl J Med 2006;
        354: 2112-21.
        [http://dx.doi.org/10.1056/NEJMoa054065]

[56]    Bhat RY, Hannam S, Pressler R, *et al.* Effect of prone and supine position on sleep, apneas, and
        arousal in preterm infants. Pediatrics 2006; 118: 101-7.
        [http://dx.doi.org/10.1542/peds.2005-1873]

[57]    Al-Saif S, Alvaro R, Manfreda J, *et al.* A randomized controlled trial of theophylline *versus* CO2
        inhalation for treating apnea of prematurity. J Pediatr 2008; 153: 513-8.
        [http://dx.doi.org/10.1016/j.jpeds.2008.04.025]

[58]    Edwards BA, Sands SA, Feeney C, *et al.* Continuous positive airway pressure reduces loop gain and
        resolves periodic central apneas in the lamb. Respir Physiol Neurobiol 2009; 168: 239-49.
        [http://dx.doi.org/10.1016/j.resp.2009.07.006]

[59]    Bloch-Salisbury E, Indic P, Bednarek F, *et al.* Stabilizing immature breathing patterns of preterm
        infants using stochastic mechanosensory stimulation. J Appl Physiol 2009; 107: 1017-27.
        [http://dx.doi.org/10.1152/japplphysiol.00058.2009]

[60]    Philippi H, Bieber I, Reitter B. Acetazolamide treatment for infantile central sleep apnea. J Child
        Neurol 2001; 16: 600-3.
        [http://dx.doi.org/10.1177/088307380101600813]

[61]    Zagol K, Lake DE, Vergales B, *et al.* Anemia, apnea of prematurity, and blood transfusions. J Pediatr
        2012; 161: 417-421.e1.
        [http://dx.doi.org/10.1016/j.jpeds.2012.02.044]

[62]    Szollosi I, Jones M, Morrell MJ, *et al.* Effect of CO2 inhalation on central sleep apnea and arousals
        from sleep. Respiration 2004; 71: 493-8.
        [http://dx.doi.org/10.1159/000080634]

[63]    Khayat RN, Xie A, Patel AK, *et al.* Cardiorespiratory effects of added dead space in patients with
        heart failure and central sleep apnea. Chest 2003; 123: 1551-60.
        [http://dx.doi.org/10.1378/chest.123.5.1551]

[64]    Shore ET, Millman RP. Central sleep apnea and acetazolamide therapy. Arch Intern Med 1983; 143:
        1278-80.
        [http://dx.doi.org/10.1001/archinte.1983.00350060210040]

[65]    Nakayama H, Smith CA, Rodman JR, *et al.* Effect of ventilatory drive on carbon dioxide sensitivity
        below eupnea during sleep. Am J Respir Crit Care Med 2002; 165: 1251-60.
        [http://dx.doi.org/10.1164/rccm.2110041]

# CHAPTER 14

# Practical Considerations in the Treatment of Pediatric Obstructive Sleep Apnea

**Amal Isaiah** and **Seckin O. Ulualp**[*]

*Department of Otolaryngology— Head and Neck Surgery, University of Texas Southwestern Medical Center, Dallas, Texas, USA*

**Abstract:** Obstructive sleep apnea syndrome (OSAS), affecting about 5% of all children, has positioned itself to be a major epidemiological problem in the United States. The prevalence of this condition appears to be increasing over time, in parallel with the growth in childhood obesity. Pediatric OSAS belongs to a spectrum of respiratory disorders called sleep-disordered breathing (SDB), caused by varying degrees of paroxysmal upper airway obstruction during sleep. Left untreated, OSAS has potential to progress over time, leading to not just fragmented sleep, but also neurocognitive problems, and in the most severe instances, serious cardiopulmonary adverse effects. The treatment of OSAS involves a structured series of steps spanning medical and surgical approaches, including adenotonsillectomy, which is considered the gold standard for management of childhood OSAS. This chapter provides a review of the epidemiology of OSAS, followed by a discussion of natural history, treatment and follow up.

**Keywords:** Adenotonsillectomy, Obesity, Pediatric obstructive sleep apnea, Snoring.

## INTRODUCTION

Sleep is a physiological state of quiescence that facilitates recovery of body functions. Most cardiopulmonary parameters are minimized to conserve energy expenditure during sleep. As a consequence, ventilatory drive reaches an expected nadir compared to wakefulness. Relaxation of upper airway musculature also increases the preponderance towards airflow obstruction. These changes principally manifest in an overall reduction in ventilatory volumes [1].

Previous studies have clearly shown that despite the tendency towards upper airway obstruction, healthy infants and children still maintain normal airflow

---
[*] **Corresponding author Seckin O. Ulualp**: Department of Otolaryngology—Head and Neck Surgery, University of Texas Southwestern Medical Center, Dallas, Texas, USA; Tel: (214) 456-3862; Fax: (214) 648-9122; Email: Seckin.ulualp@utsouthwestern.edu

without significant hindrance. However, as function of age, development and changes in body physiology, the tendency towards obstruction is not uniform across all age groups [2].

Sleep-disordered breathing (SDB) represents a broad spectrum of clinical disorders, all of which have pathologic upper airway obstruction as the common factor. SDB has continued to grow in prevalence over time, and accounts for a significant amount of public health burden [3], with estimates ranging from 1-15% by various studies [4]. It is therefore of paramount importance to maintain a strong degree of clinical suspicion when children present with history of snoring.

## Sleep-Disordered Breathing

The term SDB encompasses three principal categories, based on the severity of upper airway obstruction, and includes (i) primary snoring, (ii) upper airway resistance syndrome (UARS) and (iii) obstructive sleep apnea syndrome (OSAS). It is to be noted that accurate distinction between these three conditions requires diagnostic testing, specifically polysomnography (PSG), also called a sleep study [5].

In the mildest form of SDB, called primary snoring, there is intermittent nocturnal airflow obstruction that results in turbulence (snoring); however there are no clinical features that suggest that duration and architecture of sleep are abnormal. Primary snoring has a conservative estimate of around 7% according to one study based on administration of a questionnaire to parents of children in primary school [6]. In the same study, the authors also described an association of the condition with (i) presence of asthma and (ii) exposure to cigarette smoking. However, the utility of clinical history alone to distinguish between primary snoring alone and more severe forms of SDB has been questioned in the past [7], and this is important given that snoring seems to be associated with significant neurobehavioral deficits in a subset of children, possibly related to increased susceptibility to sleep fragmentation [8]. Others have demonstrated that primary snoring does not progress significantly over time [9].

Upper airway resistance syndrome occupies an intermediate position in the spectrum of SDB. This term was coined to describe a subset of patients who do not meet the criteria for OSAS by PSG standards, yet they present with symptoms that most closely resemble chronic upper airway obstruction. The pathophysiology of UARS has been related to abnormal maxillomandibular anatomy, and may respond to orthodontic treatment [10].

## Epidemiology

The prevalence of pediatric SDB and OSAS continue to grow since there has been a recent increase in awareness of the problem, yet the vast majority remain undiagnosed. Epidemiologic estimates place the population burden to be at about 7.45% when estimated by examining the prevalence by parental reports of snoring [11]. The same meta-analysis by strict criteria of *always snoring* reported SDB to be in the range of 1.5-6% and when the criteria changed to *often*, the prevalence increased to 3.2-14.8%. It is to be noted that the prevalence of OSAS parallels the prevalence of SDB, as the latter requires a PSG for diagnosis.

Race is an independent risk factor for SDB, with African-American children having greater preponderance towards developing the condition [12]. Hormonal influence on SDB manifests in a slight increase in prevalence among prepubertal boys, however this association has not been consistently demonstrated [6]. Despite a paucity of data from very young children, it is generally regarded that SDB decreased over time between 4 and 12 years of age [13].

The association between obesity and SDB and/or OSAS is unambiguous. Most studies that investigated this relationship have generally concluded that obesity increases the risk of SDB as well as the non-response to treatment [14, 15].

Environmental factors play a role in increased susceptibility to pediatric OSAS, and generally also include indicators of neighborhood disadvantage—specifically factors that span (i) second hand smoke exposure and (ii) low socioeconomic status [16]. These factors remained even after controlling for the effects of prematurity and obesity.

## Pathophysiology of OSA

A complex interplay of anatomical and physiologic factors is hypothesized to contribute to development of upper airway obstruction as seen in pediatric OSAS. Fixed anatomical obstruction may be attributed to narrowing at the level of the lumen, soft tissue or the craniofacial skeleton [17]. Secondary risk factors originate from disordered control of neuromuscular tone responsible for maintaining upper airway patency during sleep.

The upper airway in children with pediatric OSAS is thought to be modeled as a *Starling* resistor [18], in which airflow obstruction occurs as a function of the closing pressure within the airway lumen, termed critical closing pressure ($P_{crit}$). This index is a composite measure of both viscoelastic and neuromuscular properties of the upper airway. When $P_{crit}$ falls below threshold, airflow obstruction occurs consistently. Children with OSAS are known to have higher

$P_{crit}$ values compared to normal children without OSAS.

Maintenance of neuromuscular tone is essential to prevention of upper airway collapsibility during sleep. Pharyngeal dilator muscles act together to improve airflow by dilation of the upper airway. Abnormalities of neuromuscular tone as seen in conditions such as Down syndrome may contribute to the increased prevalence of OSAS in that population [19].

Narrowing at the level of the lumen is most consistently associated with hypertrophy of lymphoid tissues at the level of oropharynx (tonsils) and nasopharynx (adenoids). This finding has a robust association with tonsillectomy and adenoidectomy (T&A) leading to significant improvement of OSAS in most children [20]. Normal age-related increase in lymphoid tissue that trails the expansion of upper airway may play a role in the increased incidence seen in children under the age of 5 [21]. When examined under general anesthesia, the overall cross-section of the pharyngeal airway in children with OSAS has been shown to be significantly reduced in comparison with normal children without OSA [22].

## Clinical Features of Pediatric OSAS

Clinical evaluation for suspected OSAS is based primarily on parental reporting of symptoms. It is important to screen for OSAS even in healthy children given the reported increase in prevalence in recent years.

Standardized questionnaires have shown that untreated OSAS may be considerably detrimental for quality of life (QOL), and that timely treatment such as T&A provides relief [23]. The burden of pediatric OSAS on QOL is estimated to be similar to that of juvenile rheumatoid arthritis.

The symptoms of OSAS proceeds can be varied across different age groups as shown in Table **1**. Snoring, daytime sleepiness and abnormal behavior are present more consistently than other symptoms in children over the age of 12 months. Although snoring is a hallmark of upper airway obstruction, it is important to note that the presence of snoring alone cannot predict the presence of OSAS as opposed to primary snoring alone [7]. Although excessive daytime sleepiness has been shown to be associated with undiagnosed OSAS, this is observed more frequently in adults as children appear to present with hyperactivity rather than sleepiness. In these children, the spectrum of behavioral problems spans lack of attention, aggression and poor academic performance [24]. Nocturnal enuresis is also known to occur with an increased frequency in children with OSAS, and this may attributed to the effect of OSAS on the arousal response, bladder pressure or urinary hormone secretion [25]. The alteration in vascular responses to untreated

OSAS may progress to hypertension with a potential increase in risk of future cardiovascular disease [26]. Few case series have documented decreased growth, right ventricular dysfunction as well as metabolic syndromes including insulin resistance.

**Table 1. Comparison of various surgical procedures indicated for treatment of OSAS, with their ideal population and benefits/risks. Modified from Gungor *et al.* [51]**

| Therapy | Population | Benefits | Risks/challenges |
|---|---|---|---|
| Tonsillectomy and Adenoidectomy | Children with enlarged tonsils and/or adenoids | Highly effective; well-tolerated in most children | Common: pain, decreased oral tolerance; rarely hemorrhage, respiratory complications, *etc.* |
| Partial tonsillectomy and adenoidectomy | Children with enlarged tonsils±adenoids | Shorter recovery time than extracapsular tonsillectomy | Efficacy in treating OSAS less-established; effect of tonsillar regrowth on OSAS unknown |
| Lingual tonsillectomy | Persistent OSAS after AT with enlarged lingual tonsils | Definitive therapy for residual OSAS in | Concentric scarring in airway; efficacy/ideal population not well-established in OSAS |
| Tracheostomy | Children with severe OSAS and no other therapeutic option | Highly effective | Requires increased monitoring at home; increased risk of significant complications |
| Bariatric surgery | Select obese teenagers that have failed other therapies | Small studies show high short term success rate in select populations | Significant complications; no long-term efficacy data; success varies by center/type of surgery |
| Craniofacial surgery | Select children with craniofacial conditions | Highly effective in select populations | Minimal long-term follow-up data; success varies by center/type of surgery; significant morbidity |

Notwithstanding the heterogeneous nature of symptoms associated with pediatric OSAS, the constantly increasing role of obesity merits discussion. Several large population studies have demonstrated clear association, and screening for OSAS in obese children is of paramount importance. Using relatively conservative criteria, the prevalence of OSAS is between 22 and 40% in obese, yet otherwise healthy children [27].

The most resilient association between OSAS and physical examination findings has been seen in the form of hypertrophy of lymphoid tissue within the palatine tonsils (Fig. **1**) and the nasopharynx, which manifests as adenotonsillar hypertrophy [1].

This reflects favorably in treatment response to T&A, even in patients with other potential obstruction, such as obese children. Objective assessments of potential sites of upper airway obstruction have substantial value in determining the pre-test probability of OSAS, as well as to gauge potential response to first line treatment in the form of T&A.

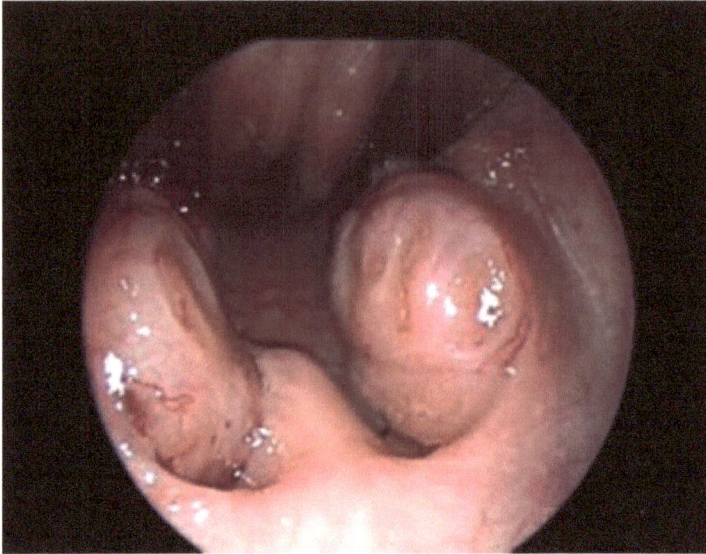

**Fig. (1).** Hypertrophy of tonsillar tissue. The grading of tonsillar hypertrophy ranges from 0 (no tonsillar tissue) to 4+ (tonsillar hypertrophy with midline contact).

A routine head and neck examination should be performed in all children suspected to have OSA. The first site of obstruction is the nasal cavity as well as the nasopharynx; more commonly, nasal airflow obstruction could occur as a result of nasal septal deviation as well as inferior turbinate hypertrophy. Nasal airflow obstruction occurring very early in life should prompt evaluation for obstruction resulting from congenital masses or anatomical malformations such as choanal atresia and congenital pyriform aperture stenosis. In older children with history of allergies, anterior rhinoscopy may reveal nasal polyposis in combination with inferior turbinate hypertrophy.

Standardized scales exist for assessment of tonsil size (0-4+) as well as palate position [28]. Although these have a subjective component based on interpretation by the examining clinician, objective assessments from patients undergoing T&A have been demonstrated to be significantly predictive of OSA severity.

Early onset of upper airway obstruction resulting in stridor may point to laryngomalacia, which is related to structural immaturity of the laryngeal framework. Poor weight gain, cyanotic spells and apneic events may follow, which may require a flexible endoscopic assessment for confirmation of diagnosis [29]. In addition, most children with disorders of tone resulting in upper airway obstruction present early in life, and OSAS is more likely to persist even after appropriate treatment is initiated [30].

Structural variation of craniofacial morphology as determined by radiological studies using standard metrics of facial growth have highlighted a role for screening for certain facial features that occur with increasing frequency in OSAS. The combination of a long face, reduced nasal prominence and width, and a retrognathic mandible represent a constellation of craniofacial features of SDB that may warrant a referral to specialists for the evaluation of other clinical symptoms [31].

## Diagnostic Testing

Diagnosis of pediatric OSAS follows clinical suspicion, history and physical examination findings, with confirmation using standard overnight polysomnography (PSG).

Numerous diagnostic tools have been proposed for confirmation of diagnosis of OSAS. The role of PSG has been considered to be the gold standard for this purpose. Although other diagnostic modalities continue to be devised, they are often abbreviated derivatives of PSG and their utility has never been completely proven. Consensus statements [32] have been established consolidating respiratory indications for performing PSG in children [33] as well as normative values in this population [34].

Polysomnography for children includes several modifications intended to improve the reliability and validity of diagnosis. These include a child-friendly approach atmosphere and approach, smaller and specialized equipment, and comprise age-adjusted ruled for scoring and interpretation of PSGs [35]. Polysomnography does record from multiple channels of physiologic information, including electroencephalography, electromyography, electrooculography, cardiac rhythm, pulse oximetry arterial oxygen saturation ($SpO_2$), chest wall and abdomen motion, oral and nasal airflow, and end-tidal $PCO_2$ ($PEtCO_2$).

The principal parameter used to determine the severity of OSAS from a PSG is called the apnea-hypopnea index (AHI). The manner in which AHI is determined in children is slightly different when compared with adults, owing to the faster respiratory rate as observed in the pediatric population [35]. Obstructive apnea is complete cessation of airflow over two respiratory cycles, and hypopnea is defined as a 50% reduction in airflow associated with an arousal, or $\geq 3\%$ desaturation. Obstructive events occur more frequently during REM sleep, and hence a sufficient proportion of REM sleep needs to be present to accurately determine the presence and severity of OSAS. Although there are not enough studies determining the prognostic significance of AHI on morbidity, for all practical purposes, an AHI $\geq 1$ but $< 5$ is considered mild OSAS, with moderate and severe OSAS being AHI $\geq 5$ and $\geq 10$ respectively. Most practitioners choose to treat OSAS when AHI $>1$.

The value of PSG in the setting of treatment of OSAS needs to be carefully weighed against costs as well as availability. If all children with SDB were to get PSG for confirmation of diagnosis, this can force a substantial amount of stress on economic resources. Although almost all guidelines generally take this into consideration, consensus statements from different organizations do have slight differences in their approach towards indications for pediatric PSG.

The clinical practice guidelines from the American Academy of Pediatrics [32] recommends PSG as the first line diagnostic test in *all patients* with snoring *or with suspicion* for pediatric OSA. These guidelines also suggest referral to a specialist, such as a sleep physician or an otolaryngologist for further evaluation and management. The American Academy for Otolaryngology—Head and Neck Surgery [36] on the other hand determined that the first step in the management of childhood SDB is T&A, with PSG indicated in patients presenting with medical comorbidities, or in whom the diagnosis is uncertain due to discordance between parental reporting and physical examination findings (*e.g.* tonsil size).

Abbreviated testing derived from full-panel PSGs continue to undergo validation *via* several studies. Unfortunately, their value in the diagnosis of OSAS has not been fully established. However, in the ideal setting, and specifically in otherwise healthy children, tests such as nocturnal oximetry could establish a definitive diagnosis for straightforward OSAS due to adenotonsillar hypertrophy in older children, or at least identify those children who can undergo definitive diagnosis with PSG.

Screening methods using questionnaires have been described in literature. Chervin *et al.* [37] first described the pediatric sleep questionnaire (PSQ), which has been shown to have moderate correlation with a diagnosis of OSAS, but only to be of utility for research applications, and not for individual patients.

There are several methods are used to determine the degree of obstruction within the upper airway. These include (i) cephalometry [38], (ii) drug induced sleep endoscopy [39] and (iii) cine magnetic resonance imaging [40]. Due to the additional costs, use of anesthesia or exposure to ionizing radiation in these methods, they are only used in the context of persistent OSAS after initial treatment with T&A (Fig. **2**).

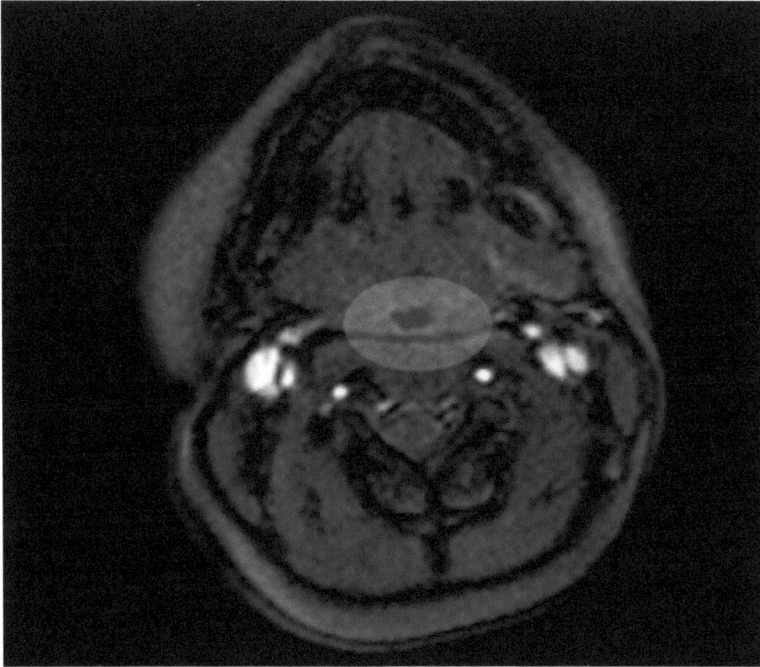

**Fig. (2).** Cine MRI for localization of upper airway obstruction. In this T1-weighted sequence from a child with persistent OSA after T&A, the highlighted area shows narrowing of the upper airway from pharyngeal fat deposition.

## Treatment of Pediatric OSAS

Due to the risk of morbidity as a result of untreated OSAS, most clinicians choose to treat even mild OSAS. A large number of treatment options do exist, and may be broadly categorized as medical or surgical.

The first line treatment option for OSA is T&A. There is robust evidence that shows substantial therapeutic response to T&A even when comorbidities are present. Unless clear surgical contraindications exist, T&A should be considered in every child with OSA. In a study of 79 children who underwent T&A for OSA showed dramatic improvement in respiratory parameters as measured by PSG in the majority of children, with resulting increase in quality of life [20]. This was confirmed by a large randomized controlled trial, which also demonstrated that early T&A leads to greater improvements in behavioral, quality of life and PSG findings, when compared with watchful waiting [41].

Tonsillectomy and adenoidectomy is performed by an otolaryngologist under general anesthesia, with a variety of techniques ranging from cold dissection of the tonsils to use of electrocautery or even radiofrequency ablation. Alternating doses of ibuprofen and acetaminophen provided an effective treatment for post-tonsillectomy pain in the majority of children and did not increase rate of bleeding [42]. Due to alterations in ventilatory control in children with OSAS, opioids are generally not prescribed for pain control currently. Titrated dosing of opioids as part of modified anesthetic protocols has also been shown to improve recovery following T&A [43]. The overall risk of bleeding is about 5-10% [44], unaffected by the surgical technique or perioperative medications. Any significant bleeding in the postoperative period requires hospital-based observation at the minimum, and control in the operating room when clinically appropriate.

Although most T&As are performed as outpatient surgical procedures, some children with risk factors for perioperative obstructive events require admission to the hospital for observation following the procedure.

A subset of patients are at risk of recidivism despite T&A. Teenagers and children with obesity, comorbidities including neurological/developmental/craniofacial abnormalities alone or in combination with asthma, or severe OSA have a high risk of residual OSA [45]. These patients are subsequently referred to the sleep physician for potentially considering continuous positive air pressure (CPAP) therapy. Although CPAP is highly effective in the management of residual OSAS, compliance is very low [46]. In some instances, inhaled nasal corticosteroids in combination with systemic anti-inflammatory therapy (*e.g.* oral leukotriene inhibitors) are successful for treatment of mild residual OSA [47].

Other surgical methods used for the treatment of pediatric OSAS are summarized in Table **1**. These are most commonly used for persistent OSAS despite T&A. Additional evaluation using one of the methods described in the section on diagnosis is essential prior to determining surgical candidacy. Tracheostomy is the most definitive therapy for OSAS and leads to complete resolution in 100% of patients. It is reserved for intractable and very severe OSAS with downstream cardiopulmonary complications with increased risk of mortality.

Although T&A is still highly efficacious even in patients with obesity [48] and the necessity for repeat post-tonsillectomy PSG has not been established, it should be considered in patients with higher risk of persistence, including obese patients, children with severe OSAS, craniofacial malformations and Down syndrome.

There is clear evidence from adult patients with OSAS to suggest that upper airway collapsibility is improved following weight control, with a corresponding increase in airflow as well as decrease in pharyngeal closing pressures [49]. With the robust relationship between obesity and OSAS, weight management should be considered in these children, and should be the mainstay, along with CPAP therapy in whom OSAS is persistent despite T&A [50, 51].

# CONCLUSION

With rising prevalence, pediatric OSAS continues to contribute to significant epidemiologic burden in the U.S. and elsewhere. Screening is critical to prevent cardiopulmonary and neurobehavioral adverse effects of the condition. Most children with OSAS are treated effectively by T&A, which addresses the most likely site of upper airway obstruction due to adenotonsillar hypertrophy. Although success rates are very high, the rising proportion of children with obesity is causing an increase in number of children with persistent OSAS. Treatment options for persistent OSAS continue to evolve and are primarily based on a trial of CPAP therapy initially and options such as multi-level sleep surgery exercised for non-compliance with CPAP therapy. Anti-inflammatory medications and nasal corticosteroids have an adjunctive role.

With an alarming increase in the prevalence of childhood obesity, the economic and public health costs of childhood OSAS will be unsustainable by the present health care system. It is therefore of paramount importance to examine options for primary prevention of the condition.

## CONFLICT OF INTEREST

The authors declare no conflict of interest, financial or otherwise.

## ACKNOWLEDGMENTS

Declared none.

## REFERENCES

[1]     Marcus CL. Sleep-disordered breathing in children. Am J Respir Crit Care Med 2001; 164(1): 16-30.

[2]     Tabachnik E, Muller NL, Bryan AC, Levison H. Changes in ventilation and chest wall mechanics during sleep in normal adolescents. J Appl Physiol 1981; 51(3): 557-64.

[3]     Redline S, Tishler P V, Schluchter M, Aylor J, Clark K, Graham G. Risk factors for sleep-disordered breathing in children. Associations with obesity, race, and respiratory problems Am J Respir Crit Care Med 1999 May; 159(5 Pt 1): 1527-32.

[4]     Bonuck KA, Chervin RD, Cole TJ, *et al.* Prevalence and persistence of sleep disordered breathing symptoms in young children: a 6-year population-based cohort study. Sleep 2011; 34(7): 875-84.

[5]     Marcus C L, Omlin K J, Basinki D J, *et al.* Normal polysomnographic values for children and adolescents. Am Rev Respir Dis 1992 Nov; 146(5 Pt 1): 1235-9.

[6]     Ersu R, Arman AR, Save D, *et al.* Prevalence of snoring and symptoms of sleep-disordered breathing in primary school children in Istanbul. Chest 2004; 126(1): 19-24.

[7]     Carroll JL, McColley SA, Marcus CL, Curtis S, Loughlin GM. Inability of clinical history to distinguish primary snoring from obstructive sleep apnea syndrome in children. Chest 1995; 108(3): 610-8.

[8] O'Brien LM, Mervis CB, Holbrook CR, *et al.* Neurobehavioral implications of habitual snoring in children. Pediatrics 2004; 114(1): 44-9.

[9] Marcus CL, Hamer A, Loughlin GM. Natural history of primary snoring in children. Pediatr Pulmonol 1998; 26(1): 6-11.

[10] Guilleminault C, Khramtsov A. Upper airway resistance syndrome in children: a clinical review. Semin Pediatr Neurol 2001; 8(4): 207-15.

[11] Lumeng JC, Chervin RD. Epidemiology of pediatric obstructive sleep apnea. Proc Am Thorac Soc 2008; 5(2): 242-52.

[12] Johnson EO, Roth T. An epidemiologic study of sleep-disordered breathing symptoms among adolescents. Sleep 2006; 29(9): 1135-42.

[13] Zhang G, Spickett J, Rumchev K, Lee AH, Stick S. Snoring in primary school children and domestic environment: a Perth school based study. Respir Res 2004; 5: 19.

[14] Capdevila OS, Kheirandish-Gozal L, Dayyat E, Gozal D. Pediatric obstructive sleep apnea: complications, management, and long-term outcomes. Proc Am Thorac Soc 2008; 5(2): 274-82.

[15] null Delasnerie-Laupretre, null Patois, null Valatx, null Kauffmann, and null Alperovitch, "Sleep, snoring and smoking in high school students. J Sleep Res 1993; 2(3): 138-42.

[16] Spilsbury JC, Storfer-Isser A, Kirchner HL, *et al.* Neighborhood disadvantage as a risk factor for pediatric obstructive sleep apnea. J Pediatr 2006; 149(3): 342-7.

[17] Katz ES, D'Ambrosio CM. Pathophysiology of pediatric obstructive sleep apnea. Proc Am Thorac Soc 2008; 5(2): 253-62.

[18] Fregosi R F, Quan S F, Morgan W L, *et al.* Pharyngeal critical pressure in children with mild sleep-disordered breathing J Appl Physiol Bethesda Md 1985 2006 Sep; 101(3): 734-9.

[19] Maris M, Verhulst S, Wojciechowski M, Van de Heyning P, Boudewyns A. Prevalence of Obstructive Sleep Apnea in Children with Down Syndrome. Sleep 2016; 39(3): 699-704.

[20] Mitchell RB. Adenotonsillectomy for obstructive sleep apnea in children: outcome evaluated by pre- and postoperative polysomnography. Laryngoscope 2007; 117(10): 1844-54.

[21] Arens R, Marcus CL. Pathophysiology of upper airway obstruction: a developmental perspective. Sleep 2004; 27(5): 997-1019.

[22] Isono S, Shimada A, Utsugi M, Konno A, Nishino T. Comparison of static mechanical properties of the passive pharynx between normal children and children with sleep-disordered breathing Am J Respir Crit Care Med 1998 Apr; 157(4 Pt 1): 1204-12.

[23] Baldassari CM, Mitchell RB, Schubert C, Rudnick EF. "Pediatric obstructive sleep apnea and quality of life: a meta-analysis," Otolaryngol.-Head Neck Surg. Off. J. Am. Acad. Otolaryngol Head Neck Surg 2008; 138(3): 265-73.

[24] Gottlieb DJ, Chase C, Vezina RM, *et al.* Sleep-disordered breathing symptoms are associated with poorer cognitive function in 5-year-old children. J Pediatr 2004; 145(4): 458-64.

[25] Brooks LJ, Topol HI. Enuresis in children with sleep apnea. J Pediatr 2003; 142(5): 515-8.

[26] Kang K-T, Chiu S-N, Weng W-C, Lee P-L, Hsu W-C. Analysis of 24-Hour Ambulatory Blood Pressure Monitoring in Children With Obstructive Sleep Apnea: A Hospital-Based Study Medicine (Baltimore) 2015 Oct; 94(40): e1568.

[27] Alonso-Álvarez ML, Cordero-Guevara JA, Terán-Santos J, *et al.* Obstructive sleep apnea in obese community-dwelling children: the NANOS study. Sleep 2014; 37(5): 943-9.

[28] Howard NS, Brietzke SE. "Pediatric tonsil size: objective vs subjective measurements correlated to overnight polysomnogram," Otolaryngol.-Head Neck Surg. Off. J. Am. Acad. Otolaryngol Head Neck Surg 2009; 140(5): 675-81.

[29]　Zafereo ME, Taylor RJ, Pereira KD. Supraglottoplasty for laryngomalacia with obstructive sleep apnea. Laryngoscope 2008; 118(10): 1873-7.

[30]　Goldberg S, Shatz A, Picard E, *et al.* Endoscopic findings in children with obstructive sleep apnea: Effects of age and hypotonia. Pediatr Pulmonol 2005; 40(3): 205-10.

[31]　Al Ali A, Richmond S, Popat H, *et al.* The influence of snoring, mouth breathing and apnoea on facial morphology in late childhood: a three-dimensional study. BMJ Open 2015; 5(9): e009027.

[32]　Marcus C L, Brooks L J, Draper K A, *et al.* American Academy of Pediatrics. Diagnosis and management of childhood obstructive sleep apnea syndrome.Pediatrics 2012; 130(3): e714-55.

[33]　Aurora R N, Zak R S, Karippot A, *et al.* American Academy of Sleep Medicine. Practice parameters for the respiratory indications for polysomnography in children.Sleep 2011; 34(3): 379-88.

[34]　Montgomery-Downs HE, Gozal D. Snore-associated sleep fragmentation in infancy: mental development effects and contribution of secondhand cigarette smoke exposure. Pediatrics 2006; 117(3): e496-502.

[35]　Beck SE, Marcus CL. PEDIATRIC POLYSOMNOGRAPHY. Sleep Med Clin 2009; 4(3): 393-406.

[36]　Roland PS, Rosenfeld RM, Brooks LJ, *et al.* Clinical Practice Guideline Polysomnography for Sleep-Disordered Breathing Prior to Tonsillectomy in Children. Otolaryngol Head Neck Surg 2011; 145(1) (Suppl.): S1-S15.

[37]　Chervin RD, Weatherly RA, Garetz SL, *et al.* Pediatric sleep questionnaire: prediction of sleep apnea and outcomes. Arch Otolaryngol Head Neck Surg 2007; 133(3): 216-22.

[38]　Ozdemir H, Altin R, Söğüt A, *et al.* Craniofacial differences according to AHI scores of children with obstructive sleep apnoea syndrome: cephalometric study in 39 patients. Pediatr Radiol 2004; 34(5): 393-9.

[39]　Ulualp SO, Szmuk P. Drug-induced sleep endoscopy for upper airway evaluation in children with obstructive sleep apnea. Laryngoscope 2013; 123(1): 292-7.

[40]　Slaats MA, Van Hoorenbeeck K, Van Eyck A, *et al.* Upper airway imaging in pediatric obstructive sleep apnea syndrome. Sleep Med Rev 2015; 21: 59-71.

[41]　Marcus C L, Moore R H, Rosen C L, *et al.* Childhood Adenotonsillectomy Trial (CHAT). A randomized trial of adenotonsillectomy for childhood sleep apnea.N Engl J Med 2013; 368(25): 2366-76.

[42]　Liu C, Ulualp SO. Outcomes of an Alternating Ibuprofen and Acetaminophen Regimen for Pain Relief After Tonsillectomy in Children. Ann Otol Rhinol Laryngol 2015; 124(10): 777-81.

[43]　Isaiah A, Pereira KD. Outcomes after adenotonsillectomy using a fixed anesthesia protocol in children with obstructive sleep apnea. Int J Pediatr Otorhinolaryngol 2015; 79(5): 638-43.

[44]　Riggin L, Ramakrishna J, Sommer DD, Koren G. "A 2013 updated systematic review & meta-analysis of 36 randomized controlled trials; no apparent effects of non steroidal anti-inflammatory agents on the risk of bleeding after tonsillectomy," Clin. Otolaryngol. Off. J. ENT-UK Off. J. Neth. Soc. Oto-Rhino-Laryngol. Cervico-Facial Surg 2013; 38(2): 115-29.

[45]　Imanguli M, Ulualp SO. Risk factors for residual obstructive sleep apnea after adenotonsillectomy in children. Laryngoscope 2016.

[46]　Marcus CL, Rosen G, Ward SL, *et al.* Adherence to and effectiveness of positive airway pressure therapy in children with obstructive sleep apnea. Pediatrics 2006; 117(3): e442-51.

[47]　Kheirandish L, Goldbart AD, Gozal D. Intranasal steroids and oral leukotriene modifier therapy in residual sleep-disordered breathing after tonsillectomy and adenoidectomy in children. Pediatrics 2006; 117(1): e61-6.

[48]    Costa DJ, Mitchell R. "Adenotonsillectomy for obstructive sleep apnea in obese children: a meta-analysis," Otolaryngol.-Head Neck Surg. Off. J. Am. Acad. Otolaryngol Head Neck Surg 2009; 140(4): 455-60.

[49]    Schwartz A R, Gold A R, Schubert N, *et al.* Effect of weight loss on upper airway collapsibility in obstructive sleep apnea Am Rev Respir Dis 1991; 144(3 Pt 1): 494-8.

[50]    Guilleminault C, Lee JH, Chan A. Pediatric obstructive sleep apnea syndrome. Arch Pediatr Adolesc Med 2005; 159(8): 775-85.

[51]    Cielo CM, Gungor A. Treatment options for pediatric obstructive sleep apnea. Curr Probl Pediatr Adolesc Health Care 2016; 46(1): 27-33.

# CHAPTER 15

# State of the Art of the Diagnosis and Management of Gastroesophageal Reflux Disease

**Ricardo Medina-Centeno** and **Rinarani Sanghavi**[*]

*Department of Pediatrics, Division of Gastroenterology and Hepatology, University of Texas Southwestern Medical Center, Dallas, TX, USA*

**Abstract:** Involuntary passage of gastric contents into the esophagus may be physiologic (Gastroesophageal Reflux-GER) or may be associated with troublesome symptoms (Gastroesophageal Reflux disease-GERD). GER is common in infants and is related to immature anti reflux mechanisms. On the other hand, GERD needs further evaluation. Presenting features of both include esophageal symptoms like vomiting and extra esophageal symptoms such as irritability, reflux laryngitis, pharyngitis and dental erosions. Upper GI series is not recommended for diagnosing GERD. Traditional pH probe examinations have been replaced largely by combined multi-channel Impedance –pH monitoring which helps establish a temporal relationship between symptoms and pathological reflux, as well as ascertain the acidic *versus* non acidic, solid *versus* liquid or gas nature of the refluxate. Proton pump inhibitors remain the mainstay of treatment, along with H2 receptor antagonists and prokinetic agents. Surgical intervention should be reserved for selected severe cases.

**Keywords:** Antacids, Bravo pH monitoring, Combined Multiple Intraluminal Impedance (MII) and pH Monitoring, Endoscopy, Esophageal manometry, GER, GERD, Lifestyle changes, Manifestations, PH monitoring, Prevalence, Prokinetics, Upper GI imaging.

## Definitions

Gastroesophageal reflux (GER) is a normal physiological process in which there is an involuntary passage of gastric contents into the esophagus. Most of the reflux episodes are asymptomatic, having short duration, occurring several times per day, particularly after meals and limited to the distal esophagus. Commonly, a reflux episode results from a transient relaxation of the lower esophageal sphincter (LES). Other causes include increased abdominal pressure not accompanied by an increase in the pressure of the LES or conditions when the

[*] **Corresponding author Rinarani Sanghavi**: Department of Pediatrics, Division of Gastroenterology and Hepatology, University of Texas Southwestern Medical Center, Dallas, TX, USA; Tel: (214) 456-3862; Fax: (214) 648-9122; Email: rina.sanghavi@utsouthwestern.edu

**Seckin Ulualp (Ed.)**

LES pressure is reduced. Physiologic GER is a reflux episode associated with regurgitation or occasionally vomiting during the first months of life or in the absence of symptoms. GER is a frequently encountered problem in infancy and tends to self-resolve [1]. Gastroesophageal reflux disease (GERD) is when reflux of gastric contents is the cause of troublesome symptoms and/or complications such as esophagitis, nutritional compromise, respiratory complications or poor weight gain. Pathologic GERD may be primary or secondary. Secondary GERD is associated with a number of genetic syndromes such as Cornelia de Lange, chromosomal abnormalities such as Trisomy 21, birth defects such as congenital diaphragmatic hernia, omphalocele and gastroschisis, and neurologic conditions such as myotonic dystrophy [2].

Regurgitation, a common manifestation of reflux in infant and older children, is defined as effortless passage of refluxed gastric contents into the oropharynx or above, while vomit is defined as forceful expulsion of the refluxed gastric contents from the mouth [3]. On the other hand, rumination is defined as voluntary contraction of the abdominal muscles resulting in regurgitation of recently ingested food that is subsequently spitted up or re-swallowed. This requires a different diagnostic and treatment algorithm than reflux and is beyond the scope of this review. The reader is referred to the Rome III criteria for further reading on rumination in children [3].

## Epidemiology

GER is extremely common in healthy infants occurring 30 or more times a day [4, 5].

Many, but not all, episodes of these reflux episodes result in regurgitation into the oral cavity. Commonly, the frequency of reflux episodes decreases with increasing age, and is unusual in children older than 18 months old [1, 6, 5]. The prevalence of GER in older children and adolescent is estimated to be as high as 10% with 6% having GERD [7]. There is a higher prevalence of GERD in patients with neuromuscular disorders such as muscular dystrophy and cerebral palsy.

## Pathophysiology

Transient lower esophageal sphincter relaxations (TLESRs) or inadequate adaptation of the sphincter tone due to changes in abdominal pressure are the most common mechanisms causing GER at any age [8]. This relaxation is a neural reflex, through the vagal nerve causing activation of intramural inhibitory neurons, releasing nitric oxide locally promoting relaxation of the LES. GER is influenced by genetic (Table 1), environmental (alcohol, smoking, drugs, food, weight), anatomic, hormonal and neurogenic factors. In infants, GER is most common as they ingest more than twice the volume than adults per kilogram body weight and feed more frequent causing more TESLRs. Delayed gastric emptying, abnormal gastric accommodation has been described in patients with GERD [9, 10]. Anatomical causes include hiatal hernia which increases the number of reflux episodes and delays esophageal clearance.

**Table 1. Genetic factors.**

| 1 | Increased GER-symptoms in relatives of GERD patients [11] |
|---|---|
| 2 | Concordance for GER is higher in monozygotic compared to dizygotic twins [12] |
| 3 | Some studies have suggested association with chromosomes 9 and 13 [13] |

There are three major tiers of defense that serve to limit the degree of GER and minimize the risk of reflux-induced injury. The first line is the antireflux barrier consisting of the LES, diaphragmatic pinchcock and angle of His. The second line is the esophageal clearance consisting of gravity, esophageal peristalsis, salivary and esophageal secretions. The third line is the esophageal mucosal defense (bicarbonate, mucin, prostaglandin E2, tight junctions, *etc.*).

## Clinical features of GERD

Symptoms of GERD may be divided into esophageal and extra esophageal symptoms. (Table **2**). Esophageal symptoms include typical symptoms such as heartburn, vomiting, water brash (sour taste at the back of mouth), and epigastric abdominal pain especially worse after eating spicy foods. Dysphagia is also thought to be a symptom of GERD, especially common in younger children (< 1 year of age). Arching of the back (Sandifer syndrome) is a common presentation of GERD in infants. It is difficult to rely on symptoms in children less than 1 year of age due to their inability to accurately verbalize symptoms. These symptoms also do not always resolve with acid suppression therapy in the first year of life, making the diagnosis even more challenging [14].

Extra esophageal symptoms of GERD have been documented for several years now. Irritability, coughing [15, 16]. Choking, wheezing, sore throat, voice hoarseness, dental erosions and reflux associated laryngitis or pharyngitis have been implicated in various studies [17 - 20].

In any patient with suspected GERD not responding to adequate therapy, particularly in children with dysphagia and choking, eosinophilic esophagitis should be considered in the differential diagnosis. Eosinophilic esophagitis has a clinical presentation similar to GERD, and as of the writing of this paper, the only reliable means to diagnose this entity remains history (*i.e.* clinical symptoms) along with increased intra esophageal eosinophils on 5 or more esophageal biopsy specimens obtained *via* endoscopy. It is important to note that the patient should have received 6-8 weeks of good acid suppression therapy prior to this evaluation to rule out any confounding role that acid may play in esophageal eosinophilia [21]. Ensuring that the child is not solely on an elemental formula before the endoscopy is an important clinical consideration as this may confound normal results.

**Table 2. Clinical manifestation of GERD.**

| Age | Esophageal symptoms | Extra esophageal symptoms |
|-----|---------------------|---------------------------|
| <1 year of age | Recurrent vomiting, feeding refusal, painful swallowing | Arching of back, poor weight gain, irritability, sleep disturbance, respiratory symptoms |
| 1-5 years of age | Vomiting, abdominal pain, feeding refusal | Cough, nocturnal cough, pneumonia, choking, sore throat, voice hoarseness, dental erosions, laryngitis, pharyngitis, worsening of sub glottis stenosis |
| > 5 years of age | Heartburn, non-cardiac chest pain, nocturnal abdominal epigastric pain, dysphagia, water brash (sour burps), nausea | Above as well as vocal cord nodules, tooth structure loss and chronic sinusitis in certain patients |

Adolescents and older children should be asked about their symptoms directly rather than asking their parents. In a study, adolescents were significantly more likely to report symptoms of nausea or sour burps themselves as compared to asking their parents [5].

**Diagnosis of GERD**

The key point in diagnosis is to establish if the patient has GER *vs* GERD. This can be established with a good clinic history and physical examination in most cases. In older children and adults, the diagnosis of GERD is mainly based on clinical history, however in younger children, the history is difficult to elicit and found to be poorly reliable up to the age of at least 8 [22]. Because of this difficulty in obtaining the history, diagnostic procedures are used for better evaluation including pH probe, multichannel impedance probe, Bravo, manometry and endoscopy. This should be reserved for evaluation of children where GERD is manifesting mainly *via* extra esophageal symptoms or in children not responding to usual management of GERD. Not all tests need to be performed in all children as different tests provide different diagnostic information. In cases of continued doubt of diagnosis, it is recommended that the patient be seen at a multidisciplinary aerodigestive clinic.

## History

A good and thorough history and clinical examination remains the first diagnostic step for GERD, and in most cases is sufficient to establish a diagnosis. A number of validated questionnaires have been developed for GERD, and may be used for documenting and monitoring parent reported GERD symptoms [23].

## Upper GI Imaging

The use of upper GI tract imaging such as a barium upper GI series is NOT to be used to diagnose GERD. This is because in the brief duration of the study, reflux episodes may occur non-pathologically, and reflex seen on a barium study does not correlate with severity of GERD or severity of esophageal inflammation. Thus, recent guidelines state that this test is not justified to diagnose GER or GERD. Rather, this test is best used for assessing anatomic abnormalities in a selected population of patients such as those with bilious emesis [24].

## Esophageal pH Monitoring

Esophageal pH monitoring measures the incidence and duration of acid reflux, however the severity of pathologic acid reflux does not correlate consistently with symptom severity or demonstrable complications. Esophageal pH monitoring is useful in evaluating the effect of a therapeutic intervention on reducing esophageal acid exposure. It may be useful to correlate symptoms (*e.g.*, cough, chest pain) with acid reflux episodes and to select those infants and children with wheezing or respiratory symptoms in which GER is an aggravating factor. The sensitivity, specificity, and clinical utility of pH monitoring for diagnosis and management of possible extra-esophageal complications of GER are not well established. Some of the limitations of pH monitoring are that it only records acidic reflux episodes, thus missing non-acidic reflux episodes as well as that it requires the placement of a nasal catheter, which leads to patient discomfort.

## Bravo pH Monitoring

This is similar to esophageal pH monitoring in that it records acidic reflux episodes, but in this case there is a small capsule, about the size of a gel cap, that is temporarily attached to the wall of the esophagus during an upper endoscopy. The capsule measures pH levels in the esophagus and transmits readings by radio telecommunications to a receiver. It offers the benefit of being a catheter free design and allows patients to maintain their regular activities. Different to the regular esophageal pH monitoring, it requires sedation for the placement of the capsule. Age and weight restrictions further limit use in pediatrics.

## Combined Multiple Intraluminal Impedance (MII) and pH Monitoring

This test detects acid, weakly acid, and weakly alkaline reflux episodes from liquids, solids and gas reflux in the esophagus. Similar to esophageal pH monitoring, it requires a placement of a nasal catheter, however it is superior to pH monitoring alone as it allows for the evaluation of the temporal relation between symptoms and refluxate and the ability to detect full column reflux episodes which could be acidic or non-acidic. (See Fig. **1**).

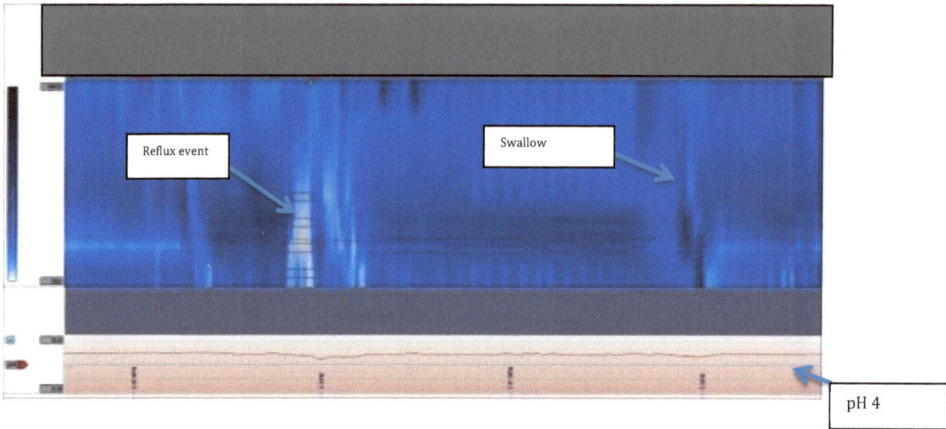

**Fig. (1).** Impedance tracing showing reflux event and a normal swallow.

Interpretation of the recording is still laborious and necessitates sufficient pediatric experience, because the automatic analysis is not standardized and is not adequate in children and infants. The major clinical application of impedance seems to be demonstration of symptom association and assessment of adequacy of acid suppression therapy in the setting of ongoing symptoms. The patient does not need to discontinue current reflux therapy while undergoing this test. This can be performed as an outpatient ambulatory test and does not require sedation. In most large centers, this test has replaced traditional esophageal pH monitoring. In some advanced centers, this test can be combined with esophageal manometry allowing detection of esophageal motility abnormalities at the same time.

## Endoscopy and Biopsies

GERD is mainly a clinical diagnosis, and as such, conservative techniques are preferred in cases needing further diagnostic testing. In children, upper GI tract endoscopy is performed using general anesthesia or conscious sedation. Risks of these need to be weighed against the benefit gained from preforming a diagnostic endoscopy. When performed, however, an endoscopy allows direct visualization of complications of GERD such as a peptic ulcer. Contributing factors to treatment resistance such as the presence of Helicobacter pylori infection could be gauged using an endoscopy. In rare cases, the presence of esophageal webs, or infectious esophagitis may be revealed on endoscopy. The most important reason today to perform an esophagogastroduodenoscopy is to assess for the presence of eosinophilic esophagitis and/or eosinophilic gastroenteritis. Both of these entities have clinical presenting features similar to GERD, but have treatments that are different from GERD and still evolving. As mentioned above, if eosinophilic esophagitis is suspected, then the patient should have received a 6-8 week course of proton pump inhibitor therapy prior to the endoscopy. Also, dietary restrictions to allergenic foods and exclusive use of an elemental formula prior to an endoscopy should be avoided as this is part of the treatment of eosinophilic esophagitis and will confound the results of the endoscopy. Clinicians should perform biopsies from at least 3 levels of the esophagus even in the setting of a normal appearing esophageal mucosa, as a large retrospective study has shown the presence of eosinophilic esophagitis in 32% of patients who had a grossly normal appearing esophagus on endoscopy [25].

## *Esophageal Manometry*

Conventional esophageal manometry has a very limited role in the diagnosis of GERD in children. In adults, it is most useful to assess for hiatal hernias. The use of combined impedance – manometry, has been helpful in assessing for an esophageal motility disorder which if present, could contribute to prolonged esophageal acid exposure. This entity is not available at all centers, and patients may need to be sent to specialized pediatric centers to have such testing performed and accurately interpreted.

## Management of GERD in Children

The management of reflux in children is dependent primarily on making the distinction between reflux disease *versus* reflux. No therapy is needed for reflux not causing symptoms or distress to patients.

## *Lifestyle Changes*

### *Infants*

For infants who are spitting up, but gaining weight well, and tolerating feeds ("happy spitters") no treatment is needed. Reassuring and educating the parents about the physiology of infant reflux and timeline is all that is needed.

For infants who are not gaining weight, who have arching of their back (Sandifer syndrome) or other symptoms of GERD treatment is needed.

Lifestyle changes may be enough for most cases of infant reflux. This includes addition of rice cereal to formula fed infants using the formula of 1 tablespoon of cereal to 1 ounce of formula and using a larger sized nipple. Cross cutting the nipple is no longer recommended. Alternatively, formulas that have pre added rice cereal are available in the market and can be used. However, commercially available thickening agents may lead to enterocolitis and as such, these are discouraged [26]. The FDA has issued a warning against using other commercially available thickeners such as 'simply thick' in babies less than 37 weeks gestation.

Keeping the baby in an upright position for 30-45 minutes after meals is recommended. Keeping the baby in a car seat is not beneficial, and in fact may worsen reflux.

Small frequent feedings and avoidance of over feeding is important.

The FDA and the AAP strongly recommend against using a reflux wedge as there have been no studies showing that it helps with reflux, but there have been documented SIDS related deaths when using this device [27].

For a certain sub set of infants, milk protein allergy is thought to play a role in the causation of reflux. In this specific subset, trying a semi elemental or even elemental formula may be beneficial. In 1 study of formula fed infants, GERD symptoms resolved in 24% of children after a 2 week trial of changing to a protein hydrolysate formula that was thickened with 1 tablespoon rice cereal and other lifestyle changes [28].

For breast fed infants, it may be recommended that the maternal diet be modified to avoid cow's milk and eggs [29]. It is important that a mother's choosing this route of therapy see a dietician herself to ensure that she receives adequate nutritional support and intake of essential vitamins and minerals such as Vitamin D.

### *Older Children and Adolescents*

For older children and adolescents, lifestyle modifications are similar to adults. Losing weight in overweight children especially reducing abdominal obesity is a key lifestyle modification. Small frequent meals, and avoidance of caffeine, chocolate, peppermint and spicy foods is recommended. Adolescents should be counseled against smoking and alcohol. There is some evidence that chewing sugarless gum may help reduce symptoms of GER [30, 31].

## Medications

There are a number of medications available to treat GERD (Table **3**). These can be divided into acid reducing /neutralizing agents and prokinetics. While there is good evidence to support the use and effectiveness of acid reducing medications [22], recent concerns about the over prescription of this group of drugs, particularly proton pump inhibitors (PPIs), necessitates understanding of guidelines for their use.

**Table 3. Medical management of GERD.**

| Mechanism of Action | Examples |
|---|---|
| Neutralization of gastric acid | Antacids such as sodium bicarbonate, aluminum hydroxide gel |
| Reduction of gastric acid secretion | 1) H2Receptor blockers such as ranitidine, famotidine<br>2) Proton pump inhibitors such as omeprazole, lansoprazole |
| Prokinetics | Metoclopramide, erythromycin<br>Bethanechol (although not strictly a prokinetic agent) |

### *Antacids*

This group of medications is used primarily to buffer acid in the stomach, and seems to be best used in an as needed basis. There is little evidence of benefit of this class of medication in infants. Antacids may be considered in mild intermittent episodes of GERD. Caution should be taken when using aluminum containing antacids as there is a risk if aluminum toxicity. Milk alkali syndrome (alkalosis, renal failure and hypercalcemia) has been reported in children taking antacids. Due to the above concerns and limited evidence of benefit, there is currently no specific recommended antacid for the chronic treatment of GERD.

### *H2 Receptor Antagonists*

This class of medications was the first to be available for the treatment of GERD and continue to be first line in the therapy of GERD.

They work by blocking histamine induced gastric secretion. All phases (basal, neurogenic and gastric) of secretion are suppressed dose dependently. In addition, secretory responses to not only histamine but also other stimuli (Acetycholine, gastrin, insulin, alcohol and food) are attenuated. Tachyphylaxis is common, limiting long term use. Side effects are generally mild and include headache, dry mouth and rashes. Cimetidine (and not other H2 receptor antagonist) has anti androgenic action (displaces dihydrotestosterone from its cytoplasmic binding site), increases plasma prolactin and inhibits degradation of estradiol by the liver. High doses over long periods of time have been associated with gynecomastia.

## Proton Pump Inhibitors

This class of medications of substituted benzimidazoles inhibits the final common step in gastric acid secretion. PPIs are inactive at neutral pH, at a pH < 5 they rearrange to 2 charged cationic forms that react covalently with the SH groups of the H+ K+ ATPase enzyme and inactivates this enzyme irreversibly. It gets concentrated in the acidic pH of the parietal cell canaliculi, because the charged forms generated there at the acidic pH are unable to diffuse back and get tightly bound to the enzyme. This factor and the specific localization of the H+ K+ ATPase confer a high degree of selectivity of action to PPIs. Acid secretion can resume only when new H+ K+ ATPase molecules are synthesized. Because of its tight binding to its target enzyme, it can be detected in the gastric mucosa long after its disappearance from plasma. Inhibition of acid secretion occurs within 1 hour, reaches a maximum at 2 hours and is still half maximal at 24 hours and lasts 3 days. With daily administration, anti-secretory effect increases until the 4th day after which is plateaus. Secretion resumes gradually over 3-5 days after stopping the drug [32].

Metabolism of PPIs tends to differ in children as compared to adults; and usually a higher dose per kilogram is needed to achieve peak serum concentrations.

Unlike H2 receptor antagonists, proton pump inhibitors can be used for long periods of time without tachyphylaxis.

Proton pump inhibitors should be initiated in moderate to severe cases of GERD in children failing H2 receptor antagonists. It is important to use appropriate doses of 1-2 mg/kg/day, and attempt to administer those 30 minutes before meals [33].

Tolia *et al* [34] found in 2007 that long term treatment with PPIs was fairly safe in children.

Recent reports on the long term implications of continuous PPI therapy have shown an increase risk for hip fractures, community acquired (but not nosocomial) pneumonias and Clostridium difficile infections and rebound symptoms of reflux in adults [35]. Hence, it is recommended that patient should be monitored for the necessity to continue PPI periodically and an attempt should be made to wean patients no longer clinically needing PPI.

## Prokinetics

Prokinetic agents such as erythromycin and metoclopramide should be reserved for cases where impedance-pH testing shows persistent full column reflux or the primary symptom is vomiting associated with poor weight gain.

## *Bethanechol*

In an adult study, bethanechol was shown to increase the Lower esophageal sphincter pressure (LESP), and improved symptoms of reflux in many, but not all patients [36]. However, Orenstein *et al*, conducted a study in children which failed to demonstrate an effect of bethanechol in the symptoms of reflux in children [37]. In our experience, using appropriate doses of 0.3mg/kg/dose given 3-4 times a day and timed 30-40 minutes prior to feeds has helped some patients with GERD. Further pediatric studies are needed to address this question accurately.

## *Surgery*

Surgical interventions, such as Nissen fundoplication, are best reserved for severe cases not responding to therapy. It is preferable to limit this therapy to a certain at risk population such as neurologically impaired children or children with severe underlying chronic lung disease who continue to have full column reflux where episodes of reflux into the lung could be associated with a high risk of morbidity and mortality.

## CONCLUSION

Physiologic reflux is common in infants and does not need diagnostic or therapeutic interventions. Patients having GERD may be treated empirically mainly based on symptoms. If treatment is not successful, or the diagnosis remains in question, then further testing may be done. An upper GI series plays no role in diagnosing GERD, rather should be used to assess for anatomic abnormalities. Multi-channel intra luminal impedance-pH studies are now the mainstay of diagnosis of GERD. Combining this with esophageal manometry is the new emerging technology in this field along with Bravo wireless capsule monitoring. Over use of medications, particularly PPIs are cautioned against. Surgical intervention such as fundoplication is not needed other than in the most severe cases of GERD posing significant morbidity and mortality risk in a selected population of patients.

## CONFLICT OF INTEREST

The authors declare no conflict of interest, financial or otherwise.

## ACKNOWLEDGEMENTS

Declared none.

## REFERENCES

[1]     Nelson SP, Chen EH, Syniar GM, Christoffel KK. One-year follow-up of symptoms of gastroesophageal reflux during infancy. Pediatric practice research group. Pediatrics 1998; 102(6): E67.
[http://dx.doi.org/10.1542/peds.102.6.e67]

[2]     Henry S. Discerning differences: gastroesophageal reflux and gastroesophageal reflux disease in infants. Adv Neonatal Care 2004; 4(4): 235-47.
[http://dx.doi.org/10.1016/j.adnc.2004.05.006]

[3]     Wood J, Grundy D, Al-Chaer E, *et al.* The functional gastrointestinal disorders Rome III. Third edit., Degnon Associates 2006.

[4]     Vandenplas Y, Goyvaerts H, Helven R, Sacre L. Gastroesophageal reflux, as measured by 24-hour pH monitoring, in 509 healthy infants screened for risk of sudden infant death syndrome. Pediatrics 1991; 88(4): 834-40.

[5]     Nelson SP, Chen EH, Syniar GM, Christoffel KK. Prevalence of symptoms of gastroesophageal reflux during infancy. A pediatric practice-based survey. Pediatric practice research group. Arch Pediatr Adolesc Med 1997; 151(6): 569-72.

[6]     Campanozzi A, Boccia G, Pensabene L, Panetta F, Marseglia A, Strisciuglio P. Prevalence and natural history of gastroesophageal reflux : Pediatric prospective survey. Pediatrics 2009; 123(3): 779-83.
[http://dx.doi.org/10.1542/peds.2007-3569]

[7]     Martigne L, Delaage PH, Thomas-Delecourt F, Bonnelye G, Barthélémy P, Gottrand F. Prevalence and management of gastroesophageal reflux disease in children and adolescents: A nationwide cross-sectional observational study. Eur J Pediatr 2012; 171(12): 1767-73.
[http://dx.doi.org/10.1007/s00431-012-1807-4]

[8]     Vandenplas Y, Hassall E. Mechanisms of gastroesophageal reflux and gastroesophageal reflux disease. J Pediatr Gastroenterol Nutr 2002; 35(2): 119-36.
[http://dx.doi.org/10.1097/01.MPG.0000018860.40775.A3]

[9]     Fonkalsrud E, Ament M. Gastroesophageal reflux in childhood. Curr Probl Surg 1996; 33(I): 1-70.

[10]    Kuiken S, Van Den Elzen B, Tytgat G, Bennink R, Boeckxstaens G. Evidence for pooling of gastric secretions in the proximal stomach in humans using single photon computed tomography discussion on celiac disease in patients with severe liver disease : Gluten-free diet may reverse hepatic failure. Gastroenterology 2002; 123(6): 2157-8.
[http://dx.doi.org/10.1053/gast.2002.37299]

[11]    Trudgill N, Kapur K, Riley S. Familial clustering of reflux symptoms. Am J Gastroenterol 1999; 94(5): 1172-8.

[12]    Cameron A, Lagergren J, Henriksson C, Nyren O, Locke G, Pedersen N. Gastroesophageal reflux disease in monozygotic and dizygotic twins. Gastroenterology 2002; 122(1): 55-9.
[http://dx.doi.org/10.1053/gast.2002.30301]

[13]    HU F. Mapping of a gene for severe pediatric gastroesophageal reflux to chromosome 13q14. JAMA 2000; 284(3): 325-34.

[14]    Sherman P, Hassall E, Fagundes-Neto U, *et al.* A global, evidence-based consensus on the definition of gastroesophageal reflux disease in the pediatric population. Am J Gastroenterol 2009; 104(5): 1278-95.
[http://dx.doi.org/10.1038/ajg.2009.129]

[15]   Jacob P, Pj K, Herzon G. Proximal esophageal pH metry in patients with ' reflux laryngitis '. PubMed commons. Gastroenterology 1991; 100(2): 305-10.

[16]   Tokayer AZ. Gastroesophageal reflux disease and chronic cough. Lung 2007; 2008(186): 29-34.
       [http://dx.doi.org/10.1007/s00408-007-9057-3]

[17]   Adhami T, Goldblum JR, Richter JE, Vaezi MF. The role of gastric and duodenal agents in laryngeal injury : An experimental canine model. Am J Gastroenterol 2004; 99(11): 2098-106.
       [http://dx.doi.org/10.1111/j.1572-0241.2004.40170.x]

[18]   Tuchman D, Boyle J, Pack A, *et al.* Comparison of airway responses following tracheal or esophageal acidification in the cat. Gastroenterology 1984; 87(5): 872-81.

[19]   Delahunty J, Cherry J. Experimentally produced vocal cord granulomas. Laryngoscope 1968; 78(11): 1941-7.

[20]   Little F, Koufman J, Kohut R, Marshall R. Effect of gastric acid on the pathogenesis of subglottic stenosis. Ann Otol Rhinol Laryngol 1985; 94(5): 516-9.

[21]   Liacouras C, Furuta G, Hirano I, *et al.* Eosinophilic esophagitis : Updated consensus recommendations for children and adults. J Allergy Clin Immunol 2011; 128(1): 3-20.
       [http://dx.doi.org/10.1016/j.jaci.2011.02.040]

[22]   Vandenplas Y, Rudolph C, Di Lorenzo C, *et al.* Pediatric gastroesophageal reflux clinical practice guidelines: Joint recommendations of the North American society for pediatric gastroenterology, hepatology, and nutrition (NASPGHAN) and the European society for pediatric gastroenterology, hepatology, a. J Pediatr Gastroenterol Nutr 2009; 49(4): 498-547.
       [http://dx.doi.org/10.1097/MPG.0b013e3181b7f563]

[23]   Kleinman L, Revicki D, Flood E. Validation issues in questionnaires for diagnosis and monitoring of gastroesophageal reflux disease in children. Curr Gastroenterol Rep 2006; 8(3): 230-6.

[24]   Lightdale JR, Gremse D. Gastroesophageal reflux: management guidance for the pediatrician. Pediatrics 2013; 131(5): e1684-95.

[25]   Liacouras CA, Spergel JM, Ruchelli E, *et al.* Eosinophilic esophagitis: A 10-year experience in 381 children. Clin Gastroenterol Hepatol 2005; 3(12): 1198-206.
       [http://dx.doi.org/10.1016/S1542-3565(05)00885-2]

[26]   Clarke P, Robinson MJ. Thickening milk feeds may cause necrotising enterocolitis. Arch Dis Child Fetal Neonatal Ed 2004; 89(3): F280.
       [http://dx.doi.org/10.1136/adc.2003.036392]

[27]   CPSC and FDA Warn Against Using Infant Sleep Positioners Because of Suffocation Risk: Initial Communication FDA 2010. http://www.fda.gov/MedicalDevices/Safety/AlertsandNotices/ucm-227301.htm.

[28]   Shalaby T, Orenstein S. Efficacy of telephone teaching of conservative therapy for infants with symptomatic gastroesophageal reflux referred by pediatricians to pediatric gastroenterologists. Pediatrics 2003; 142(1): 57-61.

[29]   Vance G, Lewis S, Grimshaw K, *et al.* Exposure of the fetus and infant to hens' egg ovalbumin *via* the placenta and breast milk in relation to maternal intake of dietary egg. Clin Exp Allergy 2005; 35(10): 1318-26.
       [http://dx.doi.org/10.1111/j.1365-2222.2005.02346.x]

[30]   Avidan B, Sonnenberg A, Schnell TG, Sontag SJ. Walking and chewing reduce postprandial acid reflux. Aliment Pharmacol Ther 2001; 15(2): 151-5.
       [http://dx.doi.org/10.1046/j.1365-2036.2001.00902.x]

[31]   Smoak B, Koufman J. Effects of gum chewing on pharyngeal and esophageal pH. Ann Otol Rhinol Laryngol 2001; 110(12): 1117-9.

[32]   Tripathy K. Gastrointestinal medications. Essentials of Medical Pharmacology. Third ed., 1985.

[33]   Rudolph CD, Mazur LJ, Liptak GS, *et al.* Guidelines for evaluation and treatment of gastroesophageal reflux in infants and children: recommendations of the North American Society for Pediatric Gastroenterology and Nutrition. J Pediatr Gastroenterol Nutr 2001; 32 (Suppl. 2): S1-S31.
[http://dx.doi.org/10.1097/00005176-200100002-00001]

[34]   Tolia V, Boyer K. Long-term proton pump inhibitor use in children: A retrospective review of safety. Dig Dis Sci 2008; 53(2): 385-93.
[http://dx.doi.org/10.1007/s10620-007-9880-7]

[35]   Thomson AB, Sauve MD, Kassam N, Kamitakahara H. Safety of the long-term use of proton pump inhibitors. World J Gastroenterol 2010; 16(19): 2323-30.
[http://dx.doi.org/10.3748/wjg.v16.i19.2323]

[36]   Miller WN, Ganeshappa KP, Dodds WJ, Hogan WJ, Barreras RF, Arndorfer RC. Effect of bethanechol on gastroesophageal reflux. Am J Dig Dis 1977; 22(3): 230-4.

[37]   Orenstein SR, Lofton SW, Orenstein DM. Bethanechol for pediatric gastroesophageal reflux: a prospective, blind, controlled study. J Pediatr Gastroenterol Nutr 1986; 5(4): 549-55.

CHAPTER 16

# Essentials of Sickle Cell Disease Management

**Jesica F. Ramirez[1]** and **Melissa Frei-Jones[2,*]**

[1] Centro Javeriano de Oncologia - Hospital Universitario San Ignacio, Bogota, Columbia

[2] Department of Pediatrics, University of Texas Health Science Center, San Antonio, Texas, USA

**Abstract:** Sickle cell disease (SCD) is the most common inherited disorder identified by newborn screening programs with an estimated 100,000 individuals living with SCD in the United States (US). The most severe phenotype of SCD is seen in patients with homozygous hemoglobin SS (HbSS) also known as sickle cell anemia. Common morbidities include invasive pneumococcal infection due to loss of splenic function, pulmonary sickling causing acute chest syndrome, cerebrovascular stroke, acute pain episodes and the development of chronic pain syndromes. Life expectancy for SCD has improved and children born with SCD today have a greater than 90% chance of survival to adulthood. Disease modifying therapies including the use of simple and chronic transfusions and oral hydroxyurea to both treat and prevent disease complications such as pain, stroke and acute chest syndrome. The only curative option for SCD remains hematopoietic stem cell transplantation with the best outcomes from a matched sibling donor.

**Keywords :** Acute chest Syndrome, Anemia, Asplenia, Avascular necrosis, Dactylitis, Electrophoresis, Hemoglobin S, Hydroxyurea, Newborn screen, Pain crisis, Pneumococcus, Prophylaxis, Sepsis, Sickle cell disease, Splenic sequestration, Stroke, Transcranial doppler ultrasound, Transfusion, Vaso-occlusive crisis.

## INTRODUCTION

Sickle cell disease (SCD) is the most common inherited red blood cell (RBC) disorder worldwide [1]. It is a life threatening condition resulting from a single base pair mutation in the β-globin gene. Hemoglobin polymerizes in its deoxygenated state, causing the RBC to take on a crescent or sickled conformation that alters blood viscosity and vascular endothelium, leading to vaso-occlusion, an exuberant inflammatory response and early death of RBC [2, 3].

---

[*] **Corresponding author Melissa Frei-Jones**: Department of Pediatrics, University of Texas Health Science Center, San Antonio, Texas, USA; Tel: 210-567-7477; Email: freijones@uthscsa.edu

**Seckin Ulualp (Ed.)**

Approximately 312,000 infants with SCD are born each year in the world. Although survival and life expectancy for children with SCD in the first world has increased due to universal newborn screening for early disease detection and initiation of prophylactic penicillin to prevent early complications, infants born in the United States (US) and Europe together represent only 2% of the annual SCD births worldwide [4]. The majority of cases of SCD are found in developing countries with limited resources for preventive care and treatment [5].

New approaches to sickle cell management with disease modifying treatments including hydroxyurea and chronic transfusions are being studied [6, 7]. Advances in early detection of complications and methods for improved survival of patients undergoing transplant have also been described [8]. In this chapter, we discuss the current guidelines for early diagnosis and management of SCD and its complications, hoping to help physicians identify the presentation of SCD, treat acute sequelae and know when to refer to a SCD specialist for chronic management.

## GENERAL CONCEPTS

### Genetics

SCD is caused by a mutation in the β-globin gene and demonstrates autosomal recessive inheritance. Given that a single HbS allele produces a phenotypic change in the hemoglobin profile, an autosomal co-dominant fashion has also been proposed [9].

"Sickle cell disease" is the term used to refer to various genotypes that cause the characteristic clinical syndrome. The most frequently occurring genotype is the homozygous state (HbSS) also known as sickle cell anemia, which has the most severe clinical phenotype. More than ten other genotypes have been described, although most are rarer [10].

### Classification of Variants

The different forms of SCD result from the coinheritance of HbS with other abnormalities in the β-globin gene. The most common variants include: Sickle-hemoglobin C disease (HbSC), Sickle-β+-thalassemia (HbSβ+), and Sickle-β--thalassemia (HbSβ0) [9].

The most severe forms of the disease are HbSS and HbSβ0. Patients with these variants have been described to have higher markers of hemolysis, lower mean hemoglobin values, and increased prevalence of complications including: vaso-occlusive pain crisis, acute chest syndrome, acute cerebrovascular stroke, leg ulcers and priapism [9, 11]. The lower the expression of β-like chains in the thalassemic allele, the more complications experienced by the patient [12]. The most common genotypes of SCD, and the associated typical peripheral blood findings in untreated SCD are shown in Table **1**.

**Table 1. Common Genotypes of Sickle Cell Disease.**

| Common Genotypes of Sickle Cell Disease | | | | | |
|---|---|---|---|---|---|
| Name /Genotype | Main Hemoglobin present | Hemoglobin level (g/dL) | Mean Corpuscular Volume (fL) | Reticulocyte % | Severity |
| Sickle cell anemia (Hb* SS) BS/BS | S | 6 to 9 | Normal | 10 to 25 | +++ |
| Sickle β0 thalassemia (Hb SB0) BS/BO | S | 6 to 9 | Decreased | 10 to 25 | +++ |
| Sickle Hb C disease (Hb SC) BS/BC | Sc | 9 to 12 | Normal | 5 to 10 | ++ |
| Sickle β+ Thalassemia (Hb SB+) BS/B+ | Sa | 10 to 13 | Decreased | 2 to 10 | + |

Most common genotypes that cause sickle cell disease are listed, resulting from one or more mutations on the β-globin gene and the laboratory findings associated with each of the presentations when left untreated.
*Abbreviations: Hb, hemoglobin. (Modified from Pediatr Clin North Am, 2013 Dec; 60(6):1363-81).

## Epidemiology

SCD is the most common genetic disorder identified through newborn screening. Approximately 300,000 infants are born with SCD-HbSS each year in the world. Sickle cell trait (SCT) is frequently found in individuals of African ancestry (sub-Saharan, equatorial Africa) but it has spread throughout the world due to migration [13]. An estimated 230,000 HbSS births occur annually in sub-Saharan Africa [4].

Approximately 100,000 people with SCD live in the US [11]. The disease is more common in African-Americans with 1 in 12 carry SCT and 1 in 365 individuals are affected with disease [11, 14]. For Hispanics the incidence is lower, 1 in every 36,000 births affected with the disease [5].

Survival to adulthood is currently between 93.9% and 95% in children enrolled in comprehensive care programs. The average age of death for patients with SCD has been estimated to be 39 years, and the mortality in pediatric patients is 0.52 per 100 patient-years. On the other hand, the developing world still has an estimated mortality rate of 50-90% before age 5; most commonly as a result of streptococcal sepsis, acute severe anemia and splenic sequestration [4, 15].

## Diagnosis and Screening

SCD is now diagnosed early in life thanks to the introduction of universal newborn screening in the US. Hemoglobin separation techniques are used, including: High Pressure Liquid Chromatography (HPLC), Isoelectric Focusing IEF, Citrate agar electrophoresis, and Cellulose acetate electrophoresis [9, 12, 13].

Sickle solubility tests are fast and easily available, they confirm the presence of sickle hemoglobin but fail to distinguish disease from trait, lacking sensitivity and specificity. High levels of HbF, and profound anemia contribute to false negative results when using sickle solubility tests [12, 16].

In addition to newborn screening, it is recommended for physicians to obtain a confirmatory test in the first clinical visit, and after 6 months, to determine the final hemoglobin phenotype [5]. Other tests, such as a complete blood count, reticulocyte count, peripheral blood morphology and family studies with genetic testing are helpful in the assessment of patients with SCD. In addition to the sickle shaped RBC Target cells and microcytosis are commonly seen in the pathology slides [9]. See Fig. **1** for Red blood cell morphology in SCA patients.

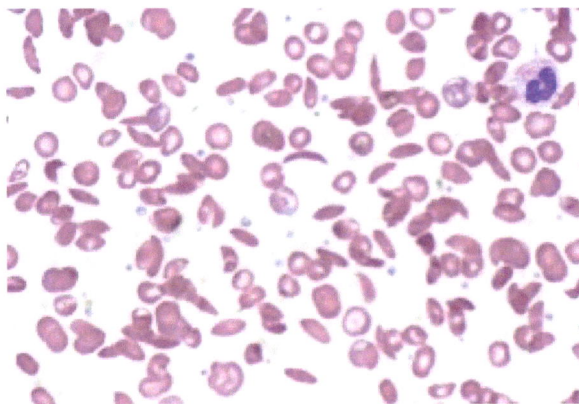

**Fig. (1).** Red blood cell morphology of a patient with Sickle Cell Anemia.

This peripheral blood smear shows normal red blood cells, fixed or irreversibly sickled cells, and target cells seen in patients with SCD. (Courtesy of Dr Frei-Jones, University of Texas Health Science Center San Antonio)

Early diagnosis and prompt referral to expert providers are essential for the efficient initiation of family education, anticipatory guidance, prophylaxis with penicillin and the prevention of common complications [5].

## PATHOPHYSIOLOGY

Due to a single-base mutation in the β-Globin gene, the hydrophilic amino acid, Glutamic acid, is substituted by the hydrophobic amino acid, Valine, changing the protein conformation. The hydrophobic end of the peptide chain is prone to interact with other hemoglobin molecules, causing polymerization in the deoxygenated state. This process is enhanced by high hemoglobin concentrations (elevated MCHC), low pH, low temperature and long capillary transit time [12, 13]. The polymerization of the hemoglobin disrupts the erythrocyte architecture, altering its flexibility and contributing to cellular dehydration, increased adhesion to the endothelium and other cells, and shortening of RBC life span. See Fig. **2** for Sickle cell pathophysiology.

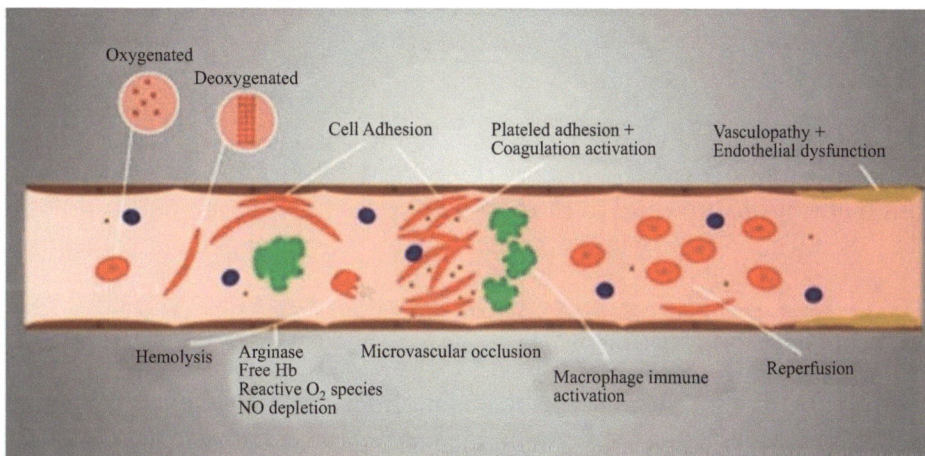

**Fig. (2).** Pathophysiology of sickle cell disease.

Binding of the red blood cells to the platelets causes platelet activation and aggregation. Additionally, the binding of red blood cells to neutrophils provokes an oxidative burst that further damages the endothelium and exposes tissue factor, involved in the coagulation cascade. The formation of heterocellular aggregates causes microvascular occlusion of the vessel lumen, local hypoxia and ischemia. Nitric oxide regulates the basal vasodilator tone, inhibiting platelet activation and transcriptional expression of nuclear factor kB dependent adhesion molecules. During hemolysis the abundant release of hemoglobin diffuses and reduces nitric oxide to nitrate, and the release of erythrocyte arginase results in the destruction of nitric oxide which contributes to the slow blood flow thought the area, allowing more sickling of the red blood cells. Restoration of blood flow further promotes tissue injury, mediated by reperfusion that causes an ongoing inflammatory response and endothelial dysfunction.

## ACUTE MANIFESTATIONS

### Vasoocclusive or Acute Pain Crisis

Nearly all individuals affected with SCD will experience a vaso-occlusive crisis (VOC) during their lifetime, especially patients with HbSS or HbSβ$^0$-thalassemia genotypes. First episodes may occur as early as 6 months of age when fetal hemoglobin levels begin to fall, with painful swelling of the hands and feet, called dactylitis.

Rapid evaluation and prompt administration of analgesics is important during acute pain crises to both treat pain and in order to distinguish pain from other sickle cell related complications such as acute chest syndrome, stroke (head pain), papillary necrosis (flank plain), splenic or hepatic sequestration (abdomen pain) [17].

Pain management should be individualized to the patient and developed through collaboration with his/her SCD team including the prescribing and monitoring of oral pain medications for mild to moderate pain and parenteral opioids for severe pain [18]. See Table **2** for general guidelines for the management of acute pain crisis.

### Acute Chest Syndrome

ACS is the most common cause of death in children with SCD and the second most common reason for hospitalization [19]. ACS is defined as a new pulmonary infiltrate on chest radiograph plus a sudden onset of 2 or more of the following: cough, shortness of breath, respiratory distress, chest pain, or fever. Children usually present with fever and upper or middle-lobe infiltrates.

Infection is the most well-known etiology. The most common pathogens include *Streptococcus pneumonia, Mycoplasma pneumonia* and *Chlamydia Sp* [5]. The exact cause of ACS is unknown but there are several conditions known to predispose to the development of ACS such as bone marrow embolism, intrapulmonary aggregates of sickle cells, atelectasis and pulmonary edema. ACS can develop as a complication during a hospitalization for pain, after a surgical procedure, and occurs with increased frequency in asthma [19].

ACS can rapidly progress to respiratory failure or death making evaluation with chest radiograph, pulse oximetry monitoring and prompt hospitalization of great importance [5, 20].

**Table 2. General recommendations for acute pain crisis assessment and management.**

| GENERAL RECOMMENDATIONS FOR ACUTE PAIN CRISIS ASSESMENT AND MANAGEMENT* | |
|---|---|
| **INITIAL APPROACH** | - Initiate analgesic therapy within 30 minutes of triage or within 60 min of registration. Start analgesia first while other diagnostic evaluations are being made.<br>- Determine characteristics, associated symptoms, location and intensity of pain based of patient report. If the characteristics of pain are atypical for the patient investigate other possible etiologies.<br>- Always assess recent analgesic use, opioid and non-opioid. Base analgesic selection on pain assessment, associated symptoms, outpatient analgesic use, patient's knowledge of effective agents and doses, and past experience with side effects. |
| **ANALGESIC ADMINISTRATION** | - In patients with mild to moderate pain who report relief with NSAIDS, in the absence of contraindications, continue treatment with NSAIDS.<br>- In patients with severe pain, rapidly initiate treatment with parenteral opioids.<br>o Calculate the parenteral (IV or SC) opioid dose based on total daily short acting opioid dose currently being taken at home to manage pain.<br>o Use the subcutaneous route when intravenous access is difficult, avoid intramuscular injections.<br>o Reassess pain and administer opioid if necessary for continued severe pain every 15-30 minutes until pain is under control per patient report.<br>o Maintain or consider escalation of the dose by 25% until pain is controlled reassess after each dose for pain relief and side effects.<br>- At discharge, evaluate inpatient analgesic requirements, wean parenteral opioids prior to conversion to oral opioids and adjust home dose of long and short acting opioid prescriptions to prevent opioid withdrawal after discharge. |
| **TO PREVENT COMPLICATIONS** | - When patients require antihistamines for itching secondary to opioid administration, prescribe agents orally, and do not re-administer with each dose of opioids in the acute management phase. Re-administer every 4 to 6 hours if needed. Avoid IV diphenhydramine due to excess sedation.<br>- To reduce the risk of acute chest syndrome, encourage use of incentive spirometry and ambulation as soon as possible.<br>- In euvolemic children, who are unable to drink fluids provide intravenous hydration at no more than maintenance rate to avoid over hydration.<br>- Do not administer a blood transfusion unless there are other indications for transfusion.<br>- In patients with pain and an oxygen saturation of <95% on room air administer oxygen. |

Listed are general recommendations for when treating patients with sickle cell disease in an acute pain crisis, to assure rapid initiation of analgesia, choosing the right medication depending on the patient profile and preventing common complications associated with pain and its management. *Abbreviations: SCD: Sickle cell disease, NSAIDS: non-steroidal anti-inflammatory drugs, IV: intravenous, SC: subcutaneous. (Modified form the Management of Sickle Cell Disease 2014 Evidence-Based Report by Expert Panel Members).

Treatment of ACS includes an intravenous cephalosporin, an oral macrolide antibiotic, supplemental oxygen to maintain oxygen saturation above 95%, bronchodilators, and pain medications to prevent atelectasis related to splinting. Current evidence suggests the use of low dose steroids (<2mg/kg/day; max: 60mg/day) of oral prednisone in patients with known asthma responsive to corticosteroids and ACS may be beneficial [19].

Blood transfusions are offered to patients with severe ACS, defined by multi-lobe disease, increased work of breathing, inability to maintain oxygen saturation above 95% even with supplemental oxygen, and pleural effusions. Simple blood transfusions of RBC 10ml/kg are indicated in patients with symptomatic ACS whose Hb concentration is at least 1g/dl below baseline [18]. Consultation with an hematologist, critical care or apheresis specialist is needed to perform urgent exchange transfusion in patients with rapid progression of ACS, oxygen saturation below 90% despite supplemental oxygen, dyspnea, progressive pulmonary infiltrates or decline in hemoglobin concentration despite simple transfusion [18]. Recurrent episodes of ACS can cause lung parenchymal scarring, progressive loss of lung function and impaired pulmonary growth [21]. Hydroxyurea is recommended for prevention of recurrent ACS.

## Fever

SCD patients are 300 times more likely to develop severe bacterial infections, such as septicemia and meningitis, than the normal population as a result of reduced or absent splenic function [22].

Prompt identification and treatment of infections is imperative. In SCD patients with a temperature >= 101.3F, consider obtaining a complete blood count (CBC) with differential, reticulocyte count, blood and urine cultures and admit the patient for further workup and initiation of IV antibiotic treatment [18, 23]. Empiric parenteral antibiotics should be started when fever is >= 39.5C/103.1F to provide coverage against *Streptococcus pneumonia* and gram negative enteric organisms.

In fever accompanied by respiratory symptoms evaluate for ACS. Bacterial osteomyelitis should be considered in SCD patients that present with fever and bone tenderness, especially when accompanied by erythema and swelling. Evaluate for infection first before assuming a VOC in patients presenting with fever and pain.

Penicillin prophylaxis has shown to decrease the risk of severe infections in patients with SCA and should be started before 2 months of age and continued through at least age 5, unless the child has had complete splenectomy or severe invasive pneumococcal infection. An oral dose of 125 mg twice daily is recommended initially with an increase to 250 mg twice daily by age 3 [24]. Penicillin prophylaxis can be withheld from patients with milder genotypes HbSC and HbSB+ Thalassemia unless they have had splenectomy. Vaccination is of limited use in children less than 2 years due to immature antibody response, but It is important to assure that all patients with SCD have completed recommended pneumococcal vaccination when discontinuing penicillin at age 5 [18, 25]. Immunization in SCD patients should be performed according to the ACIP harmonized immunization schedule. Given the increased risk of invasive pneumococcal disease (IPD) in SCD patients, a complete series of 13-valent conjugate pneumococcal vaccine should be started at 2 months and 23-valent pneumococcal polysaccharide vaccine given at age 2 with boosters every 5 years. Efforts to develop vaccines to prevent IPD continue as recently reported cases of IPD in SCD are from non-vaccine serotypes [22, 23].

It is of utmost importance to educate parents and caregivers of SCD patients to seek immediate medical attention in the case of fever.

## Stroke

Overt stroke in SCD may present as a sudden onset of focal neurological signs, altered consciousness, severe headaches, weakness, numbness, visual disturbances, dysarthria, aphasia, or ataxia [26, 27]. Overt strokes are more commonly caused by secondary stenosis or occlusion of the internal carotid or middle cerebral artery. Approximately 10% of children with SCD will experience an overt stroke [18]. Transient ischemic attacks often precede stroke and may be an indicator of cerebral vasculopathy.

Transcranial Doppler (TCD) imaging of large intracranial blood vessels to detect increased velocities secondary to stenosis can predict risk of overt stroke in children with SCA and help reduce prevalence from 10% to 1% [26, 28]. Evidence is high for annual TCD screening of patients with SCA genotypes starting at age 2 until age 16 for primary overt stroke prevention [18].

Time-averaged mean of the maximum (TAMM) velocities are consider normal <170 cm/second), conditional (170-199 cm/second) or abnormal (>200 cm/second) using non-imaging techniques. Conditional TCDs should be repeated at 3-6 month intervals, abnormal values should be repeated within 2-4 weeks of first screening [18, 26].

Consult a neurologist, perform and urgent computed tomography (CT) scan to evaluate for hemorrhage, followed by magnetic resonance imaging (MRI) of brain, cerebral veins and arteries if available, in patients with SCD in whom stroke is suspected. If confirmed, a program of monthly simple or exchange transfusions should be initiated for secondary stroke prevention. If chronic transfusion is not medically possible, initiation of hydroxyurea is recommended [18].

A sickle cell specialist should be involved in the management of patients with conditional (170-199 cm/sec) or elevated/abnormal (>200 cm/sec) TCD results or patients with acute stroke confirmed by neuroimaging.

The introduction of TCD screening and the use of chronic transfusions to prevent initial stroke in high risk patients has led to an important decline in stroke incidence. The STOP trial, a primary stroke prevention study in SCD, demonstrated a stroke risk reduction of 92% in children with abnormal TCD results >200 cm/s receiving chronic transfusions and the STOP 2 trial showed an increased risk of stroke with discontinuation of chronic transfusions [28].

A more recent study, the TWiTCH trial, compared the efficacy of hydroxyurea *versus* transfusions in the reduction of stroke risk in children with abnormal TCD velocities who have received at least one year of transfusions, and have no MRA-defined severe vasculopathy, can substitute hydroxyurea for transfusion treatment [29].

Acute stroke is managed with transfusion to prevent the progression of cerebral ischemia by reducing the percentage of HbS. When available, erythrocytapheresis is the preferred method of transfusion used for the initial treatment of stroke followed by chronic transfusion therapy to prevent a secondary stroke [17]. The SWiTCH study, a randomized phase 3 clinical trial, found chronic transfusion therapy superior to hydroxyurea as secondary stroke prevention [30].

## Priapism

Priapism is a sustained unwanted painful erection lasting four or more hours. Priapism is considered to be a urological emergency, affecting approximately 35% of boys and men with SCD. In patients with SCD, the most common causes of priapism are nocturnal erections, sexual activity, dehydration, fever, and exposure to cold.

If left untreated, priapism can cause fibrosis of the corpora cavernosa, erectile dysfunction and penile disfigurement [31]. Initial evaluation of a priapism may include color duplex ultrasonography, CBC, and C reactive protein [18].

Priapism must be evaluated and treated by specialist in a timely manner including urology and hematology teams. Initial management includes vigorous oral or intravenous hydrations and the use of analgesia. If conservative medical management does not cause detumescence, aspiration of blood from corpora cavernosa and irrigation with epinephrine should be considered. Transfusion should not be used as initial therapy for priapism due to the association of transfusion, priapism and the development of acute neurologic events that has been described [5, 18]. Although local measures such as cold packs are used for priapism in patients without SCD, cold should be avoided in SCD because it may cause further sickling and vaso-occlusion.

## Splenic Sequestration

Acute splenic sequestration occurs most often in children with severe SCD between the ages of one and four years old with sudden enlargement of the spleen and a drop in hemoglobin concentration by at least 2 g/dL below the baseline. Splenic sequestration may be triggered by fever and infection. The incidence of splenic sequestration has decreased since the introduction of newborn screening and early detection of SCD, as well as caregiver education regarding spleen palpation [24].

Splenic sequestration may be a life threatening event with left-sided abdominal pain associated with signs of hypovolemia, rapid spleen enlargement, circulatory collapse and profound anemia with levels of hemoglobin below 3 g/dL requiring emergent medical attention [5].

Management of severe acute splenic sequestration includes immediate resuscitation with IV fluids. A hematologist should be consulted for guidance in ordering transfusions in order to raise hemoglobin to a stable level but avoid over transfusion and hyperviscosity syndrome [24].

If the patient has recurrent acute splenic sequestration or symptomatic hypersplenism, surgical splenectomy should be discussed with a hematologist. Prophylactic blood transfusion has not been proven to reduce the risk of recurrent events, and puts the patient at risk of autotransfusion, caused when the spleen releases the sequestered blood leading to an increase in the hemoglobin concentration and hyperviscosity syndrome [5, 18].

## CHRONIC MANIFESTATIONS

### Chronic Pulmonary Disease

Pulmonary hypertension can be seen in sickle cell disease, secondary to chronic hemolysis and vasculopathy. Clinical presentation includes dyspnea with daily life activities, fatigue, chest pain, and palpitations. Initial echocardiography evaluation for the estimation of pulmonary artery pressure using tricuspid regurgitant jet velocity is recommended in symptomatic patients, but confirmation of pulmonary hypertension requires right heart catheterization which carries significant risk of harm reason why screening of non-symptomatic patients is not recommended [20].

For symptomatic SCD patients with an elevated TRV $\geq 2.5$ m/sec by echocardiography, a specialist referral should be made for further assessment and management [18, 32].

SCD patients with a physician diagnosis of asthma are known to be at higher risk of morbidity and mortality and more frequent episodes of ACS and VOC. Children with SCD and pulmonary symptoms should receive evaluation and management of asthma should be the same as for the general population following the NIH asthma guidelines.

Patients with SCD who have sleep disordered breathing (SDB) or obstructive sleep apnea (OSA) are at high risk of cardiopulmonary disease due to intermittent desaturation that increases vaso-occlusion. A relationship between OSA and the development of stroke, enuresis and priapism has been proposed [33].

Children with SCD are known to have adenoid and tonsillar hypertrophy that can further contribute with the SDB and apnea. It is recommended that all SCD patients with OSA be evaluated for adeno-tonsillectomy and the need for oxygen supplementation or positive airway pressure with sleep.

## Avascular Necrosis

Avascular necrosis (AVN) occurs when sickled RBCs occlude capillaries in the large joints causing ischemic necrosis. The most commonly affected bones are the humeral and femoral heads and risk factors for AVN include frequent vaso-occlusive episodes, and SCD genotype HbSS with alpha thal trait.

Clinical presentation includes severe pain that worsens with weight bearing activity and is usually relieved by resting [18, 24]. Children with SCD and intermittent or chronic hip pain should be evaluated for AVN with a thorough physical exam, x-ray and/or MRI and treated with analgesics and physical therapy. Management of advanced stages of AVN with significant compromise in daily activity, requires collaboration between orthopedic surgeons and hematologists for evaluation of possible hip arthroplasty [18].

## Proliferative Sickle Retinopathy

Patients with SCD have a higher risk for retinal disease than the normal population. Proliferative sickle retinopathy is caused by vaso-occlusion of the retinal arterioles and retinal ischemia. SCD retinopathy is associated with progressive loss of visual acuity and can lead to hemorrhage and retinal detachment. Annual screening with an ophthalmologist for dilated eye examination is recommended for individuals with SCD stating at age 10. Screening is important because therapy is available to prevent vision loss. Referral to a retinal specialist is required for further evaluation and management [18].

## Renal Disease

Nephropathy is rarely diagnosed in children with SCD. Hyposthenuria and glomerular hyperfiltration are commonly seen in young patients, but sickle nephropathy does not become clinically evident until later in life [18].

Annual screening for proteinuria should begin at age 10 years. Albumin/creatinine ratio should be performed if proteinuria is found. Modest elevations in creatinine >0.7 mg/dL and proteinuria >300 mg/24 hours in children, should be consider renal impairment prompting referral to a nephrologist for further assessment and management [18, 24].

## THERAPEUTIC CONSIDERATIONS

### Blood Transfusion in the Management of Sickle Cell Disease

Transfusion therapy has been shown to decrease the morbidity and mortality in patients with SCD by reducing the percentage of circulating HbS RBCs and improving oxygen capacity of the blood [21]. The specific threshold warranting transfusion varies with each patient but an achievement of Hb level of 10 g/dl or reduction of HbS to less than 30% are common therapy goals. Although transfusion is an important tool in both the prevention and treatment of acute and chronic complications, the current accepted indications for transfusion are based on expert consensus given the lack of clinical trials [17]. Simple transfusion or exchange transfusion is indicated in patients with symptomatic severe ACS, acute splenic sequestration accompanied by severe anemia and acute stroke. Patients who meet criteria for chronic transfusions should follow an established monitoring protocol [18].

The most common complications in SCD patients receiving transfusions are alloimmunization, with an incidence between 18-76% and iron overload. SCD patients most commonly form alloantibodies to the C, E and Kell antigens. To prevent alloantibody formation, extended cross-matching should be done [17] Iron overload occurs with as few as ten blood transfusions and is associated with hepatic, cardiac, and pituitary complications. Patients receiving chronic transfusions should have routine screening and receive treatment with iron chelators. See Table **3** for general recommendations in transfusion therapy.

Table 3. General recommendations for transfusion in Sickle cell disease patients.

| GENERAL RECOMMENDATIONS FOR TRANSFUSION IN SCD PATIENTS | |
| --- | --- |
| **PRIOR TO TRANSFUSION** | - Obtain patient transfusion history to include locations of prior transfusions and adverse effects.<br>- Obtain a RBC phenotype, type and screen. To assess the development of RBC antibodies in prior transfusions.<br>- Obtain quantitative measurement of percent HbA and percent HbS. To confirm achievement of target percentage of HbS, success of chronic transfusion<br>- Obtain complete blood count, and reticulocyte count. To help guide frequency and volume of transfusions.<br>- Confirm that all RBC units that are to be transfused to individuals with SCD should include matching for C, E, and K antigens. |
| **TRANSFUSION GOALS** | - Avoid transfusing to a target hemoglobin above 10 g/dL in patients who are not chronically transfused and therefore at risk for hyperviscosity due to high percentages of circulating HbS containing erythrocytes.<br>- In chronically transfused children with SCA, the goal of transfusion should be to maintain an HbS level of below 30 percent immediately prior to the next transfusion.<br>- If the patient has a hemoglobin higher than 8.5 g/dl, are on chronic hydroxyurea, require high risk surgery or have HbSC or HbSB$^+$-thalassemia, always consult a sickle cell expert first to confirm the indication of transfusion and method.<br>- For patients undergoing surgery or general anesthesia transfuse to an Hb of 10 g/dl to prevent postoperative complications. |
| **ASSESSMENT OF COMPLICATIONS** | - Evaluate for iron overload every 1–2 years by validated liver iron quantification methods such as liver biopsy, MRI R2 or MRI T2* or R2 techniques. Refer to a hematologist for management.<br>- Perform liver function tests annually or semiannually and Serum ferritin quarterly in individuals with iron overload, to assess iron stores and compliance with chelation therapy.<br>- Screen for hepatitis C, hepatitis B, and HIV annually in individuals receiving multiple transfusions. |

General recommendations based on the evidence base report by expert panel members for transfusing sickle cell disease patients. *Abbreviations: RBC: red blood cells, HbA: hemoglobin A, HbS: Hemoglobin S, CBC: complete blood count, SCD: Sickle cell disease, MRI: magnetic resonance imaging, HIV: Human immunodeficiency virus. (Modified form the Management of Sickle Cell Disease 2014 Evidence-Based Report by Expert Panel Members).

## Hydroxyurea Therapy

Hydroxyurea (HU) is the only FDA-approved medication for the treatment of SCD. HU increases fetal hemoglobin concentration within RBCs and reduces the number of circulating white blood cells reducing the frequency of vaso-occlusion. (6) HU was first shown to reduce hospital admission for pain and acute chest syndrome in the placebo-controlled Multi-Center Study of Hydroxyurea (MSH) in adults with severe SCD. With publication of the infant hydroxyurea study (Baby HUG), HU is now recommended for use in infants nine months of age and older with SCA regardless of clinical severity to reduce SCD-related complications [18, 34].

A CBC with differential, reticulocyte count, metabolic profile, quantitative measure of HbF and pregnancy test for women of child bearing age is recommended before the initiation of HU therapy. Starting dosage for infants and children is 20 mg/kg/day, and monitoring with CBC with reticulocyte count should be performed every four weeks when adjusting the dosage. A target of absolute neutrophil count ≥2,000/uL and platelet count ≥80,000/uL should be maintained. Referral to a hematologist should be made for further management with HU in special cases such as renal impairment or lack of response to HU therapy and inclusion of HbSC and HbSB thalassemia patients [18].

## Hematopoietic Stem Cell Transplant

Although current supportive care given to SCD patients has improved survival to adulthood, hematopoietic stem cell transplantation (HSCT) is the only available curative option for patients with SCD [35].

During HSCT, conditioning therapy is performed before the infusion of histocompatible stem cells to reduce the risk of failure of engraftment and chronic graft *versus* host disease; traditional HSCT used myeloablative regimens that were used for patients with malignancy were poorly tolerated by SCD patients. Newer transplant protocols use non-myeloablative regimens which have decreased transplant-related morbidity and mortality. The best outcomes occur with matched-sibling donors; however, a lack of matched sibling donors further reduces the options of cure for SCD patients [35].

Participation in a matched, unrelated HSCT is currently recommended as part of clinical trials for SCD patients experiencing stroke, recurrent vaso-occlusive crisis and ACS that has not improved despite receiving optimal supportive care. HSCT is recommended in symptomatic SCD patients who have a matched sibling donor [18].

Several studies to minimize early transplant related morbidity and mortality are ongoing. Due to the paucity of both related and unrelated donors, for patients with especially severe disease, studies with haploidentical donors (parent donors) offer promise of additional donor sources [36].

# CONCLUSION

SCD is a life threatening condition with childhood onset affecting individuals world-wide, causing episodes of unpredictable and severe pain with risk of multi-system complications, long hospital stays and disability. Several efforts such as newborn screening, to assure early detection, and, preventive therapies such as prophylactic penicillin and hydroxyurea therapy have improved the treatment of SCD and its complications, reducing both disease-related morbidity and mortality. Hematopoietic stem cell transplantation is the only available cure for SCD but more research is needed to reduce the associated risks and make it widely available for the SCD population.

# CONFLICT OF INTEREST

The authors declare no conflict of interest, financial or otherwise.

# ACKNOWLEDGEMENTS

Declared none.

# REFERENCES

[1]    Yawn BP, Buchanan GR, Afenyi-Annan AN, *et al.* Management of Sickle Cell Disease. Jama [Internet] 2014; 312(10): 1033. Available from: http://www.ncbi.nlm.nih.gov/pubmed/25203083 [http://dx.doi.org/10.1001/jama.2014.10517]

[2]    Manwani D, Frenette PS. Vaso-occlusion in sickle cell disease: pathophysiology and novel argeted therapies. Blood [Internet] American Society of Hematology , 2013 Dec 5; [cited 2016 Feb 12];122(24): 3892-8. Available from: /pmc/articles/PMC3854110/?report=abstract [http://dx.doi.org/10.1182/asheducation-2013.1.362]

[3]    Zhang D, Xu C, Manwani D, Frenette PS. Neutrophils, platelets, and inflammatory pathways, at the nexus of sickle cell disease pathophysiology. Blood [Internet] American Society of Hematology , 2016 Jan 12; [cited 2016 Feb 12];127(7): 801-9. Available from: http://www.bloodjournal.org/content/early/2016/01/12/blood-2015-09-618538.abstract [http://dx.doi.org/10.1182/blood-2015-09-618538]

[4]    McGann PT. Sickle cell anemia: An underappreciated and unaddressed contributor to global childhood mortality. J Pediatr [Internet] Elsevier Ltd 2014; 165(1): 18-22. Available from: http://dx.doi.org/10.1016/j.jpeds.2014.01.070

[5]    Michael E, DeBaun R, Melissa J, Frei-Jones EPV. Hemoglobinopathies, Nelson Textbook of Pediatrics [Internet]. 20th ed.. Elsevier 2016; pp. (Chapter 462): 2336-53. Available from: https://www.clinicalkey.com/#!/content/book/3-s2.0-B9781455775668004622

[6]    Wang WC, Ware RE, Miller ST, *et al.* Hydroxycarbamide in very young children with sickle-cell anaemia: A multicentre, randomised, controlled trial (BABY HUG). Lancet [Internet] 2011; 377(9778): 1663-72. Available from: http://dx.doi.org/10.1016/S0140-6736(11)60355-3

[7]    Ware RE, Davis BR, Schultz WH, *et al.* Hydroxycarbamide versus chronic transfusion for maintenance of transcranial doppler flow velocities in children with sickle cell anaemia—TCD With Transfusions Changing to Hydroxyurea (TWiTCH): a multicentre, open-label, phase 3, non-inferiority trial. Lancet [Internet] 2015; 6736(15): 1-10. Available from: http://linkinghub.elsevier.com/retrieve/pii/S0140673615010417

[8]    Du F, Zhang M, Li X, *et al.* HHS Public Access. Biochem Biophys Res Commun 2014; 452(4): 1034-9.
[http://dx.doi.org/10.1016/j.bbrc.2014.09.038]

[9]    Quinn CT. Sickle cell disease in childhood. from newborn screening through transition to adult medical care. Pediatr Clin North Am 2013; 60(6): 1363-81.
[http://dx.doi.org/10.1016/j.pcl.2013.09.006]

[10]   Rees DC, Williams TN, Gladwin MT. Sickle-cell disease. Lancet 2010; 376: 2018-31.
[http://dx.doi.org/10.1016/S0140-6736(10)61029-X]

[11]   Saraf SL, Molokie RE, Nouraie M, *et al.* Differences in the clinical and genotypic presentation of sickle cell disease around the world. Paediatr Respir Rev 2014; 15(1): 4-12.
[http://dx.doi.org/10.1016/j.prrv.2013.11.003]

[12]   Bender MA, Nielsen KR. Hemoglobinopathies [Internet] Fourth Edi Pediatric Critical Care Elsevier 2011; 1191-206. Available from: http://www.crossref.org/deleted_DOI.html

[13]   Rees DC, Williams TN, Gladwin MT. Sickle-cell disease. Lancet [Internet] Elsevier Ltd 2010; 376(9757): 2018-31.
[http://dx.doi.org/10.1016/S0140-6736(10)61029-X]

[14]   Lovett PB, Sule HP, Lopez BL. Sickle cell disease in the emergency department. Emerg Med Clin North Am [Internet] Elsevier Inc 2014; 32(3): 629-47.
[http://dx.doi.org/10.1016/j.emc.2014.04.011]

[15]   Quinn CT, Rogers ZR, Mccavit TL, Buchanan GR. Improved survival of children and adolescents with sickle cell disease. Blood J 2010; 115(17): 3447-52.
[http://dx.doi.org/10.1182/blood-2009-07-233700]

[16]   Kesse-Adu R. Inherited anaemias: sickle cell and thalassaemia. Med (United Kingdom) [Internet] Elsevier Ltd 2013; 41(4): 219-4.
[http://dx.doi.org/10.1016/j.mpmed.2013.01.012]

[17]   Chou S. Transfusion therapy for sickle cell disease: a balancing act. Hematology 2013; 2013(1): 439-46.
[http://dx.doi.org/10.1182/asheducation-2013.1.439]

[18]   Yawn BP. Evidence-bases management of sickle cell disease: expert panel report 2014. www.nhlbi.nih.gov. 2014

[19]   Ogunlesi F, Heeney MM, Koumbourlis AC. Systemic corticosteroids in acute chest syndrome: Friend or foe? Paediatr Respir Rev 2014; 15(1): 24-7. [Internet]. Elsevier Ltd.
[http://dx.doi.org/10.1016/j.prrv.2013.10.004]

[20]   Yawn BP, Buchanan GR, Afenyi-Annan AN, *et al.* Management of Sickle Cell Disease. JAMA 2014; 312(10): 1033-48.
[http://dx.doi.org/10.1001/jama.2014.10517]

[21]   Caboot JB, Allen JL. Hypoxemia in sickle cell disease: Significance and management. Paediatr Respir Rev 2014; 15(1): 17-23. [Internet]. Elsevier Ltd.
[http://dx.doi.org/10.1016/j.prrv.2013.12.004]

[22]   McCavit. Timothy L. Xuan L. Hospitalization for Invasive Pneumococcal Disease in a National Sample of Children With Sickle Cell Disease Before and After PCV7 Licensure. Pediatr Blood Cancer 2012; 58: 945-9.
[http://dx.doi.org/10.1002/pbc.23259]

[23]   McCavit TL, Quinn CT, Techasaensiri C, Rogers ZR. Increase in invasive Streptococcus pneumoniae infections in children with sickle cell disease since pneumococcal conjugate vaccine licensure. J Pediatr 2011; 158(3): 505-7. [Internet]. Mosby, Inc.
[http://dx.doi.org/10.1016/j.jpeds.2010.11.025]

[24]  Meier ER, Miller JJ. Sickle cell disease in children. Drugs 2012; 72(7): 895-906.
      [http://dx.doi.org/10.2165/11632890-000000000-00000]

[25]  Hirst C, Owusu-Ofori S. Prophylactic antibiotics for preventing pneumococcal infection in children
      with sickle cell disease. Cochrane Database Syst Rev 2012; (3):

[26]  Fasano RM, Meier ER, Hulbert ML. Cerebral vasculopathy in children with sickle cell anemia. Blood
      Cells. Mol Dis Elsevier Inc 2015; 54(1): 17-25.

[27]  Meier ER, Fasano RM, Estrada M, He J, Luban NLC, McCarter R. Early Reticulocytosis and Anemia
      Are Associated with Abnormal and Conditional Transcranial Doppler Velocities in Children with
      Sickle Cell Anemia. J Pediatr Elsevier Inc 2015; 169: 227-31.

[28]  Lee MT, Piomelli S, Granger S, Miller ST, Harkness S, Brambilla DJ, *et al.* Stroke Prevention Trial in
      Sickle Cell Anemia (STOP): Extended follow-up and final results. Blood 2006; 108(3): 847-52.
      [http://dx.doi.org/10.1182/blood-2005-10-009506]

[29]  Ware RE, Davis BR, Schultz WH, Brown RC, Aygun B, Sarnaik S, *et al.* Hydroxycarbamide versus
      chronic transfusion for maintenance of transcranial doppler flow velocities in children with sickle cell
      anaemia—TCD With Transfusions Changing to Hydroxyurea (TWiTCH): a multicentre, open-label,
      phase 3, non-inferiority trial. Lancet 2015; 6736(15): 1-10. [Internet]. Elsevier Ltd; Available from:
      http://linkinghub.elsevier.com/retrieve/pii/S0140673615010417

[30]  Ware RE, Helms RW. Stroke with transfusions changing to hydroxyurea (SWiTCH). Blood 2012;
      119(17): 3925-32.
      [http://dx.doi.org/10.1182/blood-2011-11-392340]

[31]  Donaldson JF, Rees RW, Steinbrecher HA. Priapism in children: A comprehensive review and clinical
      guideline. J Pediatr Urol 2014; 10(1): 11-25. Elsevier Ltd

[32]  Gladwin M, Vichinsky E. Pulmonary complications of sickle cell disease. N Engl J Med 2008;
      359(21): 2254-65. [Internet]. Elsevier Ltd.

[33]  Mehari A, Klings E. Pulmonary complications of sickle cell disease. Chest Elsevier Ltd 2015;
      359(21): 2254-65.

[34]  Thompson BW, Miller ST, Rogers ZR, *et al.* The pediatric hydroxyurea phase III clinical trial (BABY
      HUG). Pediatr Blood Cancer 2010; 54(2): 250-5.

[35]  Walters MC, De Castro LM, Sullivan KM, *et al.* Indications and Results of Human Leukocyte
      Antigen-identical Sibling Hematopoietic Cell Transplantation for Sickle Cell Disease. Biol Blood
      Marrow Transplant 2015; 22: 207-11.
      [http://dx.doi.org/10.1016/j.bbmt.2015.10.017]

[36]  Bolaños-Meade J, Brodsky RA. Blood and marrow transplantation for sickle cell disease: Is less more?
      Blood Rev Elsevier Ltd 2014; 28(6): 243-8.
      [http://dx.doi.org/10.1016/j.blre.2014.08.001]

# CHAPTER 17

# Management of Recurrent Epistaxis

## Kathleen R. Billings[*]

*Division of Pediatric Otolaryngology-Head and Neck Surgery, Ann & Robert H. Lurie Children's Hospital of Chicago, Chicago, IL, USA*

**Abstract:** Objective: To describe the etiology, diagnostic examination, and management options of recurrent epistaxis in children, to help clinicians better delineate which patients might benefit from conservative *versus* more aggressive therapies.

Results: Epistaxis occurs frequently in children, and affected children are often seen by primary care, emergency department, and otolaryngology physicians. Knowledge of the underlying etiology, diagnostic examination techniques, and available treatment options is essential for clinicians. A review of the current literature was performed, and this chapter provides information about epistaxis management. Most cases of epistaxis are self-limited and respond well to conservative treatments, such as lubricants and antiseptic ointments; however, some cases will require hematologic testing, diagnostic imaging, and intraoperative assessment and management.

Conclusions: Epistaxis is a common diagnosis in children. Clinicians should be familiar with the etiology and management of this condition in children.

**Keywords:** Epistaxis diagnosis, Epistaxis etiology, Epistaxis management, Pediatric epistaxis.

## INTRODUCTION

Epistaxis (nosebleed) is defined as acute bleeding from the nostril, nasal cavity, or nasopharynx [1 - 5]. The condition is very common in children, although it rarely occurs in those under 2 years of age. Reports site the incidence of at least one episode of epistaxis to be around 30% among children aged 0-5 years, 56% among those aged 6-10 years, and 64% among those aged 11-15 years. [1, 5] Most bleeding episodes are minor and self-limited, requiring no medical attention. However, bleeding can be unpredictable and may have an impact on the quality of life for the child and family. Families may fear excessive blood loss due to

---

[*] **Corresponding author Kathleen R. Billings**: Division of Pediatric Otolaryngology-Head and Neck Surgery, Ann & Robert H. Lurie Children's Hospital of Chicago, Chicago, IL, USA; Tel: 312-227-9414; Fax: 312-227-6230; Email: KBillings@luriechildrens.org

**Seckin Ulualp (Ed.)**

recurrent epistaxis [2]. Many seek medical attention from primary care or emergency department physicians and otolaryngologists for the management of epistaxis. A general understanding of the etiology, examination, and treatment options for epistaxis is essential for all clinicians caring for children. This chapter will provide a review of the current diagnostic and treatment strategies for children with recurrent epistaxis.

## ETIOLOGY

In the majority of children, spontaneous bleeding is almost always venous and arises from "Little's area," the anterior region of the nasal septum. A number of arteries anastomose in this region, forming a plexus of vessels under the thin septal mucosa called Kiesselbach's plexus. Bleeding can occur in this area when exposed to dry air or minor trauma. Crusting and scabbing in the area can cause itching, leading to repetitive trauma to the region by picking and rubbing. Recurrent epistaxis, referred to as "idiopathic epistaxis," in children is usually attributed to crusting, nasal vestibulitis and/or digital trauma, although no direct cause can be established in many cases. [1, 3 - 5] Allergic rhinitis is thought to contribute to epistaxis due to nasal mucosal inflammatory changes, leading to friable, irritated mucosa that is more apt to bleed. Nasal colonization with *Staphylococcus aureus* has been shown to be more common in children with epistaxis than in control subjects, and the bacterial colonization has been postulated to cause inflammation and new vessel formation, leading to epistaxis [6 - 8]. Irritation in the nasal cavity can lead to digital trauma and subsequent epistaxis. Kamble *et al* [7] found that the presence of *S. aureus* colonization in the anterior nasal cavity was associated with significant crusting and dilated blood vessels on the anterior septum in children with epistaxis. Other causative factors for epistaxis include trauma, anatomic abnormalities, medications, neoplasms, and coagulopathies [9, 10].

The incidence of epistaxis is thought to be greater in the cold, winter months in northern climates, when upper respiratory infections are more frequent and when indoor humidity decreases to low levels [1,11]. Nosebleeds may also occur more often in hot, dry climates with low humidity; however, given the commonality of epistaxis in children, ambient temperature may have little impact on the overall rate of bleeding.

There is no general consensus on the best approach for the evaluation of pediatric epistaxis. A thorough review of the patient's history and physical examination, including anterior rhinoscopy are recommended. History should include frequency of nose bleeds, laterality (important when considering cautery), duration of bleeding, and the presence of easy bruising or bleeding easily with other minor traumas (both possibly suggestive of coagulopathies). Documentation of prior trauma to the area, history of allergic rhinitis, and a review of medications (*i.e.*, aspirin use) may help elucidate the cause of bleeding. A family history of epistaxis is important when considering the diagnosis of hereditary hemorrhagic telangiectasia (HHT) and coagulopathies, such as hemophilia and von Willebrand disease. At physical examination, the nasal cavity is assessed for the source of bleeding. Visible vessels on the anterior septum are often apparent, in addition to drying and crusting of the nasal mucous membranes. Oral cavity examination might reveal the presence of telangiectasia in patients with HHT. Rigid or flexible nasal endoscopy is appropriate in those in whom the source is uncertain or when there is suspicion for a neoplasm, such as juvenile nasopharyngeal angiofibroma (JNA) [3, 4]. Imaging studies, such as computed tomography (CT) or magnetic resonance (MR) imaging, are not recommended in the routine examination of a child with epistaxis. When confirming or considering the diagnosis of JNA or another nasal neoplasm, imaging is necessary to assess the extent of involvement of the surrounding structures.

Knowing when more aggressive diagnostic testing should be used can be challenging. In a study by Patel *et al* [4], laboratory testing, including a complete blood count and a prothrombin time/activated partial thromboplastin time (PT/PTT), was performed in 131 of 175 (74.9%) pediatric patients with epistaxis. Twenty-seven (20.6%) patients were found to be anemic at testing, although only 2 had hemoglobin levels less than 10 mg/dL and 3 had hematocrit less than 30%. No patient required a blood transfusion for anemia or severe bleeding. A study by Elden *et al* [10] demonstrated anemia in 4 of 47 (8.5%) patients in an analysis of predictors of bleeding disorders in children with epistaxis. The study included children with severe epistaxis who had experienced medical management failure and who were undergoing intraoperative cautery. Anemia was associated with younger age in both studies mentioned (5.9 years and 6.4 years, respectively), which may reflect the impact of blood loss on lesser overall blood volume of younger children.

Sandoval *et al* [9] found duration, severity, and the presence of other bleeding symptoms to have no predictive value for the diagnosis of coagulopathy in 178 pediatric patients referred to a hematology clinic for a diagnosis of coagulopathy. The authors diagnosed coagulopathy in 59 (33.0%) of the patients analyzed (age range 15-219 months). The coagulopathies diagnosed included von Willebrand disease in 33, platelet aggregation disorders in 10, thrombocytopenia in 7, mild factor VII deficiency in 3, Bernard-Soulier syndrome in 2, and a variety of other factor deficiencies in the remaining patients. Only a family history of bleeding was predictive of the diagnosis of a bleeding disorder, and children who received a diagnosis of coagulopathy had a longer median PTT than did those without the diagnosis (33.1 *versus* 30.5, *P*=0.012) [9]. Of note, this study only included children referred to a hematology department because of the severity of their epistaxis and may not be reflective of the average child with routine idiopathic epistaxis.

When looking at the incidence of coagulopathy in children with severe epistaxis, defined as those experiencing medical management failure and requiring intraoperative cautery by an otolaryngologist, Elden *et al* [10] noted abnormal coagulation study results for 15 of 47 (31.9%) pediatric patients with epistaxis. Fifteen were referred to a hematology department for assessment, and 5 received a diagnosis of a bleeding disorder (3 cases of von Willebrand disease, 1 case of platelet aggregation disorder, and 1 case of mild factor VII deficiency). The only predictive factor for a bleeding disorder noted by the analysis of variables was a history of emergency department visit for epistaxis. Nonpredictors included additional personal history of bleeding, family history of a specific bleeding disorder, anemia due to epistaxis, history of emergent nasal interventions, prior nasal cautery, sex, age, duration of epistaxis, location of epistaxis, and frequency of epistaxis [10]. Based on these prior studies, there appears to be no definitive guideline as to which children with epistaxis might benefit from further hematologic testing. Healthcare practitioners must therefore rely on clinical judgment of the severity of a child's epistaxis, family history of bleeding disorders, and history of interventions when making decisions about ordering coagulations studies and further hematologic testing.

## MANAGEMENT

Management of idiopathic epistaxis in children often includes application of lubricants or creams to the anterior septum and/or topical nasal cautery using silver nitrate sticks. Nasal packing is less often used in the office setting and is generally reserved for emergent control of bleeding. There is no consensus on the best strategy for managing epistaxis. Lubricants like petroleum jelly, antiseptic ointments, and saline-based gels are readily available and often used for maintenance management of epistaxis. Antiseptic creams or gels are used to reduce vestibulitis and crusting. Antiseptic creams may fail to reduce vestibular irritation due to repetitive nose picking and re-colonization of the area with bacteria. However, lubricants are more easily tolerated and generally less traumatic than cautery, and they can be used daily [1, 5, 12].

Silver nitrate acts by oxidizing organic tissue and destroying the underlying blood vessels with acid, causing them to be replaced by scar tissue. There are 2 different concentrations of silver nitrate, 75% and 95%. A prospective, double-blind randomized clinical trial comparing the 2 in the management of children with idiopathic epistaxis was performed by Glynn *et al.* [13] Their results showed greater efficacy and fewer adverse effects with the 75% concentration, and this is the recommended concentration for cauterization. A double-blind, randomized controlled trial comparing children receiving silver nitrate cautery, followed by antiseptic cream for 4 weeks, with those receiving antiseptic cream only was performed by Calder *et al.* [5] The study found that a larger number of children in the silver nitrate group had improvement in their symptoms compared with those receiving antiseptic alone. In another prospective, randomized study comparing cautery to nasal antiseptic ointment, 100 children were assigned to each of the 2 groups. The authors noted recurrence of epistaxis in 38% of the silver nitrate cautery group and 52% of the nasal antiseptic group in the 3 months after treatment. The difference was not statistically significant [14]. A retrospective analysis of bilateral silver nitrate cautery of the septum noted total or near-total resolution of epistaxis in 40 of 43 (93.0%) children studied [15]. The authors reported no substantial complications of infection, perforation, long-term crusting, tattooing, or allergic reactions in their patients, and they cited the lack of evidence of risk of septal perforation in children undergoing cautery.

Concern has been raised that cautery can also lead to atrophy of the nasal mucosa, which can lead to septal crusting and perforation [1]. According to reports, cautery causes sclerosis of the vessels and thickening of the mucosa, although in children, bleeding can occur as a result of vestibulitis, which causes ulcerations in the mucosa, rather than discrete enlarged vessels, making cautery ineffective in this context. A Cochrane analysis of interventions for idiopathic epistaxis found no single treatment of epistaxis to be better than another. No serious adverse effects of the available treatment options were noted, other than pain related to silver nitrate cautery [1]. Clinical judgment must be used when making recommendations for control of bleeding with lubricants or antiseptic creams, cautery, or both in the management of simple recurrent idiopathic epistaxis in children. Active bleeding may require nasal packing. There are a variety of options when considering nasal packing, and dissolvable hemostatic options may be preferable in children.

Intraoperative management of epistaxis may be required in situations of refractory bleeding, or in cases of poor patient tolerance in the office setting. Precise localization of bleeding sites can be determined by endoscopy, and vessels can be cauterized with silver nitrate or a variety of electrocautery devices (*i.e.*, suction cautery, bipolar cautery, laser cautery). A study by Johnson *et al.* [16], compared outcomes in children undergoing bipolar electrocautery with those in children undergoing silver nitrate cautery to the anterior septum in the intraoperative setting. Of the 50 children undergoing bipolar electrocautery, 1 (2.0%) had a recurrence within 2 years, compared with 13 of 60 (22.0%) patients who underwent silver nitrate cautery. The difference was statistically significant; however, after 2 years, there was no difference between the 2 groups. More aggressive techniques, such as ligation techniques, septal surgery techniques, posterior packing, and embolization techniques, may be needed in severe cases for which less invasive options for control of bleeding have failed. These techniques are more commonly used in adults, in whom the bleeding site is more often posterior in the nasal cavity and related to underlying hypertension [17, 18]. Severity of the bleeding encountered, the ability to locate the source of bleeding, and clinician preference may affect the choice of available therapies.

## SPECIAL CONSIDERATIONS

### JNA

When evaluating teenaged boys with epistaxis, the diagnosis of JNA should be considered. In this situation, nasal endoscopy is suggested to carefully inspect the posterior nasal cavity and nasopharynx for the presence of this vascular lesion [4]. JNA is a benign, vascularized lesion that typically occurs in adolescent boys, aged 14-25 years, presenting with cpistaxis and nasal obstruction [19 - 23]. The tumor is non-encapsulated, submucosal spreading, and locally destructive. JNAs originate within the superior posterior margin of the sphenopalatine foramen and can extend into the pterygoplatine fossa, paranasal sinuses, and intracranially in 10%-20% of cases. Most patients present with minor symptoms of painless, unilateral nasal obstruction and epistaxis, although life-threatening epistaxis can occur [22]. Because of the vascular nature of these lesions, biopsy is not recommended for diagnosis; instead MR imaging, MR angiography, and/or CT scanning are used for diagnostic purposes. Staging of the lesion can be accomplished through imaging studies based on the extent of spread of the lesion [21]. Surgery is the mainstay of treatment for JNA, generally in conjunction with embolization performed before surgical resection. Surgical options, including transhyoid, transpalatal, and transfacial approaches through a lateral rhinotomy or midface degloving, and infratemporal approaches, have been described. Surgical approaches have changed through time, with the evolution of minimally invasive surgery and endoscopic approaches [19, 20]. In addition, improved surgical instrumentation and the use of CT- or MR imaging–guided surgical navigation techniques, have allowed for enhanced ability to successfully excise JNAs.

Nicolai *et al* [20] described their experience with endoscopic surgery for JNA. Fifteen patients with a mean age of 15.8 years were analyzed. All patients had 2 units of autologous blood samples collected during the 2 weeks leading up to their procedure, and all lesions were embolized prior to surgical resection. The authors concluded that the endoscopic approach was a safe and effective technique, with low morbidity, for removal of small and intermediate sized JNAs that did not have extensive involvement of the infratemporal fossa and cavernous sinus. They suggested that advanced lesions are best treated by external approaches. Scholtz *et al.* [19] suggested that the main advantage of the endoscopic approach to JNA removal was minimal disruption to soft tissue and bone without damage to external structures. Disadvantages are related to restricted access and the difficulty in shifting to alternative endoscopic approaches if complications of hemorrhaging arise. Ultimately, the surgical approach should be selected based on tumor size, tumor location, efficacy of tumor embolization, and experience of the operating surgeon. Preoperative planning for the possibility of a blood transfusion and the need to modify the approach to the lesion appear to be essential. Follow-up with endoscopic assessment and with interval MR imaging for assessment of recurrence should be established with each patient.

## HHT

HHT, or Osler-Weber-Rendu syndrome, is an autosomal dominant vascular dysplasia characterized by the presence of multiple arteriovenous malformations (AVMs) and telangiectasias. The diagnosis is made when a patient has at least 3 of 4 Curacao criteria: recurrent spontaneous epistaxis, family history of HHT, telangiectasias at characteristic sites (lips, oral cavity, nose, and fingers), and proven visceral AVMs [24 - 27]. Pathogenic variant is another consideration, because HHT is caused by pathogenic variants in a number of genes. [24, 25] Epistaxis is the most common symptom associated with HHT, with bleeding severity ranging from infrequent to severe, requiring repeated blood transfusions. Between 80% and 90% of patients with HHT will receive the diagnosis by 21 years of age, beginning at a mean age of 12 years, and almost 95% develop recurrent epistaxis at some point.

Treatment of epistaxis in patients with HHT may include humidification, topical agents, systemic hormones, oral drug therapy, laser ablation, septal dermoplasty, and nasal closure. Avoidance of vigorous nose blowing, electric or chemical cautery, and anti-inflammatory agents is recommended in patients with HHT [24, 25]. Screening for AVMs throughout the intestinal tract is important for affected patients, and appropriate genetic counseling should be provided [26].

## CONCLUSIONS

Epistaxis is common in children and is often manageable with lubricants, antiseptic gels, saline spray, and humidity. Most cases are self-limited and do not require additional examination or intervention. Nasal septal cautery with silver nitrate can be performed in the office setting and has a known favorable success rate. More aggressive cautery techniques in the operative setting can often be reserved for those with refractory bleeding that cannot be controlled with more conservative measures. Hematologic testing should also be considered in such cases. Any teenaged male presenting with epistaxis, particularly in the presence of nasal obstruction, should undergo nasal endoscopy to assess for the presence of JNA. If present, appropriate imaging and referral should be provided. Family history should be ascertained in all children with epistaxis to assess for the diagnosis of HHT in family members. Clinicians should be aware of the stress on the child and family that is associated with recurrent epistaxis and have a general understanding of the available options for management when counseling their patients.

## CONFLICT OF INTEREST

The author declares no conflict of interest, financial or otherwise.

## ACKNOWLEDGEMENTS

Declared none.

## REFERENCES

[1]    Burtan Q. Interventions for recurrent idiopathic epistaxis (nosebleeds) in children (review). Cochrane Database Syst Rev 2012; 9: 1-23.

[2]    Davies K, Kadambari K, Mehanna R, Keogh I. Pediatric epistaxis: epidemiology, management & impact on quality of life. Int J Pediatr Otorhinolaryngol 2014; 78: 1294-7.

[3]    Damrose J, Maddalozzo J. Pediatric epistaxis. Laryngoscope 2006; 116: 387-93.

[4]    Patel N, Maddalozzo J, Billings KR. An update on management of pediatric epistaxis. Int J Pediatr Otorhinolaryngol 2014; 78: 1400-4.

[5]    Calder N, Kang S, Fraser L, *et al.* A double-blind randomized controlled trial of management of recurrent nosebleeds in children. Otolaryngol Head Neck Surg 2009; 140: 670-4.

[6]    Kubba H, MacAndie C, Botma M, *et al.* A prospective, single blind, randomized controlled trial antiseptic cream for recurrent epistaxis in childhood. Clin Otolaryngol 2001; 26: 465-.

[7]    Kamble P, Saxena S, Kumar S. Nasal bacterial colonization in cases of idiopathic epistaxis in children. Int J Pediatr Otorhinolaryngol 2015; (79): 1901-4.

[8]    Whymark AD, Crampsey DP, Fraser L, *et al.* Childhood epistaxis and nasal colonization with *Staphylococcus aureus.* Otolaryngol Head Neck Surg 2008; 138: 307-10.

[9]    Sandoval C, Dong S, Visintainer P. Clinical and laboratory features of 178 children with recurrent epistaxis. J Pediatr Hematol Oncol 2002; 65: 47-9.

[10]   Elden V, Reinders M, Witmer C. Predictors of bleeding disorders in children with epistaxis: value of preoperative tests and clinical screening. Int J Pediatr Otorhinolaryngol 2012; 76: 767-71.

[11]   Mangussi-Gomes J, Enout MJ, Castro TC, *et al.* Is the occurrence of spontaneous epistaxis related to climate variables? A retrospective clinical, epidemiological and meteorological study. Acta Otolaryngol 2016. (pending)

[12]   McGarry GW. Recurrent epistaxis in children. Clin Evid 2013; 10(311): 1-9.

[13]   Glynn F, Amin M, Sheahan P, McShane D. Prospective double blind randomized clinical trial comparing 75% *versus* 95% silver nitrate cauterization in the management of idiopathic childhood epistaxis. Int J Pediatr Otorhinolaryngol 2011; 75: 81-4.

[14]   Ozmen S, Ozmen OA. Is local ointment or cauterization more effective in childhood recurrent epistaxis. Int J Pediatr Otorhinolaryngol 2012; 76(6): 783-6.

[15]   Link TR, Conley SF, Flanary V, Kerschner JE. Bilateral epistaxis in children: efficacy of bilateral septal cauterization with silver nitrate. Int J Pediatr Otorhinolaryngol 2006; 70: 1439-2.

[16]   Johnson N, Faria J, Behar P. A comparison of bipolar electrocautery and chemical cautery for control of pediatric recurrent anterior epistaxis. Otolaryngol Head Neck Surg 2015; 153(5): 851-6.

[17]   Melia L, McGarry W. Epistaxis: update on management. Curr Opin Otolaryngol Head Neck Surg 2011; 19(1): 30-5.

[18]   Soyka MB, Nikolaou G, Rufibach K, Holzman D. On the effectiveness of treatment options in epistaxis: an analysis of 678 interventions. Rhinology 2011; 49(4): 474-8.

[19]   Scholtz AW, Appenroth E, Kammen-Jolly K, Scholtz LU, Thumfart WF. Juvenile nasopharyngeal angiofibroma: management and therapy. Laryngoscope 2001; 111: 681-7.

[20]   Nicolai P, Berlucchi M, Tomenzoli D, *et al.* Endoscopic surgery for juvenile angiofibroma: when and how. Laryngoscope 2003; 113: 775-82.

[21]   Andrews JC, Fisch U, Valavanis A, Aeppli U, Makek MS. The surgical management of extensive nasopharyngeal angiofibromas with the infratemporal fossa approach. Laryngoscope 1989; (99): 429-37.

[22]   Glad H, Vainer B, Buchwald C, *et al.* Juvenile nasopharyngeal angiofibromas in Denmark 1981–2003: diagnosis, incidence, and treatment. Acta Otolaryngol 2007; 127: 292-9.

[23]   Moorthy P, Reddy B, Qaiyum H, Madhira S, Kolloju S. Management of juvenile nasopharyngeal angiofibroma: a five year retrospective study. Indian J Otolaryngol Head Neck Surg 2010; 62(4): 390-4.

[24]   Hunter BN, Timmons BH, McDonald MS, *et al.* An evaluation of the severity and progression of epistaxis in hereditary hemorrhagic telangiectasia 1 *versus* hereditary hemorrhagic telangiectasia 2. Laryngoscope 2016; 126: 786-90.

[25]   McDonald J, Pyeritz RE. Hereditary hemorrhagic telangiectasia. Gene Reviews 2000 Jun 26;

[26]   Mei-Zahav M, Letarte M, Faughnan ME, *et al.* Symptomatic children with hereditary hemorrhagic telangiectasia. Arch Pediatr Adolesc Med 2006; 160: 596-601.

[27]   Shovlin CL, Guttmacher AE, Buscarini E, *et al.* Diagnostic criteria for hereditary hemorrhagic telangiectasia. Am J Med Genet 2000; 91(1): 66-7.

**CHAPTER 18**

# Update on Management of Allergic Rhinitis

## Maria C. Veling[*]

*Department of Otolaryngology – Head and Neck Surgery, University of Texas Southwestern Medical Center, Dallas, TX, USA; Tel/Fax: 214-456-7644;*

**Abstract:** Allergic rhinitis (AR), the most common chronic disease in children, is the fifth most common chronic disease in the United States. Otolaryngologists see a large percentage of patient's whose disease process is often associated with, or caused by, upper and lower airway inflammation. Because allergy is a common contributor to airway inflammation, a working knowledge of the treatment options for pediatric allergic rhinitis is essential in the evaluation and management of children presenting to otolaryngologists.

**Keywords:** Allergic rhinitis, Allergic rhinitis and Allergic conjunctivitis, Allergic rhinitis and Asthma, Allergic rhinitis and Otitis media with effusion, Allergic rhinitis and Rhinosinusitis, Allergic rhinitis and Sleep disturbance, Allergic rhinitis comorbidities, Allergic rhinitis diagnosis, Avoidance, Environmental control, Immunotherapy, Pharmacotherapy, Subcutaneous immunotherapy, Sublingual immunotherapy.

## INTRODUCTION

Allergic rhinitis is one of several comorbid conditions often seen in patients who suffer from allergic disease (atopy). The genetic predisposition to develop allergic diseases, *i.e,* atopy, is typically associated with intensified immune responses to common allergens such as inhaled and food allergens.

The phenotype of allergy has a complicated and variable genetic contribution, hence, no single genetic test is used to identify if an individual is allergic. In the light of the genes identified, alterations in both innate and adaptive immunity are critical in allergic disease [1]. Moreover, gene-environment interactions [2], add another layer of variability to the development of allergic disease. To date exposure to cigarette smoke, higher socioeconomic level, first born or only child, and elevated total IgE (>100 IU/L) before age 6 have been identified as risk

---

[*] **Corresponding author Maria C. Veling**: Department of Otolaryngology – Head and Neck Surgery, University of Texas Southwestern Medical Center, Dallas, TX, USA; Tel/Fax: 214-456-7644; Email: maria.veling@utsouthwestern.edu

**Seckin Ulualp (Ed.)**

factors for developing allergic disease [3].

Generally, the first clinical manifestation of allergic rhinitis disease in early childhood is atopic dermatitis. A typical sequence of food allergy, rhinitis and asthma follows atopic dermatitis. The atopic march describes the progression of atopic manifestations from atopic dermatitis to allergic rhinitis and asthma. A number of cross-sectional and longitudinal studies substantiate its validity; however, more data are needed to support the atopic march hypothesis [4 - 7]. The atopic march may not be a simple progression as genetic and environmental factors influence the development of atopic dermatitis, allergic rhinitis and asthma.

## ALLERGIC RHINITIS (AR)

Allergic rhinitis, affecting 1 out of 6 Americans, is the most common chronic disease in the United States. AR and related illnesses account for 800,000 to 2 million lost school days on annual basis [8, 9].

Allergic rhinitis is a chronic disorder of the upper airways and is induced by IgE-mediated inflammation after exposure of the nasal membranes in sensitized patients to a specific allergen [10]. The symptoms of allergic rhinitis encompass nasal congestion, nasal drainage, sneezing, nasal itching, and postnasal drainage. Allergic rhinitis has a multiplicity of symptoms with varied clinical presentation in the pediatric patient, depending on the duration of allergy on exposure, age, and presence of comorbid disease. In addition, its symptoms can be similar to those of recurrent upper respiratory infections, a common occurrence in childhood, leading to under treatment of the allergic disease process.

The prevalence of AR varies with factors including, but not limited to, genetics, epigenetics, and environmental exposure. Worldwide prevalence estimates range from 1.5% to 39.7% depending on geographic location [11]. In The Pediatric Allergies in America Survey, otolaryngologists surveyed estimated that 41% of their pediatric patients, aged 4 to 17 years, were diagnosed with allergic rhinitis [12].

Although allergic rhinitis is not life threatening, it can have a significant impact on the quality of life [13], school performance, quality of sleep, and physical and emotional health [12]. In addition, it can have a substantial economic impact including both direct costs to patients and indirect costs that include absenteeism [14] and inefficient school performance [15]

## Diagnosis

Allergic rhinitis in children is diagnosed based on history, clinical assessment and allergy testing. Allergy testing in the absence of clinical likelihood of allergic disease yields unacceptable false-positive rates and is not recommended. This was illustrated by a positive skin prick test in 53.9% of 10,509 Americans randomly sampled in Third National Health and Nutrition Survey [16].

Though the recently published Clinical Practice Guideline on Allergic Rhinitis states that skin testing can be used in patients of any age [17], early sensitization to inhalant allergens in infancy occurs infrequently and there is rarely a need to test for them in children less than 4 years of age. Herr and colleagues [18] used a standardized questionnaire in 1850 infants at their 18th-month examination to identify children with allergic rhinitis-like symptoms defined as runny nose, blocked nose, and sneezing apart from a cold. Of the 1850 infants, 9.1% were found to have allergic rhinitis-like symptoms. All children were then assessed with a specific inhalant IgE screen, total IgE, and eosinophilia. There was no difference in eosinophilia or total IgE in the "allergic rhinitis-like symptoms" group compared with the "no allergic rhinitis-like symptoms" group. Only 9 of the 1850 children had both allergic rhinitis-like symptoms and elevated inhalant-specific IgE. In comparison, there were 43 of 1850 infants with elevated inhalant-specific IgE that were identified in the "no AR-like symptoms group." This suggests that allergic rhinitis is rare at 18 months of age and that screening infants for elevated specific IgE would lack specificity in identifying infants with clinical symptoms.

When there is a high degree of suspicion, testing only for indoor allergens, may identify the majority of sensitized children as demonstrated by Sahiner *et al* [19]. In their study, they looked at 432 children, less than 2 years of age, with asthma, and tested them with either a full panel of inhalant allergens, including indoor allergens *vs*. indoor allergens alone. They found the rate of sensitization to be essentially equal between the two groups concluding that in the very young, testing for indoor allergens alone, may identify the majority of affected children.

It is also important to remember that negative allergy skin testing in early childhood does not exclude sensitization and allergic symptoms at a later age [20].

## TREATMENT OF ALLERGIC RHINITIS

Treatment of allergic rhinitis in children is similar to treatment in adults, and consists of avoidance, environmental controls, pharmacologic therapy, and specific allergen desensitization.

## Avoidance and Environmental Controls

Although counseling about environmental control of allergic rhinitis is recommended, clinical efficacy in controlled studies is often disappointing [21 - 24].

Terreehorst and colleagues [25] performed a randomized placebo-control trial of dust mite mattress covers in 279 subjects allergic to dust mite. Although they were able to demonstrate a decrease in dust mite counts, no clinical improvement in AR symptoms was detected between the study and control groups. A recent Cochrane review suggested an extensive bedroom-based program including acaracides, mite impermeable covers, and high-efficiency particulate air (HEPA) filters may "be of some benefit" in improving allergic rhinitis symptoms [26].

After in-depth review of the current literature looking at the effects of environmental control in AR patients, the Clinical Practice Guideline on Allergic Rhinitis, considers allergen avoidance and environmental manipulation as an "option" for patients with identified allergens correlating with clinical symptoms [17].

## Pharmacotherapy

Pharmacotherapy for allergic rhinitis is categorized as either targeted therapy (decongestants, antihistamines, leukotriene receptor antagonists, *etc.*) or immunomodulators (steroids, immunotherapy, monoclonal antibodies). The selection of a specific medication for a patient depends on multiple factors including symptom profile, medication cost, response to previous treatment, ease of administration, associated medical conditions and side effect profile.

Intranasal steroids are strongly recommended for patients with a clinical diagnosis of allergic rhinitis and whose symptoms affect their quality of life [17]. Intranasal steroids improve the quality of life and sleep by reducing nasal symptoms including congestion, sneezing, and rhinorrhea in adults and children with allergic rhinitis [27 - 30]. A concern regarding their use in children is the effect intranasal steroids may have on growth. This has been investigated in controlled studies and although the findings are mixed, they suggest that, of the intranasal steroid preparations studied in children, fluticasone propionate and mometasone furoate showed no effects on growth compared with placebo [31, 32]. Hence, in clinical practice, it seems prudent to use the intranasal steroid preparations that have not been shown to have any negative impact on growth in children.

Oral antihistamines have been shown to be beneficial in AR patients with complaints of sneezing and itching [33]. Rapid onset of action, once daily dosing and OTC availability are advantages of oral antihistamines. Second generation antihistamines are preferred due to less sedating effect.

Intranasal antihistamines have been shown to be equal or superior to oral antihistamines for the treatment of nasal symptoms in numerous well- designed randomized studies [17]. Intranasal antihistamines have the advantage of direct delivery to the affected nasal tissues while limiting systemic effects [34], however in the pediatric patient they are limited to children 5 years old and older.

Currently, oral leukotriene receptor antagonists (LTRAs) are not recommended as primary therapy for patients with allergic rhinitis [17]. However, there is conflicting evidence as to its efficacy when these are used in combination with an oral antihistamine. Some studies have shown better clinical response when used in combination than when either medication is used alone [35, 36], while others showed no effect [37, 38].

## Immunotherapy

Overall, the majority of allergic rhinitis patients show some improvement with medical management and environmental controls. Allergic rhinitis patients who fail to have an adequate response of their symptoms to pharmacologic therapy should be offered immunotherapy. Allergen specific immunotherapy has the potential to change the natural course of AR. It is unique in its beneficial effect on allergies after the treatment is discontinued, its effect on reducing additional sensitizations, and reduction in the development of allergic asthma [39].

Both subcutaneous and sublingual immunotherapy in children has been shown to be effective [39 - 41]. Immunotherapy improves the control of comorbid conditions such as asthma and conjunctivitis, and the disease specific quality of life [17]. Risk, time, and expense of immunotherapy needs to be carefully matched to severity and ability to control allergic disease.

## COMORBIDITIES OFTEN PRESENT IN THE ALLERGIC PATIENT

The epidemiologic association among the atopic disorders has been well established and recognition of these associations has impact on both diagnosis and therapy. For instance, AR is rarely found in isolation and needs to be considered in the context of systemic allergic disease.

### Allergic Rhinitis and Allergic Conjunctivitis

There is a large overlap between AR and allergic conjunctivitis and it is often considered one disease: rhinoconjunctivitis. Bielory [42] summarizes several epidemiologic studies to estimate that there is 80% overlap, with 10% having AR alone and 10% having allergic conjunctivitis alone. The large ISAAC studies looked at rhinoconjunctivitis as single diagnosis and reported symptoms in 8.5% of 6 to 7 year old and 14.6% in 13 to 14 year old. As such, children with AR should be assessed for allergic conjunctivitis and topical antihistamine considered [42 - 44].

## Allergic Rhinitis and Rhinosinusitis

The close anatomical association between the nose and paranasal sinuses provides a great deal of influence over each other that is not limited to obstruction or spillover of inflammation. Especially in atopic individuals, rhinitis and rhinosinusitis are individual manifestations of a systemic response. Rhinitis and rhinosinusitis are characterized by inflammation with overlapping symptoms such as impaired nasal breathing and rhinorrhea. The relationship between allergic rhinitis and rhinosinusitis has been investigated in both the adult and pediatric populations. It has been reported that more than 80% of children with rhinosinusitis have a family history of allergy while in a general population allergy frequency is 15-20% [45].

Rhinosinusitis is commonly seen in patients with asthma and allergic rhinitis and has been shown to be a trigger for asthma in children and adults [46]. Allergic rhinitis has also been linked to children with asthma and otitis media with effusion, with the incidence of rhinosinusitis being higher in this patient population [47]. From the standpoint of treatment outcomes, immunotherapy before endoscopic sinus surgery in children with allergic rhinitis significantly improved the surgical success rate from 64 to 84% [48]. On the other hand, there are also studies suggesting a lack of correlation between allergic disease and pediatric rhinosinusitis [49].

## Allergic Rhinitis and Otitis Media with Effusion (OME)

The role of allergy in the pathophysiology of OME has been a matter of debate for many years. Epidemiological studies have demonstrated an association between OME and atopic conditions such as allergic rhinitis [50, 51]. The prevalence of allergic rhinitis in patients with chronic or recurrent OME varies widely, ranging from 16.3% to 89% [52], and may be higher than that of the general population [53, 54].

The studies aimed at examining the relationship between allergic rhinitis and OME have yielded incongruous results suggesting either large regional differences or bias in associating otitis and allergic disease. Furthermore, a true causative association would suggest that suppressing the inflammatory response would lead to improvement of otitis media symptoms, which has not been found.

At this time the resulting literature, including the recent Clinical Practice Guidelines on Otitis Media with Effusion update [17], do not support the treatment of isolated OME with antihistamines, decongestants, oral or topical steroids in the general population [55 - 58].

It is however important to note, that the vast majority of studies examining the relationship between AR and OME, do not consider the allergy status of the children treated for OME, and it is unknown whether the subgroup with proven allergic inflammation might respond differently. Recently age was identified as an effect modifier in patients with OME [59]. In children 6 years old or older, the presence of AR significantly increased the odds of OME and ETD. Well-designed trials, with better-defined subpopulations are needed to further evaluate the possible causality between AR and OME in the older child.

## Allergic Rhinitis and Asthma

Demonstration of a statistical association between AR and asthma does not allow us to conclude that AR causes asthma. Allergic rhinitis might be an independent risk factor for asthma [10, 60]. Although the link between AR and asthma is well-established, a causal relationship is not. It is possible that AR and asthma are both manifestations of an underlying systemic allergic tendency [61]. Nevertheless, the association between AR and asthma renders children with AR to be assessed for asthma and vice versa [62, 63].

Treatments targeting either asthma or AR may alleviate the other coexisting condition [64, 65]. Treating co-morbid allergic rhinitis may result in better asthma outcomes in terms of asthma symptoms, emergency department visits and hospitalizations, and lower overall costs [66].

The data on the effect of allergen avoidance or pharmacotherapy on the long-term natural history of respiratory allergy, in particular the development of asthma, has been limited [22, 67, 68]. Much more promising is the field of allergen specific immunotherapy. Allergen-specific immunotherapy (SIT) may alter the natural course of an allergic disease and has potential to interfere with the development of allergic asthma in some patients [69].

In the PAT study [70 - 72], children with seasonal rhinoconjunctivitis receiving subcutaneous immunotherapy with grass and/or birch standardized allergen extracts for 3 years, showed long-term ($\geq$7 years) clinical effects and a preventive effect on asthma development. Randomized controlled open trials of sublingual immunotherapy in children have also suggested a preventive asthma effect [73 - 75].

In an effort to further substantiate the disease-modifying effect of SIT on the development of asthma, the ongoing GAP (Grazax Asthma Prevention) trial represents the first double-blind, placebo controlled randomized study aiming to assess the preventive effect of SIT on asthma development [76]. Awareness of asthma is important for otolaryngologists because of the epidemiologic link between chronic upper and lower airway inflammation [10, 77].

Asthma is under diagnosed, impairs quality of life, and even mild persistent asthma is potentially life threatening [78]. The ability to identify asthma, initiate treatment, and ensure appropriate continued care should be the goal of every specialist who cares for children that are known to be at increased risk of this common disease.

## Allergic Rhinitis and Its Impact on Sleep

Sleep disturbance has been increasingly recognized as one of the major impacts of allergic rhinitis, and has been demonstrated to be more common in patients with allergic diseases than in the general population [79 - 81]. Nasal congestion is a hallmark symptom of allergic rhinitis and is considered to be the most important mechanism behind poor sleep and daytime sleepiness in AR patients. AR has been identified as a potential risk factor for sleep disordered breathing (SDB) [82].

Nasal congestion has been reported to be the cause of difficulty falling asleep in 49% of children and 48% of adults with AR. It is also reported as the cause of arousals from sleep in 49% of children and 51% of adults [83]. Epidemiological studies both support and refute the hypothesis that SDB and allergic rhinitis are interconnected in adult and pediatric populations [84 - 88].

Not all research supports the contribution of allergic rhinitis to sleep-disordered breathing (SDB). Adenotonsillectomy outcomes for treatment of OSA in over 500 children revealed that over 39.5% of children were identified as having allergic rhinitis [85]. However, a lack of a control group and the fact that the prevalence of AR was within the estimates of allergic rhinitis in the general population [89], resulted in this study not being able to identify allergic rhinitis as a factor influencing response to adenotonsillectomy for the treatment of SDB [85].

In a qualitative systematic review of the association between allergic rhinitis and SDB in children [90], two-thirds of the articles demonstrated statistically significant association between allergic rhinitis and SDB whereas one-sixth of the articles found no statistically significant correlation. The weakness of the data included lack of the use of formal polysomnography for the diagnosis of OSA and allergy testing to diagnose allergic rhinitis in the majority of the articles.

It has been previously demonstrated that sleep disorders, independent of allergic rhinitis, affect the normal balance of Th17 and T regulatory cells (Treg) [91, 92] and that the Th17/Treg ratio positively correlates with the severity of OSA [93, 94]. Th17 cells through IL17 production play critical roles in the development of auto immunity and allergic reactions. Treg cells are involved in immune tolerance by releasing anti-inflammatory cytokines. The balance between the two is critical for controlling the development of autoimmune and inflammatory responses such as allergic disease.

Recently, Ni and colleagues [95] looked at the role of Th17/Treg ratio in children with OSA and its relationship with allergic rhinitis. Their study revealed that compared to the control group, OSA children exhibited a significant increase in the number of peripheral Th17 cells (pro-inflammatory) and dramatic decreases in the number of Treg cells (involved in immune tolerance). In addition, the increase was significantly larger in OSA patients who also had allergic rhinitis compared to the OSA group without AR. They concluded that Th17/Treg imbalance may increase the risk of developing OSA, and that AR may promote the development of the disease. It seems appropriate that preoperative evaluation and proper management of AR might be considered in pediatric SDB [96].

## CONCLUSION

Because of our patient population, the pediatric otolaryngologist is in a unique position to diagnose and treat allergic rhinitis along with its frequent comorbidities [97]. The treatment modalities of allergic rhinitis include avoidance and environmental controls, pharmacotherapy and immunotherapy. Familiarity with the diagnosis and treatment of pediatric inhalant allergy offers an opportunity to substantially improve the quality of life of allergic children.

## CONFLICT OF INTEREST

The author declares no conflict of interest, financial or otherwise.

## ACKNOWLEDGEMENT

Declared none.

## REFERENCES

[1]   Holloway JW, Yang IA, Holgate ST. Genetics of allergic disease. J Allergy Clin Immunol 2010; 125(2) (Suppl. 2): S81-94.

[2]   Zambelli-Weiner A, Ehrlich E, Stockton ML, *et al.* Evaluation of the CD14/-260 polymorphism and house dust endotoxin exposure in the Barbados AsthmanGenetics Study. J Allergy Clin Immunol 2005; 115: 1203-9.

[3]   Skoner DP. Allergic rhinitis: definition, epidemiology, pathophysiology, detection, and diagnosis. J

Allergy Clin Immunol 2001; 108(1) (Suppl.): S2-8.

[4]     Kulig M, Bergmann R, Klettke U, *et al.* Natural course of sensitization to food and inhalant allergens during the first 6 years of life. J Allergy Clin Immunol 1999; 103: 1173-9.

[5]     Kapoor R, Menon C, Hoffstad O, *et al.* The prevalence of atopic triad in children with physician-confirmed atopic dermatitis. J Am Acad Dermatol 2008; 58: 68-73.

[6]     Ricci G, Patrizi A, Baldi E, *et al.* Long-term follow-up of atopic dermatitis: retrospective analysis of related risk factors and association with concomitant allergic diseases. J Am Acad Dermatol 2006; 55: 765-71.

[7]     Van der Hulst AE, Klip H, Brand PL. Risk of developing asthma in young children with atopic eczema: a systematic review. J Allergy Clin Immunol 2007; 120: 565-9.

[8]     Blaiss MS. Allergic rhinitis: Direct and indirect costs. Allergy Asthma Proc 2010; 31: 375-80.

[9]     Meltzer EO, Bukstein DA. The economic impact of allergic rhinitis and current guidelines for treatment. Ann Allergy Asthma Immunol 2011; 106: S12-6.

[10]    Bousquet J, Khaltaev N, Cruz AA, *et al.* Allergic Rhinitis and its Impact on Asthma (ARIA) 2008 update (in collaboration with the World Health Organization, GA(2)LEN and AllerGen). Allergy 2008; 63: 8-160.

[11]    Asher MI, Montefort S. Worldwide time trends in the prevalence of symptoms of asthma, allergic rhinoconjunctivitis, and eczema in childhood: ISAAC Phase One and Three repeat multicountry cross-sectional surveys. Lancet 2006; 368: 733-43.

[12]    Meltzer EO, Blaiss MS, Derebery MJ, *et al.* Burden of allergic rhinitis: results from the pediatric allergies in America survey. J Allergy Clin Immunol 2009; 124: S43-70.

[13]    Blaiss MS. Allergic rhinoconjunctivitis: burden of disease. Allergy Asthma Proc 2007; 28(4): 393-7.

[14]    Smith DH, Malone DC, Lawson KA, *et al.* A National Estimate of the Economic Costs of Asthma. Am J Respir Crit Care Med 1997; 156(3 Pt 1): 787-93.

[15]    Walker S, Khan-Wasti S, Fletcher M, *et al.* Seasonal allergic rhinitis is associated with a detrimental effect on examination performance in United Kingdom teenagers: case-control study. J Allergy Clin Immunol 2007; 120(2): 381-7.

[16]    Arbes SJ Jr, Gergen PJ, Elliott L, *et al.* Prevalences of positive skin test responses to 10 common allergens in the US population: results from the third National Health and Nutrition Examination Survey. J Allergy Clin Immunol 2005; 116(2): 377-83.

[17]    Seidman MD, Gurgel RK, Lin SY, *et al.* Clinical practice guideline: allergic rhinitis. Otolaryngol Head Neck Surg 2015; 152(1) (Suppl.): S1-S43.

[18]    Herr M, Clarisse B, Nikasinovic L, *et al.* Does allergic rhinitis exist in infancy? Findings from the PARIS birth cohort. Allergy 2011; 66(2): 214-21.

[19]    Sahiner UM. Buyuktiryaki AB, Yavuz ST, *et al.* The spectrum of aeroallergen sensitization in children diagnosed with asthma during first 2 years of life. Allergy Asthma Proc 2013; 34(4): 356-61.
        [http://dx.doi.org/10.2500/aap.2013.34.3655]

[20]    Pesonen M. Kallio MJ, Siimes MA, Ranki A. Allergen skin prick testing in early childhood: reproducibility and prediction of allergic symptoms into early adulthood. J Pediatr 2015; 166(2): 401-6.e1.
        [http://dx.doi.org/10.1016/j.jpeds.2014.10.009]

[21]    Gotzsche PC, Johansen HK. House dust mite control measures for asthma. Cochrane Database Syst Rev 2004; 18: CD001187.

[22]    Wood RA, Johnson EF, Van Natta ML, Chen PH, Peyton EA. A placebo-controlled trial of a HEPA air cleaner in the treatment of cat allergy. Am J Respir Crit Care Med 1998; 158: 115-20.

[23]    Sublett JL. Effectiveness of air filters and air cleaners in allergic respiratory diseases: a review of the recent literature. Curr Allergy Asthma Rep 2011; 11: 395-402.

[24]    McDonald E, Cook D, Newman T, Griffith L, *et al.* Effect of Air Filtration Systems on Asthma: A Systematic Review of Randomized Trials. Chest 2002; 122: 1535-42.

[25]    Terreehorst I, Hak E, Oosting AJ, *et al.* Evaluation of impermeable covers for bedding in patients with allergic rhinitis. N Engl J Med 2003; 349(3): 237-46.

[26]    Sheikh A, Hurwitz B, Nurmatov U, *et al.* House dust mite avoidance measures for perennial allergic rhinitis. Cochrane Database Syst Rev 2010; 7: CD001563.

[27]    Rodrigo GJ, Neffen H. Efficacy of fluticasone furoate nasal spray *vs.* placebo for the treatment of ocular and nasal symptoms of allergic rhinitis: a systematic review. Clin Exp Allergy 2011; 41: 160-70.

[28]    Penagos M, Compalati E, Tarantini F, *et al.* Efficacy of mometasone furoate nasal spray in the treatment of allergic rhinitis: meta-analysis of randomized, double-blind, placebo- controlled, clinical trials. Allergy 2008; 63: 1280-91.

[29]    Yamada T, Yamamoto H, Kubo S, *et al.* Efficacy of mometasone furoate nasal spray for nasal symptoms, quality of life, rhinitis-disturbed sleep, and nasal nitric oxide in patients with perennial allergic rhinitis. Allergy Asthma Proc 2012; 33: e9-e16.

[30]    Meltzer EO, Munafo DA, Chung W, *et al.* Intranasal mometasone furoate therapy for allergic rhinitis symptoms and rhinitis- disturbed sleep. Ann Allergy Asthma Immunol 2010; 105: 65-74.

[31]    Allen DB, Meltzer EO, Lemanske RF Jr, *et al.* No growth sup- pression in children treated with the maximum recommended dose of fluticasone propionate aqueous nasal spray for one year. Allergy Asthma Proc 2002; 23: 407-13.

[32]    Schenkel EJ, Skoner DP, Bronsky EA, *et al.* Absence of growth retardation in children with perennial allergic rhinitis after one year of treatment with mometasone furoate aqueous nasal spray. Pediatrics 2000; 105: E22.

[33]    Simons FE, Simons KJ. Histamine and H1-antihistmines: celebrating a century of progress. J Allergy Clin Immunol 2011; 128: 1139-50.

[34]    Nickels AS, Dimov V, Wolf R. Pharmacokinetic evaluation of Olopatadine for the treatment of allergic rhinitis and conjunctivitis. Expert Opin Drug Metab Toxicol 2011; 7: 1593-9.

[35]    Lombardo G, Quattrocchi P, Lombardo GR, *et al.* Concomitant levocetirizine and montelukast in the treatment of seasonal allergic rhinitis: influence on clinical symptoms. Italian Journal of Allergy and Clinical Immunology 2006; 16: 63-8.

[36]    Meltzer EO, Malmstrom K, Lu S, *et al.* Concomitant montelukast and loratadine as treatment for seasonal allergic rhinitis: a randomized, placebo-controlled clinical trial. J Allergy Clin Immunol 2000; 105: 917-22.

[37]    Ciebiada M, Barylski M, Gorska Ciebiada M. Nasal eosinophilia and serum soluble intercellular adhesion molecule 1 in patients with allergic rhinitis treated with montelukast alone or in combination with desloratadine or levocetirizine. Am J Rhinol Allergy 2013; 27(2): e58-62.

[38]    Watanasomsiri A, Poachanukoon O, Vichyanond P. Efficacy of montelukast and loratadine as treatment for allergic rhinitis in children. Asian Pac J Allergy Immunol 2008; 26(2-3): 89-95.

[39]    Halken S, Lau S, Valovirta E. New visions in specific immunotherapy in children: an iPAC summary and future trends. Pediatr Allergy Immunol 2008; 19 (Suppl. 19): 60-70.

[40]    Roder E, Berger MY, de Groot H, *et al.* Immunotherapy in children and adolescents with allergic rhinoconjunctivitis: a systematic review. Pediatr Allergy Immunol 2008; 19(3): 197-207.

[41]    Lin S, *et al.* Sublingual immunotherapy for the treatment of allergic rhinoconjunctivitis and asthma: A systematic review. JAMA 2013; 309(12): 1278-88.

[42]    Bielory L. Allergic conjunctivitis and the impact of allergic rhinitis. Curr Allergy Asthma Rep 2010; 10(2): 122-34.

[43]    Fok AO, Wong GW. What have we learnt from ISAAC phase III in the Asia-Pacific rim? Curr Opin Allergy Clin Immunol 2009; 9(2): 116-22.

[44]    Bjorksten B, Clayton T, Ellwood P, *et al.* Worldwide time trends for symptoms of rhinitis and conjunctivitis: phase III of the international study of asthma and allergies in childhood. Pediatr Allergy Immunol 2008; 19(2): 110-24.

[45]    Shapiro GG, Rachelesvsky GS. Introduction and definition of sinusitis. J Allergy Clin Immunol 1992; 90: 417-8.

[46]    Georgitis JW, Matthews BL, Stone B. Chronic sinusitis: characterization of cellular influx and inflammatory mediators in sinus lavage fluid. Int Arch Allergy Immunol 1995; 106: 416-21.

[47]    Brook I, Yocum P, Shah K. Aerobic and anaerobic bacteriology of concurrent chronic otitis media with effusion and chronic sinusitis in children. Arch Otolaryngol Head Neck Surg 2000; 126: 174-6.

[48]    Ramadan HH, Hinerman RA. Outcome of endoscopic sinus surgery in children with allergic rhinitis. Am J Rhinol 2006; 20: 438-40.

[49]    Leo G, Piacentini E, Incorvaia C. etal. Chronic rhinosinusitis and allergy. Pediatr Allergy Immunol 2007; 18 (Suppl. 18): 19-21.

[50]    Alles R, Parikh A, Hawk L, *et al.* The prevalence of atopic disorders in children with chronic otitis media with effusion. Pediatr Allergy Immunol 2001; 12: 102-6.

[51]    Caffarelli C, Savini E, Giordano S, *et al.* Atopy in children with otitis media with effusion. Clin Exp Allergy 1998; 28: 591-6.

[52]    Luong A, Roland PS. The link between allergic rhinitis and chronic otitis media with effusion in atopic patients. Otolaryngol Clin North Am 2008; 41(2): 311-23.

[53]    Newacheck PW, Stoddard JJ. Prevalence and impact of multiple childhood chronic illnesses. J Pediatr 1994; 124: 40-8.

[54]    Sly RM. Changing prevalence of allergic rhinitis and asthma. Ann Allergy Asthma Immunol 1999; 82: 233-48.

[55]    Griffin G, Flynn CA. Antihistamines and/or decongestants for otitis media with effusion (OME) in children. Cochrane Database Syst Rev 2011; 9: CD003423.

[56]    Simpson SA, Lewis J, van der Voort J, *et al.* Oral or topical nasal steroids for hearing loss associated with otitis media with effusion in children. Cochrane Database Syst Rev 2011; 5 CD001935.pub3

[57]    Van Zon A, van der Heijden GJ, van Dongen TM, *et al.* Antibiotics for otitis media with effusion in children. Cochrane Database Syst Rev 2012; 9: CD009163.

[58]    Williamson I, Benge S, Barton S, *et al.* A double-blind randomised placebo-controlled trial of topical intranasal corticosteroids in 4- to 11-year-old children with persistent bilateral otitis media with effusion in primary care. Health technology assessment (Winchester, England) 2009; 13(37): 1-144.

[59]    Roditi RE, Veling M, Shin JJ. Age: An effect modifier of the association between allergic rhinitis and otitis media with effusion. Laryngoscope 2015.
        [http://dx.doi.org/10.1002/lary.25682]

[60]    Togias A. Rhinitis and asthma: evidence for respiratory system integration. J Allergy Clin Immunol 2003; 111(6): 1171-83.

[61]    Van Cauwenberge P, Watelet JB, Van Zele T, *et al.* Does rhinitis lead to asthma? Rhinology 2007; 45(2): 112-21.

[62]    Georgalas C, Terreehorst I, Fokkens W. Current management of allergic rhinitis in children. Pediatr Allergy Immunol 2010; 21(1 Pt 2): e119-26.

[63]  Caimmi D, Marseglia A, Pieri G, Benzo S, Bosa L, Caimmi S. Nose and lungs: one way, one disease. Ital J Pediatr 2012; 38: 60.

[64]  Sazonov Kocevar V, Thomas J III, Jonsson L, *et al.* Association between allergic rhinitis and hospital resource use among asthmatic children in Norway. Allergy 2005; 60(3): 338-42.

[65]  Humbert M, Boulet LP, Niven RM, Panahloo Z, Blogg M, Ayre G. Omalizumab therapy: patients who achieve greatest benefit for their asthma experience greatest benefit for rhinitis. Allergy 2009; 64(1): 81-4.

[66]  Thomas M. Allergic rhinitis: evidence for impact on asthma. BMC Pulm Med 2006; 6 (Suppl. 1): S4.

[67]  Nurmatov U, van Schayck CP, Hurwitz B, Sheikh A. House dust mite avoidance measures for perennial allergic rhinitis: an updated Cochrane systematic review. Allergy 2012; 67(2): 158-65.

[68]  Bjornsdottir US, Jakobinudottir S, Runarsdottir V, Juliusson S. The effect of reducing levels of cat allergen (Fel d 1) on clinical symptoms in patients with cat allergy. Ann Allergy Asthma Immunol 2003; 91(2): 189-94.

[69]  Calderon MA, Gerth van Wijk R, Eichler I, *et al.* Perspectives on allergen-specific immunotherapy in childhood: an EAACI position statement. Pediatr Allergy Immunol 2012; 23(4): 300-6.

[70]  Jacobsen L, Niggemann B, Dreborg S, *et al.* Specific immunotherapy has long-term preventive effect of seasonal and perennial asthma: 10-year follow-up on the PAT study. Allergy 2007; 62(8): 943-8.

[71]  Niggemann B, Jacobsen L, Dreborg S, *et al.* Five-year follow-up on the PAT study: specific immunotherapy and long-term prevention of asthma in children. Allergy 2006; 61(7): 855-9.

[72]  Moller C, Dreborg S, Ferdousi HA, *et al.* Pollen immunotherapy reduces the development of asthma in children with seasonal rhinoconjunctivitis (the PATstudy). J Allergy Clin Immunol 2002; 109(2): 251-6.

[73]  Di Rienzo V, Marcucci F, Puccinelli P, *et al.* Long-lasting effect of sublingual immunotherapy in children with asthma due to house dust mite: a 10-year prospective study. Clin Exp Allergy 2003; 33(2): 206-10.

[74]  Novembre E, Galli E, Landi F, *et al.* Coseasonal sublingual immunotherapy reduces the development of asthma in children with allergic rhinoconjunctivitis. J Allergy Clin Immunol 2004; 114(4): 851-7.

[75]  Olaguibel JM, Alvarez Puebla MJ. Efficacy of sublingual allergen vaccination for respiratory allergy in children. Conclusions from one meta-analysis. J Investig Allergol Clin Immunol 2005; 15(1): 9-16.

[76]  Valovirta E, Berstad AK, de Blic J, *et al.* Design and recruitment for the GAP trial, investigating the preventive effect on asthma development of an SQ-standardized grass allergy immunotherapy tablet in children with grass pollen-induced allergic rhinoconjunctivitis. Clin Ther 2011; 33(10): 1537-46.

[77]  Tsilochristou O, Douladiris N, Makris M, Papadopoulos N. Pediatric Allergic Rhinitis and Asthma: Can the March be Halted? Paediatr Drugs 2013; 15: 431-40.

[78]  NIH Guidelines for the diagnosis and management of asthma–2007 (EPR-3) , 2007 [Accessed November 2, 2010]; Available at: http://www.nhlbi.nih.gov/guidelines/asthma/index.htm.

[79]  Liberati A, Altman DG, Tetzlaff J, *et al.* The PRISMA statement for reporting systematic reviews and meta-analyses of studies that evaluate health care interventions: explanation and elaboration. J Clin Epidemiol 2009; 62: e1-e34.

[80]  Oxford Centre for Evidence Based Medicine. Levels of evidence 2009. [Accessed November 4, 2012]. http://www.cebm.net/index. aspx = 1025.

[81]  Wells GA, Shea B, O'Connell D, *et al.* The Newcasete-Ottawa Scale (NOS) for assessing the quality of nonrandomized studies in meta-analysis , [Accessed November 4, 2012]; http://www.ohri.ca/ programs/clinical_epidemiology/ oxford.asp.

[82]   Anuntaseree W, Rookkapan K, Kuasirikul S, *et al.* Snoring and obstructive sleep apnea in Thai school-age children: prevalence and predisposing factors. Pediatr Pulmonol 2001; 32: 222-7.

[83]   Craig TJ, Ferguson BJ, Krouse JH. Sleep impairment in allergic rhinitis, rhinosinusitis, and nasal polyposis. Am J Otolaryngol 2008; 29: 209-17.

[84]   Ishman SL, Smith DF, Benke JR, *et al.* The prevalence of sleepiness and the risk of sleep-disordered breathing in children with positive allergy test. Int Forum Allergy Rhinol 2012; 2: 139-43.

[85]   Bhattacharjee R, Kheirandish-Gozal L, Spruyt K, *et al.* Adenotonsillectomy outcomes in treatment of obstructive sleep apnea in children: a multicenter retrospective study. Am J Respir Crit Care Med 2010; 182: 676-83.

[86]   Urschitz MS, Brockmann PE, Schlaud M, Poets CF. Population prevalence of obstructive sleep apnoea in a community of German third graders. Eur Respir J 2010; 36: 556-68.

[87]   Vichyanond P, Suratannon C, Lertbunnaphong P, *et al.* Clinical characteristics of children with nonallergic rhinitis *vs* with allergic rhinitis. Asian Pac J Allergy Immunol 2010; 28: 270-4.

[88]   Park CE, Shin SY, Lee KH, *et al.* The effect of allergic rhinitis on the degree of stress, fatigue and quality of life in OSA patients. Eur Arch Otorhinolaryngol 2012; 269: 2061-4.

[89]   Settipane RA, Charnock DR. Epidemiology of rhinitis: allergic and nonallergic. Clin Allergy Immunol 2007; 19: 23-34.

[90]   Lin SY, Melvin TA, Boss EF, Ishman SL. The association between allergic rhinitis and sleep-disordered breathing in children: a systematic review. Int Forum Allergy Rhinol 2013; 3: 504-9.

[91]   Bollinger T, Bollinger A, Skrum L, Dimitrov S, Lange T, Solbach W. Sleep- dependent activity of T cells and regulatory T cells. Clin Exp Immunol 2009; 155: 231-8.

[92]   Aho V, Ollila HM, Rantanen V. Partial sleep restriction activates immune response-related gene expression pathways: experimental and epidemiological studies in humans. PLoS One 2013; 8: e77184.

[93]   Ye J, Liu H, Zhang G, Li P, Wang Z, Huang S, *et al.* The Treg/Th17 imbalance in patients with obstructive sleep apnoea syndrome. Mediators Inflamm 2012; 2012: 815308.

[94]   Kim J, Bhattacharjee R, Khalyfa A, Kheirandish-Gozal L, Capdevila OS, Wang Y, *et al.* DNA methylation in inflammatory genes among children with obstructive sleep apnea. Am J Respir Crit Care Med 2012; 85: 330-8.

[95]   Ni K, Zhao L, Wu J, *et al.* Th17/Treg balance in children with obstructive sleep apnea syndrome and the relationship with allergic rhinitis. Int J Pediatr Otorhinolaryngol 2015.
[http://dx.doi.org/10.1016/j.ijporl.2015.06.026]

[96]   Kimple, Adam J.a; Ishman, Stacey L. Allergy and sleep disordered breathing. Curr Opin Otolaryngol Head Neck Surg 2013; 21: 277-81.

[97]   Veling M. The role of allergy in pediatric rhinosinusitis. Curr Opin Otolaryngol Head Neck Surg 2013; 21: 271-6.

CHAPTER 19

# The Management of Pediatric Allergic Emergencies

Olga Hardin[1] and Joshua L. Kennedy[1,2,3,*]

[1] *Department of Internal Medicine, Division of Allergy and Immunology, University of Arkansas for Medical Sciences, Little Rock, AR, USA*

[2] *Department of Pediatrics, Division of Allergy and Immunology, University of Arkansas for Medical Sciences, Little Rock, AR, USA*

[3] *Arkansas Children's Research Institute, Little Rock, AR, USA*

**Abstract:** Anaphylaxis is a dangerous condition that must be treated quickly. The prevalence is on the rise, and the diagnosis requires a low index of suspicion in someone experiencing the typical constellation of symptoms involving more than one body system after exposure to a possible allergen. Treatment involves the administration of intramuscular epinephrine before consideration of any other modalities. While treatment of anaphylaxis with epinephrine always comes first, specific laboratory tests including serum tryptase and directed specific IgE tests can be considered to help aid in the diagnosis. Finally, every patient who experiences anaphylaxis should be discharged with injectable epinephrine and an emergency action plan.

**Keywords:** Anaphylaxis, Drug Allergy, Epinephrine, Food Allergy, Histamine, Tryptase, Venom Allergy.

## INTRODUCTION

Rapid recognition of allergic emergencies is crucial to a timely and appropriate treatment. Allergic emergencies are synonymous with a complex of symptoms affecting two or more organ symptoms known as anaphylaxis. The National Institute of Allergy and Infectious Disease (NIAID) and The Food Allergy and Anaphylaxis Network (FAAN) define anaphylaxis as "a serious allergic reaction that is rapid in onset and may cause death" [1]. The incidence of anaphylaxis is increasing in the US and in other Western countries [2 - 6]. In the United States, the lifetime prevalence of anaphylaxis is estimated to be around 0.05% to 2%

* **Corresponding author Joshua L. Kennedy**: Department of Pediatrics, Division of Allergy and Immunology, University of Arkansas for Medical Sciences, Little Rock, AR, USA; Tel: 501-364-1060; Email: KennedyJoshuaL@uams.edu

[7, 8]. Despite the increase in prevalence, there continue to be examples of mis- or under-diagnosis across the United States. In fact, anaphylaxis accounted for 186-225 deaths per year according to the Multiple Cause of Death Database between the years 1999-2009 [9]. This chapter will provide an overview of common causes, pathophysiology, diagnostic criteria, treatment, complications, and follow up recommendations for children during and after anaphylaxis.

## Common Causes of Anaphylaxis in Children

### Food Allergy

Food is the most common trigger for anaphylaxis among all age groups [2], and eight major foods including peanuts, tree nuts, shell fish, fish, cow's milk, eggs, wheat, and soy are responsible for more than 90% of these reactions in children [1, 10 - 13]. While the true prevalence of food allergy is unknown, studies suggest that physician diagnosis of food allergy is on the rise in the United States affecting approximately 6-8% of children [14, 15]. According to a study done by the Centers for Disease Control and Prevention in 2013, food allergy diagnoses increased 50% between 1997 and 2011 [16]. Perceived food allergy is also on the rise, which makes the diagnosis difficult. Furthermore, the revelation that anaphylaxis to foods can be delayed by several hours when considering the carbohydrate galactose-1,3-alpha-galactose (alpha-gal) found in mammalian meat has made diagnosis even more difficult. Patients with this allergy present with delayed symptoms, including anaphylaxis for 4-6 hours after exposure, to beef, pork, lamb, and other mammalian meats [17 - 21]. This food allergy has been described in children; however, it does not seem to be a problem in infancy, but usually begins around the age of 2 [21]. Avoidance of the allergenic food is the only known treatment for this condition, and patients with known food allergy should always carry an epinephrine autoinjector.

### Venom Allergy

Venom allergy accounts for 5-13% of all anaphylaxis events presenting in children [22 - 24]. Stinging insects belong to the insect order Hymenoptera, but less than 1% of this order is responsible for human stings [25 - 27]. Honey bee, yellow jacket, wasp, and hornet stings, as well as fire ant bites can result in a wide range of symptoms ranging from temporary local reactions to anaphylaxis. While local reactions are common, life-threatening systemic reactions only occur in 0.4%-0.8% of children [28 - 31] and account for ~40 deaths annually in the US [32]. However, many clinicians remain unaware that immunotherapy (venom allergy shots) can successfully provide prophylaxis for venom allergic patients against future systemic reactions to hymenoptera [25].

## Drug Allergy

Medications account for 5%–12% of anaphylaxis cases [22 - 24]. The most common culprits of drug allergy include antibiotics (penicillin and sulfa drugs, specifically), anticonvulsants, aspirin and other nonsteroidal anti-inflammatory drugs (NSAIDs), and chemotherapy agents. Antibiotics are most common drugs to cause anaphylaxis [23, 24]. In a large study evaluating the incidence of antibiotic allergy incidence, it was found that 25% of patients requiring antimicrobial therapy reported that they had an allergy to an antimicrobial agent. 15.9% of all antibiotic allergic patients in this study reported that they were allergic to penicillin, making penicillin the most commonly reported antibiotic allergy [33]. However, it is important to note that in studies attempting to confirm penicillin allergy in patients who had a reported history of reactions to the medication, an overwhelming 96% of the subjects had negative skin testing and were able to pass an oral challenge, suggesting the number of patients with true allergy to penicillin is much lower than is suspected by the general population [34].

### Presentation and Diagnosis

The presenting symptoms of anaphylaxis can be nonspecific, and, thus, a low index of suspicion is required to properly and quickly treat patients. As defined by NIAID and FAAN, the diagnosis of anaphylaxis requires symptoms involving two or more organ systems. Cutaneous (skin) manifestations, such as urticaria (hives), pruritus (itching), erythema (redness), or angioedema (swelling), are present in up to 90% of anaphylaxis cases. Respiratory symptoms are common as well, presenting in ~70% of cases. These symptoms include dyspnea (difficulty breathing), wheezing (musical sound heard in the lungs made by excess mucus and bronchoconstriction of lower airways), cough, congestion, stridor (musical sound made by upper airway constriction), and hoarseness. Gastrointestinal (GI) upset, altered mental status, and/or cardiovascular compromise may be present as well. Many patients experiencing anaphylaxis describe a "feeling of impending doom," which should be taken seriously [35].

The diagnosis of anaphylaxis may be challenging, given the number of possible signs and symptoms and the variation of severity [7, 36 - 45]. History of events leading to presentation is very helpful in connecting nonspecific symptoms to suspected anaphylaxis. To help with the diagnosis, the NIAID and FAAN have developed diagnostic criteria that are helpful in defining anaphylaxis (Table 1). Certain conditions have been related to increased risk for severe anaphylaxis and should be considered in a patient with known triggers for anaphylaxis. These conditions include recurrent wheezing or asthma, eczema, atopic dermatitis, and mastocytosis [46].

## Pathophysiology

On a broader level, the development of systemic allergic symptoms remains somewhat of an enigma. How an exposure of one system to an allergen can lead to a multisystem response in such a coordinated and rapid fashion challenges researchers with more questions than answers. Instigation of allergic conditions and development of allergic inflammation has been more thoroughly studied, and an overview of this process follows:

Once a potential allergen comes into contact with an epithelial cell surface of the nose, skin, lung or the gastrointestinal mucosa, a cascade of inflammatory signals can initiate the beginning of allergy. If sensitization is going to occur, stimulation of various receptors on the surface of epithelial cells leads to innate cytokine release that can bias toward a T helper ($T_H2$) (allergic) response [4 - 6]. Second, dendritic cells (DCs), which function as professional antigen presenting cells (APCs), will capture the allergen and transport it to the regional lymph nodes where it will be presented to naïve T cells through major histocompatibility complex (MHC) class II receptors. In the presence of interleukin (IL)-4 or IL-13, the T cell will become a $T_H2$ cell, subsequently secreting its own IL-4, IL-5, IL-9, and IL-13, amongst others. T helper cells will then interact with B cells, which will cause the production of Immunoglobulin (Ig) E to the specific antigen that was seen at the mucosal surface [47]. This occurs when IgE binds to receptors on mast cells and basophils, the allergic effector cells. The subject is now sensitized to the allergen. The next time this individual is exposed to that allergen, there is cross linking of IgE leading to activation and degranulation of mast cells and basophils occurs with release of mediators, including histamine, tryptase, tumor necrosis factor (TNF), lipid derived mediators such as Prostaglandin (PG)$D_2$, leukotriene (LT) $B_4$, platelet-activating factor, and the cysteinyl leukotrienes $LTC_4$, $LTD_4$, and $LTE_4$. These cytokines lead to specific systemic responses such as nasal congestion, cough, wheezing, skin manifestations, and ultimately anaphylaxis [7].

## The Mediators

Histamine is one of the most widely studied and understood mediators of allergic reactions. Its action on H1 and H2 receptors causes a variety of effects throughout the body [48]. Flushing, hypotension, and headache are mediated by both H1 and H2 receptors while dyspnea, bronchospasm, pruritus and tachycardia are mediated by H1 receptors alone. Systemic release of histamine results in cardiovascular changes, while localized histamine release in the skin causes urticaria. Histamine binding to H1 receptors stimulates the conversion of amino acid L -arginine into nitric oxide (NO), which is a potent vaso- and broncho- dilator, a compensatory measure that is meant to flush the offending allergen from the system [49, 50]. This mediator also acts directly on the myocardium [48, 51, 52], causing an increase in coronary blood flow and a decrease in coronary vascular resistance and mean arterial pressure [53].

Tryptase is the most abundant secretory granule derived serine protease found in mast cells [54]. It is a marker of mast cell activation, and it can be elevated during an anaphylactic reaction, though not always. The route of exposure to the allergen may be related as to whether tryptase levels are elevated. Allergens ingested orally (*i.e.* food) are less likely to be correlated with elevated tryptase levels, while parenterally injected allergens (*i.e.* insect venom, medications) are more likely to have higher tryptase levels [55 - 57].

Platelet activating factor (PAF) is a phospholipid involved in many immune and inflammatory processes [58]. It is very potent and has been found to have significant effects at concentrations as low as 10-12 mol/L [59]. PAF can be produced by many cell types including mast cells, monocytes, platelets, eosinophils and endothelial cells. Once PAF binds to its receptor, kinases such protein kinase C lead to a release of arachidonic acid and prostaglandins including prostaglandin E2 (PGE-2) from vascular smooth muscle cells [60, 61]. In a recent study, PAF levels were shown to be correlated with anaphylaxis severity, even when tryptase and histamine levels were not elevated [62].

## Diagnosis

The diagnosis of anaphylaxis is clinical (Table **1**) and laboratory testing should not delay urgent treatment. As mentioned above, the NIAID and FAAN have provided a definition and diagnostic criteria (Table **1**) to help providers determine if anaphylaxis is present [1]. In the way of diagnostics, several lab tests have been studied and can be confirmatory of diagnosis- plasma histamine levels, serum or total tryptase levels.

There are standardized assays available to measure total serum or plasma tryptase with optimal collection time between 15 minutes to 3 hours after the onset of symptoms. Baseline tryptase levels are higher in infants under the age of six months than in older infants and children [63]. As previously discussed, tryptase levels are often normal in reactions caused by food allergens but are often elevated in parenterally injected allergens (venom, medications). Serial measurements of tryptase may increase the sensitivity and the specificity of the tests. If tryptase levels are elevated over baseline, clinical severity is directly related to the levels [64]. Current guidelines suggest that normal tryptase levels may still indicate anaphylaxis in the correct setting. Levels of tryptase during the event that indicate anaphylaxis should be determined by the formula 2+ 1.2 * (baseline tryptase). For this reason, it is necessary to obtain a tryptase level outside of the event in question. Tryptase levels that remain significantly elevated outside of the anaphylactic event could represent a diagnosis of mastocytosis.

**Table 1. Diagnostic Criteria for Anaphylaxis- requires one of the following 3 criteria[1]. Adapted from NIH NIAID and FAAN Guidelines.**

| |
|---|
| 1. Acute onset of an illness (minutes to several hours) with involvement of the skin, mucosal tissue, or both (*e.g.,* generalized hives, pruritus or flushing, swollen lips-tongue-uvula) |
| *AND AT LEAST ONE OF THE FOLLOWING* |
| a. Respiratory compromise (*e.g.,* dyspnea, wheeze-bronchospasm, stridor, reduced PEF, hypoxemia) |
| b. Reduced BP or associated symptoms of end-organ dysfunction (*e.g.,* hypotonia [collapse], syncope, incontinence) |
| 2. Two or more of the following that occur rapidly after exposure *to a likely allergen for that patient* (minutes to several hours): |
| a. Involvement of the skin-mucosal tissue (*e.g.,* generalized hives, itch-flush, swollen lips-tongue-uvula) |
| b. Respiratory compromise (*e.g.,* dyspnea, wheeze-bronchospasm, stridor, reduced PEF, hypoxemia) |
| c. Reduced BP or associated symptoms (*e.g.,* hypotonia [collapse], syncope, incontinence) |
| d. Persistent gastrointestinal symptoms (*e.g.,* crampy abdominal pain, vomiting) |
| 3. Reduced BP after exposure to *known allergen for that patient* (minutes to several hours): |
| [a.] Infants and children: low systolic BP (age specific) or greater than 30% decrease in systolic BP* |
| b. Adults: systolic BP of less than 90 mm Hg or greater than 30% decrease from that person's baseline |

*PEF*, Peak expiratory flow; *BP*, blood pressure.
* Low systolic blood pressure for children is defined as less than 70 mm Hg from 1 month to 1 year, less than (70 mm Hg + [2 × age]) from 1 to 10 years, and less than 90 mm Hg from 11 to 17 years.

Histamine levels are more likely to be elevated than tryptase in a patient with anaphylaxis [62]. However, histamine levels peak within 5-15 minutes of the onset of symptoms of anaphylaxis, and because of this timeframe, utility of this test in the setting of anaphylaxis in patients presenting from the community to the ED is limited. Histamine should be measured in plasma, not serum, due to clotting. Testing requires special precautions such as using large bore needle, keeping sample cold and centrifuging immediately to store the plasma for testing, all of which further complicate obtaining this test [65]. Urinary histamine can also be evaluated, but this is usually done by obtaining 24-hour urinary levels, which can be difficult in the outpatient or emergency department setting.

While PAF is a new and exciting mediator involved in the anaphylactic cascade, there are no commercially available laboratory tests presently available. Researchers are using this mediator in clinical studies, and it is possible that providers may have the option to use PAF to help diagnosis anaphylaxis in the future.

## Treatment-Immediate

Once a diagnosis is made based on clinical history and presenting signs and symptoms (see Table **1**), initiate treatment immediately by removing the offending allergen (ex. stopping a drug infusion at the first recognition of allergic symptoms). Protocols can be used that will help to streamline the treatment of anaphylaxis (Fig. **1**). Intramuscular epinephrine is a life-saving intervention and must be administered as soon as the diagnosis of anaphylaxis is suspected. Absorption is complete and more rapid in children who use an auto-injector in the thigh [66]. If an epinephrine auto-injector is not available, epinephrine 1:1000 dilution, 0.01 mg/kg in children up to a maximum dose, 0.3 mg should be given intramuscularly every 5 minutes until improvement in symptoms [22 - 24, 66]. Neither subcutaneous epinephrine or the use of other muscles, including deltoid muscles, are as effective as intramuscular epinephrine given in the vastus lateralis muscle of the thigh [66]. For the patient who has a poor response to several intramuscular injections, intravenous epinephrine infusion may be considered. This should be done in a closely monitored setting, where hemodynamic parameters can be closely monitored, such as the Intensive Care Unit. Epinephrine is preferably infused through a central venous line to prevent extravasation [67]. For infants and children, the recommended dose of intravenous epinephrine infusion is 0.05 to 0.5mcg/kg/min titrated to goal blood pressure in a closely monitored setting. An infusion of epinephrine is preferred over an IV bolus administration as bolus administration has been associated with increased adverse cardiovascular complications [68, 69].

In a physician supervised setting, an initial survey to ensure airway, breathing, circulation, and mental status should be performed. The patient should be placed in the recumbent position and supplemental oxygen should be delivered to maintain appropriate oxygenation status. If stridor or impending airway compromise is present, intubation should be performed. Intubation may be difficult due to the presence of laryngeal edema thus precautions should be in place as cricothyroidotomy may be required for the more severe cases. At least two large bore IVs should be placed and intravenous (IV) fluid resuscitation should be started due to massive fluid shifts that occur due to vasodilation.

In hypotensive children, normal saline boluses of 20 mL/kg over 5-10 minutes should be provided, which may be repeated as needed. In normotensive patients, maintenance fluids should be started at appropriate volumes. Bronchodilators may be used adjunctively although intramuscular epinephrine remains the primary modality to improve the overall systemic response.

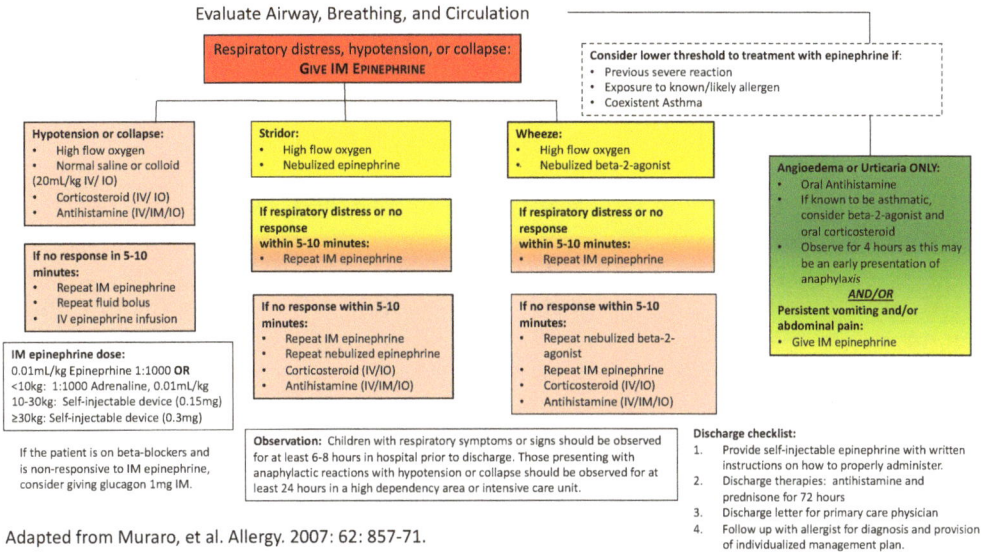

**Fig. (1).** Protocol for management of pediatric allergic emergencies. (Muraro, Allergy, 2007).

There are no published guidelines regarding the use of $H_1$-antihistamines, $H_2$-antihistamines, or glucocorticoids [43]. Several attempts have been made to review the data available regarding the use of glucocorticoids in anaphylaxis and no recommendations have been made due to lack of appropriate trials and data [70, 71]. However, glucocorticoids may prevent biphasic anaphylaxis in some patients. Similarly, uncertainty exists with regard to use of H1 and H2-antihistamines for anaphylaxis [71, 72]. Although, antihistamines should be used if needed for other symptoms such as urticaria or itching.

## Complications

There have been reports of anaphylaxis recurring approximately 6-10 hours after the resolution of initial presentation of anaphylaxis, without known exposure to an allergen [73, 74]. This is known as biphasic anaphylaxis, and it has been reported to occur in 4.5-11% of children with anaphylaxis [73, 75]. For this reason, patients experiencing anaphylaxis should be monitored for 4-6 hours after the event to ensure safety.

Protracted anaphylaxis is failure of symptomatic improvement with standard treatments of epinephrine and requires escalation of care into the intensive care setting. There are no published guidelines regarding the treatment of protracted anaphylaxis. Methylene blue has been used in case reports in adults [76] but studies are available in the pediatric population. In patients who do not respond to epinephrine, it is important to perform a thorough inspection of home medications to determine if the patient is on beta-blockers. If beta-blockers are used on a regular basis, the patient can be non-responsive to epinephrine and in this case, intramuscular glucagon (1 mg) should be given, followed by more epinephrine [77].

Empty ventricle syndrome is a deadly complication that was described after review of fatal anaphylaxis cases in which death occurred in patients who were moved to an upright position during the episode. The condition is thought to be caused by reduced venous return in a setting of already compromised hemodynamics (*e.g.,* vasodilation) [78]. For this reason, it is important to keep patients with suspected anaphylaxis in a recumbent position.

**Follow-up Recommendations**

There are no recommendations regarding the minimal required observation period for patients who present anaphylaxis. The accepted norm is a minimum of 4-8 hours, although this decision would be based on the clinical judgment of physicians and institutional standards. Overnight observation in the hospital should be considered for those patients who experience hypotension or laryngeal edema, those who require 2 or more epinephrine injections, those with a history of asthma, and those who ingest the allergen due to an increased risk for biphasic anaphylaxis [45, 75]. All anaphylaxis patients should be discharged with an emergency action plan and an epinephrine auto-injector, even if the offending allergen is unknown. Determination of the offending allergen is important to prevent further exposure, either from history, directed skin prick testing or serum IgE testing. Patients who have had anaphylaxis are at risk for recurrent anaphylaxis unless preventative care is initiated [7, 44], and patients and their caregivers should be educated about anaphylaxis. SAFE is a mnemonic recommended for this purpose and stands for: **S**eek support, **A**llergen identification and avoidance, **F**ollow-up for specialty care, and **E**pinephrine for emergencies [79]. In the pediatric population, it is important that all who are participating in their care- *i.e.* daycare, school or babysitter are aware of the child's allergy and emergency action plan. These facilities should also have access to injectable epinephrine and be instructed on appropriate indications and use of this medication.

**CONCLUSION**

Anaphylaxis is a dangerous condition that must be treated quickly. The prevalence is on the rise, and the diagnosis requires a low index of suspicion in someone experiencing the typical constellation of symptoms involving more than one body system after exposure to a possible allergen. Treatment involves the administration of intramuscular epinephrine before consideration of any other modalities. While treatment of anaphylaxis with epinephrine always comes first, specific laboratory tests including serum tryptase and directed specific IgE tests can be considered to help aid in the diagnosis and reveal any possible allergic triggers. Finally, every patient who experiences anaphylaxis should be discharged with auto-injectable epinephrine and an emergency action plan.

## CONFLICT OF INTEREST

Neither Dr. Kennedy nor Dr. Hardin disclose any conflicts of interest that pertain to this manuscript.

## ACKNOWLEDGEMENTS

Special thanks to Dr. Sheva Chervinskiy and Dr. Ashley Stoner for their generous edits of the manuscript.

## REFERENCES

[1]　Boyce JA, Assa'ad A, Burks AW, *et al.* Guidelines for the Diagnosis and Management of Food Allergy in the United States: Summary of the NIAID-Sponsored Expert Panel Report. J Allergy Clin Immunol 2010; 126: 1105-18.

[2]　Decker WW, Campbell RL, Manivannan V, Luke A, St Sauver JL, Weaver A. The etiology and incidence of anaphylaxis in Rochester, Minnesota: a report from the Rochester Epidemiology Project. J Allergy Clin Immunol 2008; 122: 1161-5.

[3]　Liew WK, Williamson E, Tang ML. Anaphylaxis fatalities and admissions in Australia. J Allergy Clin Immunol 2009; 123: 434-42.

[4]　Lin RY, Anderson AS, Shah SN, Nurruzzaman F. Increasing anaphylaxis hospitalizations in the first 2 decades of life: New York State, 1990 -2006. Ann Allergy Asthma Immunol 2008; 101: 387-93.

[5]　Poulos LM, Waters AM, Correll PK, Loblay RH, Marks GB. Trends in hospitalizations for anaphylaxis, angioedema, and urticaria in Australia, 1993-1994 to 2004-2005. J Allergy Clin Immunol 2007; 120: 878-84.

[6]　Sheikh A, Hippisley-Cox J, Newton J, Fenty J. Trends in national incidence, lifetime prevalence and adrenaline prescribing for anaphylaxis in England. J R Soc Med 2008; 101: 139-43.

[7]　Lieberman P, Nicklas RA, Oppenheimer J, Kemp SF, Lang DM, Bernstein DI. The diagnosis and management of anaphylaxis practice parameter: 2010 update. J Allergy Clin Immunol 2010; 126: 477-80. e1-42

[8]　Wood RA, Camargo CA Jr, Lieberman P, Sampson HA, Schwartz LB, Zitt M. Anaphylaxis in America: the prevalence and characteristics of anaphylaxis in the United States. J Allergy Clin Immunol 2014; 133: 461-7.

[9]　Ma L, Danoff TM, Borish L. Case fatality and population mortality associated with anaphylaxis in the United States. J Allergy Clin Immunol 2014; 133: 1075-83.

[10]　Liu AH, Jaramillo R, Sicherer SH, Wood RA, Bock SA, Burks AW. National prevalence and risk factors for food allergy and relationship to asthma: results from the National Health and Nutrition

Examination Survey 2005-2006. J Allergy Clin Immunol 2010; 126: 798-806 e13.

[11]    May CD. Objective clinical and laboratory studies of immediate hypersensitivity reactions to foods in asthmatic children. J Allergy Clin Immunol 1976; 58: 500-15.

[12]    Panel NI-SE. Guidelines for the diagnosis and management of food allergy in the United States: report of the NIAID-sponsored expert panel. J Allergy Clin Immunol 2010; 126: S1-S58.

[13]    Sicherer SH, Munoz-Furlong A, Sampson HA. Prevalence of seafood allergy in the United States determined by a random telephone survey. J Allergy Clin Immunol 2004; 114: 159-65.

[14]    Gupta RS, Springston EE, Warrier MR, Smith B, Kumar R, Pongracic J, *et al.* The prevalence, severity, and distribution of childhood food allergy in the United States. Pediatrics 2011; 128: e9-e17.

[15]    Sampson HA. Update on food allergy. J Allergy Clin Immunol 2004; 113: 805-19.

[16]    Jackson KD, Howie LD, Akinbami LJ. Trends in allergic conditions among children: United States, 1997-2011. NCHS Data Brief 2013; 1-8.

[17]    Commins SP, James HR, Kelly LA, Pochan SL, Workman LJ, Perzanowski MS. The relevance of tick bites to the production of IgE antibodies to the mammalian oligosaccharide galactose-alpha-1-3-galactose. The Journal of allergy and clinical immunology 2011; 127: 1286-93 e6.

[18]    Commins SP, Platts-Mills TA. Anaphylaxis syndromes related to a new mammalian cross-reactive carbohydrate determinant. J Allergy Clin Immunol 2009; 124: 652-7.

[19]    Commins SP, Platts-Mills TA. Allergenicity of carbohydrates and their role in anaphylactic events. Curr Allergy Asthma Rep 2010; 10: 29-33.

[20]    Commins SP, Satinover SM, Hosen J, *et al.* Delayed anaphylaxis, angioedema, or urticaria after consumption of red meat in patients with IgE antibodies specific for galactose-alpha-1,3-galactose. J Allergy Clin Immunol 2009; 123: 426-33.

[21]    Kennedy JL, Stallings AP, Platts-Mills TA, Oliveira WM, Workman L, James HR. Galactose-alph--1,3-galactose and delayed anaphylaxis, angioedema, and urticaria in children. Pediatrics 2013; 131: e1545-52.

[22]    Braganza SC, Acworth JP, McKinnon DR, Peake JE, Brown AF. Paediatric emergency department anaphylaxis: different patterns from adults. Arch Dis Child 2006; 91: 159-63.

[23]    de Silva IL, Mehr SS, Tey D, Tang ML. Paediatric anaphylaxis: a 5 year retrospective review. Allergy 2008; 63: 1071-6.

[24]    Russell S, Monroe K, Losek JD. Anaphylaxis management in the pediatric emergency department: opportunities for improvement. Pediatr Emerg Care 2010; 26: 71-6.

[25]    Lockey RF, Turkeltaub PC, Olive ES, Hubbard JM, Baird-Warren IA, Bukantz SC. The Hymenoptera venom study. III: Safety of venom immunotherapy. J Allergy Clin Immunol 1990; 86: 775-80.

[26]    Moffitt JE, Golden DB, Reisman RE, *et al.* Stinging insect hypersensitivity: a practice parameter update. J Allergy Clin Immunol 2004; 114: 869-86.

[27]    Schwartz HJ, Golden DB, Lockey RF. Venom immunotherapy in the Hymenoptera-allergic pregnant patient. J Allergy Clin Immunol 1990; 85: 709-12.

[28]    Bilo BM, Bonifazi F. Epidemiology of insect-venom anaphylaxis. Curr Opin Allergy Clin Immunol 2008; 8: 330-7.

[29]    Golden DB, Marsh DG, Kagey-Sobotka A, Freidhoff L, Szklo M, Valentine MD. Epidemiology of insect venom sensitivity. JAMA 1989; 262: 240-4.

[30]    Settipane GA, Boyd GK. Prevalence of bee sting allergy in 4,992 boy scouts. Acta Allergol 1970; 25: 286-91.

[31]    Settipane GA, Newstead GJ, Boyd GK. Frequency of Hymenoptera allergy in an atopic and normal population. J Allergy Clin Immunol 1972; 50: 146-50.

[32]    Graft DF. Insect sting allergy. Med Clin North Am 2006; 90: 211-32.

[33]    Lee CE, Zembower TR, Fotis MA, Postelnick MJ, Greenberger PA, Peterson LR, *et al.* The incidence of antimicrobial allergies in hospitalized patients: implications regarding prescribing patterns and emerging bacterial resistance. Arch Intern Med 2000; 160: 2819-22.

[34]    Park M, Markus P, Matesic D, Li JT. Safety and effectiveness of a preoperative allergy clinic in decreasing vancomycin use in patients with a history of penicillin allergy. Ann Allergy Asthma Immunol 2006; 97: 681-7.

[35]    Webb L, Greene E, Lieberman PL. Anaphylaxis: A review of 593 cases. J Allergy Clin Immunol 2004; 113: S241.

[36]    Brown SG, Mullins RJ, Gold MS. Anaphylaxis: diagnosis and management. Med J Aust 2006; 185: 283-9.

[37]    Ewan PW, Dugue P, Mirakian R, Dixon TA, Harper JN, Nasser SM, *et al.* BSACI guidelines for the investigation of suspected anaphylaxis during general anaesthesia. Clin Exp Allergy 2010; 40: 15-31.

[38]    Kemp SF, Lockey RF. Anaphylaxis: a review of causes and mechanisms. J Allergy Clin Immunol 2002; 110: 341-8.

[39]    Muraro A, Roberts G, Clark A, Eigenmann PA, Halken S, Lack G, *et al.* The management of anaphylaxis in childhood: position paper of the European academy of allergology and clinical immunology. Allergy 2007; 62: 857-71.

[40]    Oswalt ML, Kemp SF. Anaphylaxis: office management and prevention. Immunol Allergy Clin North Am 2007; 27: 177-91. [vi.].

[41]    Sampson HA, Munoz-Furlong A, Bock SA, Schmitt C, Bass R, Chowdhury BA. Symposium on the definition and management of anaphylaxis: summary report. J Allergy Clin Immunol 2005; 115: 584-91.

[42]    Sampson HA, Munoz-Furlong A, Campbell RL, Adkinson NF Jr, Bock SA, Branum A. Second symposium on the definition and management of anaphylaxis: summary report--Second National Institute of Allergy and Infectious Disease/Food Allergy and Anaphylaxis Network symposium. J Allergy Clin Immunol 2006; 117: 391-7.

[43]    Simons FE. Anaphylaxis. J Allergy Clin Immunol 2010; 125: S161-81.

[44]    Simons FE, Ardusso LR, Bilo MB, El-Gamal YM, Ledford DK, Ring J. World Allergy Organization anaphylaxis guidelines: summary. J Allergy Clin Immunol 2011; 127: 587-93. e1-22

[45]    Soar J, Pumphrey R, Cant A, *et al.* Emergency treatment of anaphylactic reactions--guidelines for healthcare providers. Resuscitation 2008; 77: 157-69.

[46]    Simons FE, Sampson HA. Anaphylaxis: Unique aspects of clinical diagnosis and management in infants (birth to age 2 years). J Allergy Clin Immunol 2015; 135: 1125-31.

[47]    Lambrecht BN, Hammad H. Allergens and the airway epithelium response: Gateway to allergic sensitization. J Allergy Clin Immunol 2014; 134: 499-507.

[48]    Kaliner M, Sigler R, Summers R, Shelhamer JH. Effects of infused histamine: analysis of the effects of H-1 and H-2 histamine receptor antagonists on cardiovascular and pulmonary responses. J Allergy Clin Immunol 1981; 68: 365-71.

[49]    Mitsuhata H, Shimizu R, Yokoyama MM. Role of nitric oxide in anaphylactic shock. J Clin Immunol 1995; 15: 277-83.

[50]    Palmer RM, Ferrige AG, Moncada S. Nitric oxide release accounts for the biological activity of endothelium-derived relaxing factor. Nature 1987; 327: 524-6.

[51].   Marone G, Patella V, de Crescenzo G, Genovese A, Adt M. Human heart mast cells in anaphylaxis and cardiovascular disease. Int Arch Allergy Immunol 1995; 107: 72-5.

[52] Triggiani M, Patella V, Staiano RI, Granata F, Marone G. Allergy and the cardiovascular system. Clin Exp Immunol 2008; 153 (Suppl. 1): 7-11.

[53] Vigorito C, Giordano A, De Caprio L, Vitale DF, Maurea N, Silvestri P, *et al.* Effects of histamine on coronary hemodynamics in humans: role of H1 and H2 receptors. J Am Coll Cardiol 1987; 10: 1207-13.

[54] Schwartz LB, Bradford TR, Rouse C, Irani AM, Rasp G, Van der Zwan JK, *et al.* Development of a new, more sensitive immunoassay for human tryptase: use in systemic anaphylaxis. J Clin Immunol 1994; 14: 190-204.

[55] Lieberman P. Anaphylaxis. In: Adkinson NF, Ed. Middleton's Allergy: Principles and Practice. 7th ed. St. Louis: Mosby 2009; p. 1027.

[56] Mertes PM, Laxenaire MC, Alla F, Groupe d'Etudes des Reactions Anaphylactoides P. Anaphylactic and anaphylactoid reactions occurring during anesthesia in France in 1999-2000. Anesthesiology 2003; 99: 536-45.

[57] Schwartz LB. Effector cells of anaphylaxis: mast cells and basophils. Novartis Found Symp 2004; 257: 65-74. discussion -9, 98-100, 276-85

[58] Venable ME, Zimmerman GA, McIntyre TM, Prescott SM. Platelet-activating factor: a phospholipid autacoid with diverse actions. J Lipid Res 1993; 34: 691-702.

[59] Benveniste J, Le Couedic JP, Polonsky J, Tence M. Structural analysis of purified platelet-activating factor by lipases. Nature 1977; 269: 170-1.

[60] Chao W, Olson MS. Platelet-activating factor: receptors and signal transduction. Biochem J 1993; 292(Pt 3): 617-29.

[61] Thivierge M, Parent JL, Stankova J, Rola-Pleszczynski M. Modulation of human platelet-activating factor receptor gene expression by protein kinase C activation. J Immunol 1996; 157: 4681-7.

[62] Vadas P, Perelman B, Liss G. Platelet-activating factor, histamine, and tryptase levels in human anaphylaxis. J Allergy Clin Immunol 2013; 131: 144-9.

[63] Komarow HD, Hu Z, Brittain E, Uzzaman A, Gaskins D, Metcalfe DD. Serum tryptase levels in atopic and nonatopic children. J Allergy Clin Immunol 2009; 124: 845-8.

[64] Sala-Cunill A, Cardona V, Labrador-Horrillo M, *et al.* Usefulness and limitations of sequential serum tryptase for the diagnosis of anaphylaxis in 102 patients. Int Arch Allergy Immunol 2013; 160: 192-9.

[65] Simons FE, Frew AJ, Ansotegui IJ, *et al.* Risk assessment in anaphylaxis: current and future approaches. J Allergy Clin Immunol 2007; 120: S2-S24.

[66] Simons FE, Roberts JR, Gu X, Simons KJ. Epinephrine absorption in children with a history of anaphylaxis. J Allergy Clin Immunol 1998; 101: 33-7.

[67] Le A, Patel S. Extravasation of Noncytotoxic Drugs: A Review of the Literature. Ann Pharmacother 2014; 48: 870-86.

[68] Campbell RL, Bellolio MF, Knutson BD, *et al.* Epinephrine in anaphylaxis: higher risk of cardiovascular complications and overdose after administration of intravenous bolus epinephrine compared with intramuscular epinephrine. J Allergy Clin Immunol Pract 2015; 3: 76-80.

[69] Simons KJ, Simons FE. Epinephrine and its use in anaphylaxis: current issues. Curr Opin Allergy Clin Immunol 2010; 10: 354-61.

[70] Choo KJ, Simons E, Sheikh A. Glucocorticoids for the treatment of anaphylaxis: Cochrane systematic review. Allergy 2010; 65: 1205-11.

[71] Choo KJ, Simons FE, Sheikh A. Glucocorticoids for the treatment of anaphylaxis. Cochrane Database Syst Rev 2012; 4: CD007596.

[72]    Sheikh A, Ten Broek V, Brown SG, Simons FE. H1-antihistamines for the treatment of anaphylaxis: Cochrane systematic review. Allergy 2007; 62: 830-7.

[73]    Rohacek M, Edenhofer H, Bircher A, Bingisser R. Biphasic anaphylactic reactions: occurrence and mortality. Allergy 2014; 69: 791-7.

[74]    Tole JW, Lieberman P. Biphasic anaphylaxis: review of incidence, clinical predictors, and observation recommendations. Immunol Allergy Clin North Am 2007; 27: 309-26. [viii.].

[75]    Mehr S, Liew WK, Tey D, Tang ML. Clinical predictors for biphasic reactions in children presenting with anaphylaxis. Clin Exp Allergy 2009; 39: 1390-6.

[76]    Jang DH, Nelson LS, Hoffman RS. Methylene blue for distributive shock: a potential new use of an old antidote. J Med Toxicol 2013; 9: 242-9.

[77]    Cheng A. Emergency treatment of anaphylaxis in infants and children. Paediatr Child Health 2011; 16: 35-40.

[78]    Pumphrey RS. Fatal posture in anaphylactic shock. J Allergy Clin Immunol 2003; 112: 451-2.

[79]    Lieberman P, Decker W, Camargo CA Jr, Oconnor R, Oppenheimer J, Simons FE. SAFE: a multidisciplinary approach to anaphylaxis education in the emergency department. Ann Allergy Asthma Immunol 2007; 98: 519-23.

# CHAPTER 20

# Autism Spectrum Disorder: What a Pediatrician Should Know

**Jayne Bellando**\*, **Jaimie Flor** and **Maya Lopez**

*Section of Pediatric Psychology, University of Arkansas for Medical Sciences, Little Rock, Arkansas, USA*

**Abstract:** It is important for pediatricians to increase their expertise in the area of Autism Spectrum Disorders (ASD). With the increase prevalence rate of ASD and the emphasis on early detection, pediatricians need to be familiar with diagnostic criteria for ASD and know when to refer for a comprehensive evaluation. After a formal diagnosis is given, pediatricians will be "front line" in the medical management of co-morbid medical/psychiatric symptoms of ASD for their patients. They will serve as the medical home for families to guide evidence-based treatment options and to help find community resources for the child with ASD. The goals of this chapter are to provide an overview of ASD diagnostic criteria; to increase knowledge in early detection and diagnosing ASD; provide information about common medical comorbidities for individuals with ASD; and build knowledge in guiding families as they find evidenced-based therapeutic resources for their child with ASD.

**Keywords:** Alternative treatments for autism, Autism, Autism Spectrum Disorder, Autism early screening, Autism evaluation, Autism identification, Autism interventions, Autism toolkits, Complementary and Alternative treatments, DSM-5, Pediatrician knowledge, Medical co-morbidities, Vaccines.

## INTRODUCTION

Autism is a neurodevelopmental disorder that typically presents very early in life [1]. Autism Spectrum Disorders (ASD) have increased in public awareness and in prevalence, based upon most recent estimates of 1 in 68 children [2]. The American Academy of Pediatrics [3, 4] and the American Academy of Neurology [5] have published on the importance of early screening and early detection of ASD in order to obtain services that will yield best outcomes for the child and their families.

\* **Corresponding author Jayne Bellando**: Section of Pediatric Psychology, University of Arkansas for Medical Sciences, Little Rock, Arkansas, USA; Tel: 501 364-1021; Fax: 501 364-1095; Email: BellandoJayne@uams.edu

**Seckin Ulualp (Ed.)**

Given the increased prevalence in ASD, it is certain that pediatricians will encounter children with ASD in their practice. Pediatricians are often the first professionals to assess for developmental concerns and guide the family in obtaining appropriate services. Given that there is no blood test or specific medical markers for an autism diagnosis, the pediatrician is charged with the daunting task of screening and providing consultation for a disorder that is currently diagnosed by behavioral measures and skilled observation. The pediatrician also needs to be able to help guide caregivers as they decide upon treatment options and ways to access and pay for treatments for their child. This in itself can be overwhelming for the family as well as for the pediatrician. Given the ubiquitous access to electronic information, the pediatrician must also be aware of controversial treatments and pop culture information about autism so questions can be appropriately discussed with families.

This chapter attempts to provide information on key diagnostic features of ASD, review screening guidelines and the recommended assessment process for ASD. Information about common co-morbid medical conditions will also be discussed. Resources to find evidenced based information about well-established treatments for ASD will be presented as well as providing resource sites for more alternative interventions for ASD. The goals of this chapter are to help the busy pediatrician build knowledge in identifying and diagnosing ASD; provide information about common medical comorbidities for individuals with ASD; and build knowledge in guiding families as they find therapeutic resources for their child with ASD.

## DIAGOSTIC CRITERIA FOR AUTISM SPECTRUM DISORDER

The most recent Diagnostic and Statistical Manual (DSM-5) was published in May 2013 and significantly changed the way autism was classified [6]. Autism was first introduced to the DSM-III under the term Pervasive Developmental Disorder [7] and this has remained until DSM-5. Pervasive Developmental Disorder has been replaced with the term Autism Spectrum Disorder (ASD), which now subsumes the former DSM-IV diagnoses of Autistic Disorder, Asperger Disorder and Pervasive Developmental Disorder, Not Otherwise Specified (PDD, NOS). Given its genetic etiology, Rett's disorder is now included as an associated feature of ASD but does not have its own diagnostic code. The diagnosis of Childhood Disintegrative Disorder has also been eliminated from the DSM-5. Another difference is in diagnostic criteria. Instead of three factors, the DSM-5 has two diagnostic factors: "persistent deficits in social communication and social interactions across multiple contexts and restricted, repetitive patterns of behaviors, interests or activities" [6 p50-59]. Studies have shown that the two factor model is a better fit than the DSM-IV three factor model for a diagnosis of autism [8 - 10]. Like other diagnostic codes in the DSM-5, ASD has specifiers to capture associated features (language impairment, cognitive impairment) and to indicate severity of symptoms. Severity level ratings can change over time to reflect the trajectory of the patient's course. To receive an ASD diagnosis, differences in development must be seen within the early developmental period; however, the DSM-5 acknowledges that for some individuals the deficits may not manifest until social demands exceed their ability or deficits may be minimized by strategies that have been learned [6]. Criteria now can also be met by current symptom presentation or by history. If a diagnosis based upon DSM-IV criteria has already been given and is well established, the new diagnosis of ASD should be applied. The DSM-5 is also clear that specifiers should not be used to determine eligibility for or for the provision of services [6].

Ozonoff [11] provides a well-articulated rationale behind the research that guided the criteria and theoretical changes for the DSM-5. In the time leading up to the publication of the DSM-5, some studies showed good sensitivity and specificity with the new DSM-5 criteria [12, 13] while other studies reported concerns about the DSM-5's ability to correctly classify individuals with ASD [14 - 16] The rebuttal to studies that were not complementary to the new criteria stated that the final DSM-5 criteria were not used in these studies [17, 18]. Since the publication of the DSM-5 is still relatively recent, some studies have been published to help answer questions about specificity and sensitivity [19 - 21]. with differing results. More research is needed to determine if there are groups of individuals by age or symptom presentation that might be less likely to be captured in the new criteria. The Autism Spectrum Disorder Task Force has described the DSM-5 ASD criteria as a "living document" [6] so it is assumed that new research findings will guide future updates of the Autism Spectrum Disorder diagnostic criteria.

## SCREENING AND ASSESSMENT OF ASD

While it is important for pediatricians to know the diagnostic criteria for ASD, it is just as important to apply it to children in your practice to screen for ASD/developmental concerns. In a study of screening practices of PCPs for ASD, it was reported that only 8% of general pediatric providers screened specifically for ASD [22]. Among the reasons cited for this low rate is PCPs' perception that they lack experience with screening tools or that they do not have adequate time to screen within the confines of a PCP visit [22]. The AAP has outlined an algorithm specifically for the identification of ASD in all children [4]. The process involves: surveillance, screening and implementation of an action plan

Surveillance entails listening to parent's concerns about development, actively eliciting developmental concerns from parents, taking a good developmental history, making behavioral observations in the clinic, and identifying risk factors for the child [23]. Johnson and Myers [4] specified the following risk factors of significance: sibling(s) diagnosed with ASD, an ASD concern raised by a parent, caregiver or someone familiar with the child (such as school personnel), or the pediatrician.

All children should be screened for ASD at either the 18-month or 24 -month old health maintenance visit. Screening involves a screening tool that assesses for age-appropriate social communication milestones (for children less than 18 months of age), or a measure that is more ASD-specific (for children who are 18 months or older). However, if any risk factor is identified, ASD or social development screening should be done, regardless of age [4]. One of the more commonly used screening tools is the MCHAT (Modified Checklist for Autism in Toddlers), an ASD-specific parent completed screening tool that is reasonably quick and easy to administer, and is free and available online [24]. The MCHAT is appropriate for children from 16 to 30 months of age. When screening tools reveal an ASD concern, or if 2 or more risk factors for ASD are identified, then PCPs are urged to take action.

An action plan involves: Initiating a referral to ASD specialists and referring the child for education services. For a child less than 3 years of age, refer to the state's Early Intervention (EI) program and for a child 3 years of age or older, refer to the Early Childhood (EC) program of the local public school. An Audiology assessment should also be ordered to rule out hearing loss. PCP's should also schedule interval visits with the family to also ensure the referral process to an ASD specialist is well coordinated between involved parties [4].

The following clinical pearls are critical in the recognition of autism in young children. First, PCPs must be knowledgeable about the "red flags" for an ASD diagnosis. The perspective of "wait-and-see" is not recommended [4]. Early detection leads to better outcomes for these children. Second, children can qualify for developmental therapy services under other diagnoses without a formal autism diagnosis [25]. Thus, referral for education services or therapies should never be deferred for the reason that a formal autism diagnosis has not been made yet or that the child has not yet seen an autism specialist.

## Components of a Comprehensive ASD Evaluation

If there is enough evidence of suspicion, the pediatrician should refer for a comprehensive evaluation for ASD. According to the Committee on Children With Disabilities, a comprehensive evaluation for ASD should be conducted "by a specialist or, preferably, a multidisciplinary team of specialists with expertise in ASD to make the definitive diagnosis and search for possible etiological disorders" [3 p1222]. This team of specialists typically includes medicine (pediatrician, developmental behavioral pediatrician or psychiatrist), psychology, social work, a speech/language pathologist, educators and other allied health professionals such as occupational or physical therapists. While some assessments occur by professionals working individually, it has become more common to see interdisciplinary or transdisciplinary groups of professionals assessing the child [26]. According to Johnson and Myers [4] the primary goals of a comprehensive evaluation are: making the diagnosis of an ASD; recognizing the child's overall level of functioning; and assessing for co-morbid medical conditions and other associated etiology. Correct diagnosis also helps make appropriate recommendations for interventions.

The history provided by caregivers is critical in the diagnostic evaluation. The diagnostic interview reviews a child's developmental history (current skills and history of skill acquisition), behavioral history and genetic/family history. Ideally, information from various sources who know the child well and in different settings is critical to obtaining behavioral information from different contexts. Specific questions that relate to core features of ASD should be discussed in depth. Johnson and Myers give a very thorough description of the medical/ developmental diagnostic interview for an ASD evaluation [4]. Some clinicians will use a structured interview tool to ensure standardization in the diagnostic interview (*i.e.* the Autism Diagnostic Interview-Revised) [27].

The direct testing of the child typically includes assessment of intelligence (developmental level for younger children), expressive/receptive language, pragmatic language, adaptive behavior, fine and gross motor, sensory processing, and academic skills. The use of an autism specific assessment tool is critical to a comprehensive evaluation. Autism specific questionnaires can be completed by adults who know the child well, but these questionnaires are still classified as screening tools [28]. Best practice should include a direct observation of the child by a trained clinician of behavior that is consistent with an autism spectrum disorder. The Autism Diagnostic Observation Tool-2nd Edition [29] is the "gold-standard" for this direct observation. The ADOS-2 is a semi-structured play based measure that assesses communication, social interactions, imagination/play skills and stereotyped behaviors and restricted interests. Research has shown that including the ADOS-2 in a comprehensive assessment increases sensitivity of an ASD diagnosis to 82-91% [29, 30].

The comprehensive evaluation for ASD should also include consideration of differential diagnosis, existing co-morbid conditions. It should also include discussion with the family/patient to suggest components of a treatment plan for the child and to give family information about available resources. Referral to other sub-specialists, to educational and allied health professionals, and state/federal agencies for financial support are often recommendations that stem from the comprehensive autism evaluation [4].

## MEDICAL CO-MORBITITIES OF AUTISM SPECTRUM DISORDER

A child may be referred to a specialty team for a comprehensive evaluation and possible medical follow up, but the child's pediatrician continues to be the child's medical home. Because of this, it is imperative that pediatricians understand the medical co-morbidities that will likely present in their clinic. Just like typically developing children, children with ASD should receive basic primary medical care, such as health supervision visits and immunizations [31]. It is important for pediatricians to recognize that there are several co-morbid medical, psychiatric or behavioral conditions that can potentially occur in children with ASD. Pediatricians are often faced with the challenges of managing these conditions in the context of the child's ASD [31]. These common medical and behavioral co-morbidities include seizures/epilepsy, gastrointestinal problems, sleep disorders and challenging behaviors. Seizure disorder occurs at a higher rate in children with ASD, compared to that of the general population, with the prevalence even greater in children with *both* ASD and profound developmental delays [23]. The peak onset of epilepsy is bimodal, usually between ages 1 to 5, or in the adolescent period [31]. Gastrointestinal complaints that are seen in ASD children include: frequent abdominal pain, chronic constipation, chronic diarrhea, and gastroesophageal reflux (GER). Because many children with ASD are not able to verbalize their distress, gastrointestinal conditions can present as behavioral symptoms and acting out behavior [32]. Sleep disturbances are also common in children with ASD and may include problems with sleep onset and sleep maintenance, early awakening, or insomnia. Sleep problems can also be present due to behavior factors such as lack of caregiver's limit setting or the child learning inappropriate sleep associations. Pediatricians should also be aware that possibly, medical or psychiatric factors can result in sleep disturbances (for example, reflux, obstructive sleep apnea, anxiety) [23, 31].

Challenging behaviors and mental health issues are also frequently seen in children with ASD. Examples of this include: emotional lability or irritability, extreme tantrums, aggression to others, self-injurious behaviors, ADHD symptoms, anxiety, depression, repetitive and rigid behaviors (perseverative or OCD-like symptoms), pica, and feeding difficulties (very restricted food choices, or oral texture aversions to certain foods) [23]. If these challenging behaviors in ASD children are acute in onset or different from their baseline behavior, an underlying etiology should be considered and treated if identified [30, 33]. For instance, a nonverbal autistic child who suddenly presents with irritability is not able to convey to care providers a location of body pain, such as a dental infection. At times challenging behaviors might serve a purpose for the child, such as a means of obtaining attention or gaining access to a desired item or conversely to avoid an unfavorable situation or task [23, 33].

It is beyond the scope of this chapter to discuss in detail the medical management of each of these conditions, but excellent resources exist in the literature for the treatment of these medical, behavioral and mental health issues [3, 30, 32 - 35].

## THE ONGOING MANAGEMENT OF AN AUTISM SPECTRUM DISORDER

The management goal of the pediatrician for their patient with autism goes beyond basic medical care, and expands to helping the family navigate and access appropriate services for their child across healthcare, education and community systems.

### Family Feedback on their Pediatric Care

Two studies have shown that families with children with developmental disabilities are less than satisfied with the care that they receive. Surveys conducted by Liptak show families perceive deficits in PCP's ability to answer questions about their child's condition and in the PCP's ability to connect them with other families who have similar issues. Connecting with other families is an important way to understand the impact of their child's chronic condition on the family [36]. Additionally, families with children with ASD volunteered negative comments regarding their PCP's knowledge of complementary and alternative medicine (CAM) and the community support around them [36]. Carbone conducted parent/provider focus groups, where parents commented that PCPs did not act early enough on their child's symptoms and the care they received is lacking in comprehensiveness and family centeredness. Providers, on the other hand, cite lack of time, little resources and minimal training provided as barriers in the provision of health care [37].

### Resources for Evidence-based Treatments

Based on the families' feedback, PCPs would benefit from educating themselves on issues commonly raised by families of children and adolescents with ASD. The American Academy of Pediatrics has published *Autism: Caring for Children with Autism Spectrum Disorders: A Resource Toolkit for Clinicians DVD* [38]. This publication provides handouts for families and brief discussions about many topics, such as vaccines, behavioral treatments, toilet training, seizures, insomnia, behavior principles, psychopharmacology, eating and nutrition, seizures and epilepsy, and many others. In addition, the Autism Speaks website features many tool kits on various topics, including behavior treatments for autism, dental visits, blood draws, first 100 days (from diagnosis), feeding issues, insomnia and many others [35]. Another value resource is the National Standards Project (Phase 1 and 2) published by the National Autism Center [44]. In 2009 the National Autism Center established a set of standards for research-validated educational and behavioral treatments for children with ASD. Treatments are rated using the following classification: established evidence-based; emerging treatments; and unestablished treatments. In 2015 an update of the National Standards report was published which includes research from 2007 to 2012 as well as treatments for adults, which have not been studies in the past. This website and down-loadable documents can provide valuable guidelines for pediatricians but also parents, educators and service providers as treatment options are evaluated [44].

## A note on Complementary and Alternative Medical Treatments (CAM Treatments)

A significant number of children (11.6%) in the United States use yet to be scientifically proven treatments as complement (in addition to conventional treatments) or as an alternative (substitute for conventional treatments) [39]. In several ASD populations, frequency of CAM usage is at a much higher ranging from 28 to 82% [40]. Despite these numbers, parents of children with ASD usually do not discuss CAM treatments with their primary care providers. Parents perceive their providers to have little knowledge and interest in CAM [36, 41]. Parents have experienced their provider to be unwilling to discuss and accept CAM use [42].

Healthcare providers for children with ASD should be aware about CAM treatments and have regular discussions with families about CAM to help them negotiate the different treatments and make decisions. The National Center for Complementary and Alternative Medicine (NCCAM), aims to promote CAM discussion among providers and patients through their program Time to Talk (www.nccih.nih.gov/timetotalk/) [43]. This program offers providers free material, such as posters, tip sheets, patient wallet cards, and other resource information to help encourage discussion of CAM use.

## Vaccines as a Cause of Autism

The question of vaccines continues to be raised by parents so it is important that pediatricians know how to respond to this question. There is no link between vaccines and autism. In 1998, a small study in England was published that suggested a causal relationship between the MMR vaccine and the onset of autism [45]. This had a polarizing effect, with many parents challenging established vaccination practice to the point of delaying or refusing vaccines for their children. Reports from the Institutes of Medicine (IOM) in 2011 [46] concluded that there is no association between the MMR vaccine and onset of autism. In addition, the data was deemed to favor rejection of any causal relationship. In 2004, the IOM reviewed published data on thiomersal as a vaccine ingredient and onset of autism. Similarly, the data was deemed to favor rejection of any causal relationship [47]. There are no new studies that would challenge these reports adequately since their publication.

## CONCLUSION

Feeling prepared to help identify and manage ASD for your patients and their families can be a daunting task. Proficiency seems to be a function of medical training and proactively preparing yourself and your practice. The first step of this process is knowing what is available for patients with ASD and their families in your area. The more you know about local and state resources, the better you are able to serve the families in your clinic. Another important task is creating relationships with these providers of ASD services. These relationships can help you and your staff know the correct people to contact for treatment. These relationships can streamline the accessing of treatment and services for your patients and their families. Another important task is to take the time to have handouts and printed resources readily available at your clinic. The following suggestions may help provide some structure for this process:

1. Take time to create a mechanism in your medical record system to flag patients for an 18 and a 24-month developmental/autism screening. Have screening instruments printed and easily accessible so this process becomes part of your daily clinical practice. Standardizing this process is not only for you but also for the team of individuals working in your office.
2. Create relationships with agencies in your community that directly serve children and families with ASD. This may mean asking agencies such as Early Intervention (EI) and Early Childhood (EC) to meet with you and your staff. Agencies can bring written information about their programs that you can pass along to families. These relationships also help families since you are creating the bridge to find the right professionals for their child's needs.
3. Identify professionals in your city, region or state who conduct comprehensive evaluations for ASD. Having a list to give to families of these clinicians/ teams and, if possible, having the referral/intake forms from these professionals in your office. If a referral can be made before the family leaves your office, you have created confidence for families in your care. It is also a way to potentially streamline the referral process.
4. Create a resource center (hard copies and/or electronic) that you and your staff can access quickly in order to educate the families you serve. Most of the

resources discussed in this chapter can be accessed with no cost and can provide valuable information about ASD, related conditions and best practice treatment options. Taking the time to put this information into an easy to access format and location can yield great benefits to yourself and the patients in your practice.

Research in the area of ASD is growing exponentially and it will be important to find ways to keep up with new information. The final goal of this chapter is to provide evidence based resources which a busy pediatrician can have access to in order to keep abreast of updates in the field of Autism Spectrum Disorders. Some of the references for this chapter can provide excellent information as the field of ASD diagnosis, treatment and research continues to unfold.

## CONFLICT OF INTEREST

The authors declare no conflict of interest, financial or otherwise.

## ACKNOWLEDGEMENTS

Declared none.

## REFERENCES

[1]     Ibanez LV, Stone WL, Coonrod EE. Screening for autism in young children. In: Volkmar FR, Rogers SJ, Paul R, Pelphrey KA, Eds. Handbook of Autism and Pervasive Developmental Disorders-. 4th ed. New Jersey: Wiley Press 2014; p. 585.

[2]     CDC. Prevalence of autism spectrum disorder among children aged 8 years-autism and developmental disabilities monitoring network, 11 sites, United States, 2010. MMWR 2014; 63(2): 21p.

[3]     Committee on Children with Disabilities. The pediatrician's role in the diagnosis and management of autism spectrum disorder in children. Pediatrics 2001; 107(5): 1221-6.
        [http://dx.doi.org/10.1542/peds.107.5.1221]

[4]     Johnson CP, Myers SM. Identification and Evaluation of Children with Autism Spectrum Disorders. Pediatrics 2007; 120(5): 1183-215.
        [http://dx.doi.org/10.1542/peds.2007-2361]

[5]     Filipek PA, Accardo PJ, Ashwal S, Baranek GT, Cook EH Jr, Dawson G. Practice parameter: Screening and diagnosis of autism. Neurology 2000; 55(4): 468-79.
        [http://dx.doi.org/10.1212/WNL.55.4.468]

[6]     American Psychiatric Association. Diagnostic and statistical manual of mental disorders. 5th ed. Arlington, VA: American Psychiatric Publishing 2013; pp. 50-9.

[7]     American Psychiatric Association. Diagnostic and statistical manual of mental disorders. 3rd ed., Washington, DC: American Psychiatric Association 1980.

[8]     Frazier TW, Youngstrom EA, Speer L, *et al.* Validation of proposed DSM-5 criteria for autism spectrum disorder. J Am Acad Child Adolesc Psychiatry 2012; 51(1): 28-40.
        [http://dx.doi.org/10.1016/j.jaac.2011.09.021]

[9]     Mandy WP, Charman T, Skuse DH. Testing the construct validity of proposed criteria for DSM-5 autism spectrum disorder. J Am Acad Child Adolesc Psychiatry 2012; 51(1): 41-50.
        [http://dx.doi.org/10.1016/j.jaac.2011.10.013]

[10]   Guthrie W, Swineford LB, Wetherby AM, Lord C. Comparison of DSM-IV and DSM-5 factor structure models for toddlers with autism spectrum disorder. J Am Acad Child Adolesc Psychiatriy 2013 August; 52(8): 797-805e2.

[11]   Ozonoff S. Editorial perspective: Autism Spectrum Disorder in DSM-5-An historical perspective and the need for change. J Child Psychol Psychiatry 2012; 53(10): 1092-4.
[http://dx.doi.org/10.1111/j.1469-7610.2012.02614.x]

[12]   Huerta M, Bishop SL, Duncan A, Hus V, Lord C. Application of DSM-5 criteria for autism spectrum disorder to three samples of children with DSM-IV diagnoses of pervasive developmental disorders. Am J Psychiatry 2012; 169(10): 1056-64.
[http://dx.doi.org/10.1176/appi.ajp.2012.12020276]

[13]   Regier Darrel A, Narrow William E, Clarke Diana E, *et al.* DSM-5 Field Trials in the United States and Canada, Part II: Test-Retest Reliability of Selected Categorical Diagnoses. Am J Psychiatry 2013; 170(1): 59-70.

[14]   Mattila M, Kielinen M, Linna S, Jussila K, Ebeling H, Bloigu R. Autism spectrum disorders according to DSM-IV-TR and comparison with DSM-5 draft criteria: An epidemiological study. J Am Acad Child Adolesc Psychiatry 2011 June; 50(6): 583-592e11.

[15]   Matson J, Kozlowski A, Hattier M, Horovitz M, Sipes M. DSM-IV *vs* DSM-5 diagnostic criteria for toddlers with Autism. Dev Neurorehabil 2012; 15(3): 185-90.
[http://dx.doi.org/10.3109/17518423.2012.672341]

[16]   McPartland JC, Reichow B, Volkmar FR. Sensitivity and specificity of proposed DSM-5 diagnostic criteria for autism spectrum disorder. J Am Acad Child Adolesc Psychiatry 2012; 51(4): 368-83.
[http://dx.doi.org/10.1016/j.jaac.2012.01.007]

[17]   Swedo SE, Baird G, Cook EH Jr, Happe FG, Walker JC, Kaufman WE. Commentary from the DSM-5 workgroup on neurodevelopmental disorders. J Am Acad Child Adolesc Psychiatry 2012; 51(4): 347-9.
[http://dx.doi.org/10.1016/j.jaac.2012.02.013]

[18]   American Psychiatric Association [internet].. Commentary takes issue with criticism of new autism definition: DSM-5 experts call study flawed American Psychiatric Association news release 2014 March 4; Available from http://www.psychiatry.org/newsroom/news-releases/ commentary-take--issue-with-criticsm.

[19]   Kim YS, Fombonne E, Koh Y, *et al.* A Comparison of DSM-IV Pervasive Developmental Disorder and DSM-5 Autism Spectrum Disorder Prevalence in an Epidemiologic Sample. J Am Acad Child Adolesc Psychiatry 2014; 53(5): 500-8.
[http://dx.doi.org/10.1016/j.jaac.2013.12.021]

[20]   Smith IC, Reichow B, Volkmar FR. The effect of DSM-5 criteria on number of individuals diagnosed with autism spectrum disorder: A systematic review. J Autism Dev Disord 2015; 45: 2541-52.
[http://dx.doi.org/10.1007/s10803-015-2423-8]

[21]   Christiansz JA, Gray KM, Taffe J, Tongue BJ. Autism spectrum disorder in the DSM-5: Diagnostic sensitivity and specificity in early childhood. J Autism Dev Disord [internet] , 2016 Feb 9; [cited Feb 25]; Available from http://link.springer.com/article/10.1007/s10803-016-2734-4

[22]   Dosreis S, Weiner C, Johnson L, Newschaffer C. Autism spectrum disorder screening and management practices among general pediatric providers. J Dev Behav Pediatr 2006; 27 (Suppl. 2): S88-94.
[http://dx.doi.org/10.1097/00004703-200604002-00006]

[23]   Myers S, Challman T. Autism spectrum disorders. In: Voight RG, Macias MM, Myers SM, Eds. Developmental and Behavioral Pediatrics. 1st ed. Elk Grove Village, Ill: American Academy of Pediatrics 2011; pp. 249-91.

[24]   M-CHAT [internet]. M_CHATorg , 2016 [cited 2016 March 6]; Available from: https://m-chat.org

[25]   American academy of pediatrics; National center on birth defects and developmental disabilities at the centers for disease control and prevention (US). Autism A.L.A.A.R.M. [internet]. American Academy of Pediatrics (US) 2012. [cited 2016 Feb 7]. Available from http://aap.org/en-isabilities/ Documents/AutismAlarm.pdf

[26]   Volkmar FR, Booth LL, McPartland JC, Wiesner LA. Clinical evaluation in multidisciplinary settings. In: Volkmar FR, Rogers SJ, Paul R, Pelphrey KA, Eds. Handbook of Autism and Pervasive Developmental Disorders-. 4th ed. New Jersey: Wiley Press 2014; pp. 661-72.
[http://dx.doi.org/10.1002/9781118911389.hautc26]

[27]   Lord C, Rutter M, LeCouteur A. The autism diagnostic interview-revised: A revised version of a diagnostic interview for caregivers of individuals with possible pervasive developmental disorders. J Autism Dev Disord 1994; 24(5): 659-85.
[http://dx.doi.org/10.1007/BF02172145]

[28]   Bishop SL, Luyster R, Richler J, Lord C. Diagnostic assessment. In: Chawarska K, Klin A, Volkmar FR, Eds. Autism Spectrum Disorders in Infants and Toddlers: Diagnosis, assessment and treatment. New York: The Guilford Press 2008; pp. 34-8.

[29]   Lord C, Rutter M, DeLavore P, Risi S, Gotham K, Bishop S. Autism Diagnostic Observation Schedule, Second Edition (ADOS-2) Manual (Part 1): Modules 1-4. Torrance, CA: Western Psychological Services 2012; p. 446 p.

[30]   Risi S, Lord C, Gotham K, *et al.* Combining information from multiple sources in the diagnosis of autism spectrum disorders. J Am Acad Child Adolesc Psychiatry 2006; 45(9): 1094-103.
[http://dx.doi.org/10.1097/01.chi.0000227880.42780.0e]

[31]   Myers SM, Johnson CP. Management of children with autism spectrum disorders. Pediatrics 2007; 120(5): 1162-82.
[http://dx.doi.org/10.1542/peds.2007-2362]

[32]   Buie T, Fuchs GJ, Furuta GT, *et al.* Recommendations for evaluation and treatment of common gastrointestinal problems in children with ASDs. Pediatrics 2010; 125 (Suppl. 1): S19-29.
[http://dx.doi.org/10.1542/peds.2009-1878D]

[33]   McGuire K, Fung T K, Hagopian L, *et al.* Irritability and problem behavior in autism spectrum disorder: A practice pathway for pediatric primary care. Pediatrics 2016; 137 (Suppl. 2): S136-48.
[http://dx.doi.org/10.1542/peds.2015-2851L]

[34]   Malow BA, Katz T, Reynolds AM, *et al.* Sleep difficulties and medications in children with autism spectrum disorders: A registry study. Pediatrics 2016; 137 (Suppl. 2): S105-14.
[http://dx.doi.org/10.1542/peds.2015-2851H]

[35]   Bellando BJ, Fussell JJ, Lopez ML. Autism Speaks toolkits: Resources for busy physicians. Clin Pediatr (Phila) 2016; 55(2): 171-5.
[http://dx.doi.org/10.1177/0009922815594587]

[36]   Liptak G, Orlando M, Yingling J, *et al.* Satisfaction With Primary Health Care Received by Families of Children With Developmental Disabilities. J Pediatr Health Care 2006; 20(4): 245-52.
[http://dx.doi.org/10.1016/j.pedhc.2005.12.008]

[37]   Carbone P, Behl D, Azor V, Murphy N. The medical home for children with autism spectrum disorders: Parent and pediatrician perspectives. J Autism Dev Disord 2009; 40(3): 317-24.
[http://dx.doi.org/10.1007/s10803-009-0874-5]

[38]   American Academy of Pediatrics. Autism: Caring for children with autism spectrum disorders: A resource toolkit for clinicians. Elk Grove Village, Ill: American Academy of Pediatrics Press 2012.

[39]   Black L, Clarke T, Barnes P, Stussman B, Nahin R. Use of complementary health approaches among children aged 4–17 years in the United States: National health interview survey, 2007–2012. National

Center for Health Statistics 2015; 1-8.

[40] Perrin J, Coury D, Hyman S, Cole L, Reynolds A, Clemons T. Complementary and alternative medicine use in a large pediatric autism sample. Pediatrics 2012; 130 (Suppl.): S77-82.
[http://dx.doi.org/10.1542/peds.2012-0900E]

[41] Huang A, Seshadri K, Matthews T, Ostfeld B. Parental perspectives on use, benefits, and physician knowledge of complementary and alternative medicine in children with autistic disorder and attention-deficit/hyperactivity disorder. J Altern Complement Med 2013; 19(9): 746-50.
[http://dx.doi.org/10.1089/acm.2012.0640]

[42] O'Keefe M, Coat S. Increasing health-care options: The perspectives of parents who use complementary and alternative medicines. J Paediatr Child Health 2010; 46(6): 296-300.
[http://dx.doi.org/10.1111/j.1440-1754.2010.01711.x]

[43] NCCIH. Be an Informed Consumer 2013. [cited 4 March 2016]. Available from: http://nccam.nih.gov/timetotalk

[44] National Autism Center. National Standards Project 2015. [cited 7 March 2016]. Available from http://www.nationalautismcenter.org/national-standards-project

[45] Wakefield AJ, Murch SH, Anthony A, *et al.* RETRACTED: Ileal-lymphoid-nodular hyperplasia, non-specific colitis, and pervasive developmental disorder in children. Lancet 1998; 9103: 637-41.
[http://dx.doi.org/10.1016/S0140-6736(97)11096-0]

[46] Adverse Effects of Vaccines 2012. [cited 9 March 2016]. Available from: http://www.nap.edu/read/13164/chapter/1

[47] Immunization Safety Review 2004. [cited 9 March 2016]. Available from: http://www.nap.edu/catalog/10997/immunization-safety-review-vaccines-and-autism

# CHAPTER 21

# Treating Anxiety in Children

**Kristine Schmitz[1,*], Mi-Young Ryee[2] and Leandra Godoy[2]**

[1] *Department of General and Community Pediatrics, Children's National Health System, Washington DC, USA*

[2] *Department of Psychology, Children's National Health System, Washington DC, USA*

**Abstract:** Pediatric providers can play a key role in the early identification and treatment of anxiety. Brief screening tools can be used to enhance detection and differentiation of anxiety symptoms. Once identified, providers can triage concerns to determine the best course of action, including treatment setting (primary care *versus* referral to an outpatient provider) and intervention approach (cognitive-behavioral therapy, medication management). Distraction and parent education can be effective tools to reduce short-term anxiety associated with office-based procedures. More long-term treatment of anxiety, either within primary care or in community-based settings, can vary depending on presenting concerns and the child's age. However, evidence-based approaches typically include psychoeducation, cognitive behavioral therapy, recognition and management of physical cues of anxiety, cognitive restructuring, exposures, relapse prevention, and collaboration with parents and schools. Medication may be a useful way to augment treatment in certain circumstances.

**Keywords:** Anxiety in children, Anxiety treatment, Co-located mental health, Cognitive-behavioral therapy, Pediatrics, Selective serotonin reuptake inhibitor (SSRI).

## INTRODUCTION

Anxiety is one of the most common mental health disorders [1, 2]. Lifetime prevalence of anxiety disorders is 28%, surpassing depression and impulse-control disorders, such as attention deficit hyperactivity disorder [1]. Anxiety disorders present earlier than many other childhood mental health disorders [1] and are associated with later development of depression, substance abuse, and other socio-emotional disorders [1, 2]. Early identification of anxiety and intervention is critical to treating anxiety and preventing co-morbidity.

* **Corresponding Author Kristine Schmitz:** 111 Michigan Ave, NW, Washington, DC 20010, USA; Tel: (202) 854-0769; Fax: 202-476-3386; Email: KSchmitz@childrensnational.org

**Seckin Ulualp (Ed.)**

## Identifying Anxiety

To facilitate identification of anxiety concerns, pediatricians can combine their observations and clinical interview with a more structured screening tool. Use of a standardized screening tool can be beneficial given that providers often overlook mental health issues and many parents of children with mental health problems do not independently report concerns about their children's behavior [3]. Anxiety may have even lower sensitivity rates of provider identification because the perceived burden on parents and functional impairment can appear less severe than for disruptive behavior disorders [4]. Routine, universal screening can help to identify potential mental health concerns, such as anxiety, earlier among a wider range of families and has therefore been increasingly encouraged within primary care as a way to reduce unmet mental health needs [5, 6]. Screening tools should not be used diagnostically, but rather are most appropriate when used in combination with provider's clinical interview, observations, and judgment.

Several brief screening tools exist and can be been used in primary care to assess for anxiety. These include broad-based screening tools that have questions about anxiety, as well as anxiety-specific tools (Table **1**). Broad-based screening tools are more appropriate for universal screening efforts as a way to identify possible mental health concerns across a large group of children and a variety of areas. In contrast, anxiety-specific screening tools are more appropriate when used as a second stage screener (*e.g.*, when broad-based tool raises concerns about anxiety) or when parents or providers raise concerns about anxiety. For anxiety in particular, it may be important to obtain youth report in addition to parent reported symptoms [7].

Once concerns about anxiety have been raised, either *via* screening tools or clinical interview, providers can triage concerns by asking questions about symptom severity (*e.g.*, frequency, intensity, and duration of anxiety symptoms) and functional impairment—or the extent to which anxiety symptoms get in the way of the child's ability to function at home, at school, and in the community. For younger children in particular, assessing the impact of anxiety symptoms on parents and family members is also important (*e.g.*, determining if parent has had to change work schedule to accommodate child's behaviors). The level of severity and impairment, as well as the provider's own skills and the availability of community-based resources will inform decisions about referral to an outside provider.

## Brief Office Interventions

Children can experience significant anxiety during their medical interactions, including both routine preventive care and procedural care. Numerous approaches may reduce acute anxiety within the office setting, including distraction techniques and parental presence and training. While distraction can exacerbate anxiety symptoms in the long-term, it is a mainstay for addressing acute anxiety caused by medical procedures. Audiovisual approaches, such as offering video cartoons or three-dimensional glasses during immunizations or medical procedures, have demonstrated significant reductions in anxious behavior in children and parental report of their child's anxiety [8 - 11]. Use of cold and vibration during intravenous catheter insertion or immunizations can also reduce anxiety and pain [11, 12]. Use of music appears to be less effective, but may be preferred by patients [13].

Table 1. Sample anxiety screening tools suitable for use in primary care.

| Tool | Domains | Ages | Forms/ Questions | Availability |
|------|---------|------|------------------|--------------|
| Screen for Anxiety and Related Disorders (SCARED) [73] | Panic/somatic symptoms, generalized anxiety, social anxiety, school avoidance, total anxiety | 8-18 years | Parent: 41 Youth: 41 | Free |
| Spence Children's Anxiety Scale (SCAS) [74] | Panic/agoraphobia, social anxiety, separation anxiety, generalized anxiety, obsessions/compulsions, physical injury, total anxiety | 2.5-12 years | Parent: 38 Youth: 44 | Free |
| Revised Children's Manifest Anxiety Scale—2nd Edition (RCMAS-2) [75] | Physiological anxiety, worry, social anxiety, defensiveness, inconsistent responding, total anxiety | 6-19 years | Youth: 49 | $ (Pro-Ed: www.proedinc.com/) |
| Beck Youth Inventories –2nd Edition (BYI—II) | School performance, the future, negative reactions of others, fears including loss of control, and physiological symptoms | 7-18 years | Parent: 20 Youth: 20 | $ (www.pearsonclinical.com/) |
| Multidimensional Anxiety Scale for Children (MASC 2) [76] | Separation anxiety, phobias, generalized anxiety, social anxiety, obsessions & compulsions, physical symptoms, harm avoidance, inconsistency index | 8-19 years | Parent: 50 Youth: 50 | $ (www.mhs.com/) |

Partnering with a parent to reduce their child's anxiety can yield good results, particularly for younger children, though success can depend on the parent's own anxiety. When a parent is calm at the start of an operative procedure and they accompany the child into the operating room, their child may feel significantly less anxious and have fewer anxious behaviors at the onset of anesthesia, even without other behavioral or pharmacological interventions [14]. However, parental presence alone may not reduce a child's anxiety, and the presence of an anxious parent may actually increase the child's anxiety [14, 15].

Incorporating parents in procedure preparation, helping parents address their own anxieties, and providing them with tools they can use to reduce their child's anxiety can lead to significant improvement in their child's pain and distress during a medical procedure. Additionally, since a parent's anxiety is often mediated by the child's anxiety, there is benefit to the family unit when the child's anxiety is addressed [16]. Tools for practice may include informal psychoeducation and teaching or a more structured intervention such as using a computerized program to teach parent's coaching strategies, such as deep breathing and distraction techniques [17]. Careful assessment of how anxious a child and his or her parents are helps clinicians determine if parental training needs to be coupled with professional support, such as in-person support by a therapist at the time of the procedure or, in more severe cases, preparatory work prior to the procedure [18].

## Co-Located Mental Health Services

Increasingly, mental health is being integrated within medical settings, including primary care and relevant specialty care clinics (*e.g.*, gastroenterology). Mental health concerns are often comorbid with medical illnesses and integrated approaches to care can lead to improved engagement in services and destigmatization of mental health problems. Additionally, while mental health care services can be difficult to access and are often underused, access to primary care is better with most youth seeing a primary care practitioner (PCP) annually [19]. Children with mental health care needs have more health care visits and expenditures than children without these needs [20, 21]. PCPs are often the first professional to whom parents express concerns about mental health issues [22]. Despite the key gatekeeping role that PCPs play in identifying and linking children with needed mental health care, many report feeling ill-equipped to do this on their own [23]. Thus, integrated mental health professionals can support PCPs in identifying and addressing concerns by providing the training and support to identify, triage, and address mental health concerns in a number of ways that vary in intensity and approach. When mental health staff cannot provide adequate in-house services to meet the demand, referral to outpatient mental health providers is warranted, though these referrals can be enhanced *via* targeted care coordination. Considered to be an essential component of the medical home [24, 25], care coordination can improve outcomes for children with special health care needs by improving family engagement in services [25, 26]. However, ideally, mental health services are available within the primary care clinic. Research has found higher rates of treatment initiation and completion as well as greater reductions in mental health symptoms and parental stress when mental health care is provided on site as compared to facilitated specialty care referral [27]. Integrated mental health professionals, who benefit from warm hand-offs and shared trust, can serve in a range of roles. For example, they can provide brief consultations to triage concerns, clarify diagnoses, inform treatment planning, and facilitate referrals. They can also provide ongoing intervention services [28 - 30].

In the many practices that do not have access to integrated mental health professionals, child mental health access programs, in which a team of mental health professionals (*e.g.,* psychiatrists, social workers, care coordinators) provide real-time phone consultation to PCPs, offer an innovative way to improve access to care. Such programs support PCPs as they triage and address concerns in primary care or *via* referral to community-based resources. Started over a decade ago in Massachusetts, child mental health access programs are growing in popularity with over 30 states now implementing these programs [31]. Research suggests that such access programs may help increase providers' feelings of competency in meeting the needs of children with mental health concerns [32].

## Psychotherapy Interventions for Anxiety

When the need for on-going therapy for anxiety is determined, a number of treatment modalities may be employed. Cognitive-behavioral therapy (CBT) is the gold-standard, evidence-based treatment for anxiety disorders in youth [33, 34]. CBT has been shown to be effective in treating anxiety with comorbid conditions as well [35]. This is important as an estimated 75% of youth diagnosed with anxiety have multiple anxiety disorders, approximately 50% - 60% may have a comorbid affective disorder [36, 37], and 25% - 33% a comorbid externalizing disorder [38].

With a course of CBT treatment (typically 12 to 16 weeks), approximately two out of three children will be diagnosis-free [39]. Table **2** provides a list of anxiety disorders and the treatments that have been found to be most helpful. The majority of interventions include some form of CBT, but there are some other treatment approaches included as well. The classification system is based on the works of Chambless *et al* [40] and Southam-Gerow & Prinstein [41], which includes distinct methodological and evidence criteria to determine the degree of empirical support for a treatment. Of note, due to limited research of some disorders, treating interventions may not yet meet the evidence-based criteria of more established treatments. For example, cognitive-behavioral techniques are often used to treat selective mutism, however, there is a paucity of randomized controlled studies to evaluate efficacy [42].

Specific programs for treating anxiety can vary, especially by the type of anxiety disorder being treated, but the following are some common elements of CBT for pediatric anxiety [43] – psychoeducation about anxiety and CBT, recognition and management of physical cues of anxiety (*e.g.*, diaphragmatic breathing, imagery, progressive muscle relaxation), cognitive restructuring (*e.g.*, recognizing and challenging negative thoughts, positive self-talk), exposures (imaginal or in-vivo exposures to anxiety-provoking stimuli with desensitization), relapse prevention (through use of booster sessions), and collaboration with parents and schools. Additionally, Seligman and Ollendick [39] highlight a focus on building skills and developing a strong therapeutic alliance with patients and families as important components of CBT. While many specific manuals have been developed and studied, Kendall and colleagues recommend flexibility, clinical thoughtfulness, and consideration of developmental context in the use of CBT for pediatric anxiety [44, 45]. This is important as availability and accessibility of manualized treatments may be more limited for families. Greater flexibility in treatment application is also necessary for more complex cases including those with comorbidities and management of individual and familial psychosocial stressors that may present during the course of care.

Table 2. Evidence-based anxiety treatment modalities.

|  | Best Support / Well-Established Treatments | Good Support / Probably Efficacious Treatments | Moderate Support / Possibly Efficacious Treatments |
|---|---|---|---|
| Anxiety (general symptoms) [77] | CBT Exposure Modeling CBT with Parents Education CBT + medication | Family Psychoeducation Relaxation Assertiveness Training Attention Control CBT for Child and Parent Cultural Storytelling Hypnosis | Contingency Management Group Therapy |
| Obsessive-Compulsive Disorder (OCD) [78] |  | Individual CBT Family Focused Individual CBT **For OCD, the CBT that has been shown to be the most effective includes Exposure and Response Prevention (EX/RP or ERP) [79] | Family-Focused Group CBT Group CBT |

*(Table 2) contd.....*

| | Best Support / Well-Established Treatments | Good Support / Probably Efficacious Treatments | Moderate Support / Possibly Efficacious Treatments |
|---|---|---|---|
| Posttraumatic Stress Disorder [80] | Trauma-Focused CBT (TF-CBT) | School-Based Group CBT for Anxiety | Resilient Peer Treatment Cognitive Processing Therapy Client Centered Therapy Eye Movement Desensitization and Reprocessing Therapy (EMDR) Family Therapy for PTSD Child-Parent Psychotherapy |
| Social Phobia and Specific Phobia [18] | | Individual CBT Group CBT for Social Phobia Social Effectiveness Training for Social Phobia | Emotive imagery (specific phobia of darkness) In-vivo behavioral exposures with EMDR (for specific phobia of spiders) Exposures plus contingency management for specific phobia One-session exposure treatment for specific phobia One-session exposure treatment with parents for specific phobia Individual CBT for school refusal behavior Parent/Teacher Training for School refusal behavior |
| Body-Focused Repetitive Behavior Disorders (BFRBs) [81] | | Individual behavior therapy for cheek biting and thumb sucking | Individual behavior therapy for trichotillomania ****Behavior therapy for trichotillomania typically includes awareness training, stimulus control and competing responses [82]. |

(*For the purposes of this chapter, Levels 1-3 (Well-Established, Probably Efficacious and Possibly Efficacious) of the 5-level system have been included (Levels 4 and 5 being Experimental and Of Questionable Efficacy).

## Medications to Treat Anxiety

In conjunction with other therapies, medications, such as selective serotonin reuptake inhibitors (SSRIs), can be important tools for treating moderate to severe anxiety disorders in children. Medications are more effective when used with behavioral interventions and may be considered when the symptoms are severe or when behavioral interventions have been trialed and unsuccessful after 3-4 months of good engagement in therapy.

## Selective Serotonin Reuptake Inhibitors

Selective serotonin reuptake inhibitors (SSRIs) have demonstrated effectiveness in treatment of anxiety for children [46, 47], however, few medications are FDA approved, requiring frequent off-label use (Table **3**). Literature supports SSRI use in obsessive-compulsive disorder (OCD), generalized anxiety disorder, social anxiety [48, 49], and less so for post-traumatic stress disorder (PTSD), although they may be a helpful component of trauma treatment [50, 51]. Two large multisite studies, the POTS and CAMS, demonstrated that a combination of cognitive behavioral therapy and SSRIs were most effective in treating anxiety disorders [52 - 56].

**Table 3. SSRI dosing parameters [47].**

| Generic (Brand) | FDA Approval for Children and Adolescents | Initial Dose | Titration | Maximum Recommended Dose | Dosage Forms |
|---|---|---|---|---|---|
| Citalopram (Celexa) | None | 20mg/day | 10mg | 40mg/day | 10 mg/5 mL; 10mg, 20mg, 40mg tablets |
| Escitalopram (Lexapro) | ≥12yo* with depression | < 12yo: 5mg/day ≥12yo: 10mg/day | <12 yo: 5mg ≥12 yo:10mg | 20mg/day | 5mg/5ml; 5mg and10mg tablets |
| Fluoxetine Hydrochloride (Prozac) | ≥8yo with depression ≥7yo with OCD | < 12yo: 5mg/day ≥12yo: 10mg/day | <12 yo: 5mg ≥12 yo:10mg | 40mg/day | 20 mg/5 mL; 10-, 20-, and 40mg capsules 10-, 20-, and 60mg tablets 90mg delayed release capsule |

*(Table 3) contd.....*

| Generic (Brand) | FDA Approval for Children and Adolescents | Initial Dose | Titration | Maximum Recommended Dose | Dosage Forms |
|---|---|---|---|---|---|
| Fluvoxamine (Luvox) | ≥8yo with OCD | 25mg/day | 25mg (divide BID for doses > 50mg/day) | <12 yo: 200mg/day ≥12 yo: 300mg/day | 25-, 50-, and100mg tablets 100- and 150mg extended release capsules |
| Sertraline (Zoloft) | ≥6yo with OCD | <12yo 12.5mg/day ≥12yo 25mg/day | <12 yo:25mg ≥12 yo:50mg | 200mg/day | 20mg/ml; 25-, 50-, and 100mg tablets |

*OCD = Obsessive Compulsive Disorder **yo = years old

The use of SSRIs in youth has come into question due to concerns for increased suicidal thoughts and behaviors in children and adolescents. This prompted a Food and Drug Administration (FDA) black box warning. While this risk is low (1-2% of children experience increased suicidality), prescribers and caregivers need to be vigilant about the possible risk [57 - 59]. The risk is highest in the first two weeks of treatment and when starting doses higher than usual [60 - 62]. The risks and benefits of using these medications should be made on an individualized basis and discussed with the child and their caregivers.

## Other Medications to Treat Anxiety Disorders

Venlafaxine [63, 64], a selective norepinephrine reuptake inhibitor (SNRI) shows effectiveness for generalized anxiety disorder and social anxiety disorder. Like SSRIs, venlafaxine is likely most effective when combined with cognitive behavioral therapy. For children with co-morbid attention deficit hyperactivity disorder (ADHD) and anxiety, atomoxetine, another SNRI, may be more effective than other ADHD medications [47]. Benzodiazepines [65, 66] and buspirone have shown mixed results for generalized anxiety [67]. Clonazepam, a benzodiazepine, showed no significant effect on separation anxiety disorder [68] and is associated with oppositional behavior and paradoxical reactions, such as disinhibition and exacerbations of symptoms. When prescribing these medications, it's important to consider the risk of a paradoxical reaction, which occur more often in children than adults [69].

## Medications for Acute Anxiety

While benzodiazepines are not considered a first-line treatment for anxiety disorders, they may provide some benefit in the immediate treatment of acute anxiety in children. Thus, for brief, anxiety-provoking procedures, benzodiazepines such as lorazepam and alprazolam may be offered when a child's anxiety is severe or when their anxious behaviors significantly interfere with the procedure. They have also been used as a bridge therapy while awaiting SSRI's effect in panic disorder [70]. In addition to benzodiazepines, melatonin shows some promise in reducing anxiety and pain compared to placebo while having the benefit of fewer side effects than those associated with benzodiazepines [71, 72]. Non-benzodiazepine medications, such as melatonin, warrant further investigation.

## CONCLUSION

Pediatric providers play a key role in early identification and treatment of anxiety in children. Integrating brief screening tools along with co-located mental health services and basic knowledge of psychopharmacology can aide pediatricians in addressing anxiety and preventing co-morbid conditions.

## CONFLICT OF INTEREST

The authors declare no conflict of interest, financial or otherwise.

## AKNOWLEDGEMENTS

Declared none.

## REFERENCES

[1]     Kessler RC, Berglund P, Demler O, Jin R, Merikangas KR, Walters EE. Lifetime prevalence and age-of-onset distributions of DSM-IV disorders in the National Comorbidity Survey Replication. Arch Gen Psychiatry 2005; 62(6): 593-602.

[2]     Kessler RC, Avenevoli S, Costello J, *et al.* Severity of 12-month DSM-IV disorders in the National Comorbidity Survey Replication Adolescent Supplement. Arch Gen Psychiatry 2012; 69(4): 381-9.

[3]     Sheldrick RC, Merchant S, Perrin EC. Identification of developmental-behavioral problems in primary care: a systematic review. Pediatrics 2011; 128(2): 356-63.

[4]     Mian ND. Little children with big worries: addressing the needs of young, anxious children and the problem of parent engagement. Clin Child Fam Psychol Rev 2014; 17(1): 85-96.

[5]     Weitzman C, Wegner L. Promoting optimal development: screening for behavioral and emotional problems. Pediatrics 2015; 135(2): 384-95.

[6]     Committee on Psychosocial Aspects of Child and Family Health and Task Force on Mental Health. Policy statement--The future of pediatrics: mental health competencies for pediatric primary care. Pediatrics 2009; 124(1): 410-21.

[7]     WREN FJ. BRIDGE JA, BIRMAHER B. Screening for Childhood Anxiety Symptoms in Primary Care: Integrating Child and Parent Reports. J Am Acad Child Adolesc Psychiatry 2004; 43(11): 1364-71.

[8]     Cerne D, Sannino L, Petean M. A randomised controlled trial examining the effectiveness of cartoons as a distraction technique. Nurs Child Young People 2015; 27(3): 28-33.

[9] Guinot Jimeno F, Mercadé Bellido M, Cuadros Fernández C, Lorente Rodríguez AI, Llopis Pérez J, Boj Quesada JR. Effect of audiovisual distraction on children's behaviour, anxiety and pain in the dental setting. Eur J Paediatr Dent Off J Eur Acad Paediatr Dent 2014; 15(3): 297-302.

[10] Nuvvula S, Alahari S, Kamatham R, Challa RR. Effect of audiovisual distraction with 3D video glasses on dental anxiety of children experiencing administration of local analgesia: a randomised clinical trial. Eur Arch Paediatr Dent 2015; 16(1): 43-50.

[11] Canbulat N, Ayhan F, Inal S. Effectiveness of external cold and vibration for procedural pain relief during peripheral intravenous cannulation in pediatric patients. Pain Manag Nurs Off J Am Soc Pain Manag Nurses 2015; 16(1): 33-9.

[12] Moadad N, Kozman K, Shahine R, Ohanian S, Badr LK. Distraction using the BUZZY for children during an IV insertion. J Pediatr Nurs 2016; 31(1): 64-72.

[13] Aitken JC, Wilson S, Coury D, Moursi AM. The effect of music distraction on pain, anxiety and behavior in pediatric dental patients. Pediatr Dent 2002; 24(2): 114-8.

[14] Kain ZN, Caldwell-Andrews AA, Maranets I, Nelson W, Mayes LC. Predicting which child-parent pair will benefit from parental presence during induction of anesthesia: a decision-making approach. Anesth Analg 2006; 102(1): 81-4.

[15] Hickmott KC, Shaw EA, Goodyer I, Baker RD. Anaesthetic induction in children: the effects of maternal presence on mood and subsequent behaviour. Eur J Anaesthesiol 1989; 6(2): 145-55.

[16] Bearden DJ, Feinstein A, Cohen LL. The influence of parent preprocedural anxiety on child procedural pain: mediation by child procedural anxiety. J Pediatr Psychol 2012; 37(6): 680-6.

[17] Cohen LL, Rodrigues NP, Lim CS, Bearden DJ, Welkom JS, Joffe NE, et al. Automated parent-training for preschooler immunization pain relief: a randomized controlled trial. J Pediatr Psychol 2015; 40(5): 526-34.

[18] McCarthy AM, Kleiber C, Hanrahan K, Zimmerman MB, Ersig A, Westhus N, et al. Matching doses of distraction with child risk for distress during a medical procedure: a randomized clinical trial. Nurs Res 2014; 63(6): 397-407.

[19] FastStats , [cited 2016 Mar 11]; [Internet]. Available from: http://www.cdc.gov/nchs/fastats/physician-visits.htm

[20] Guevara J, Lozano P, Wickizer T, Mell L, Gephart H. Utilization and cost of health care services for children with attention-deficit/hyperactivity disorder. Pediatrics 2001; 108(1): 71-8.

[21] Newacheck PW, Kim SE. A national profile of health care utilization and expenditures for children with special health care needs. Arch Pediatr Adolesc Med 2005; 159(1): 10-7.

[22] Ellingson KD, Briggs-Gowan MJ, Carter AS, Horwitz SM. Parent identification of early emerging child behavior problems: predictors of sharing parental concern with health providers. Arch Pediatr Adolesc Med 2004; 158(8): 766-72.

[23] Horwitz SM, Storfer-Isser A, Kerker BD, Szilagyi M, Garner A, O'Connor KG, et al. Barriers to the identification and management of psychosocial problems: changes from 2004-2013. Acad Pediatr 2015; 15(6): 613-20.

[24] Brown NM, Green JC, Desai MM, Weitzman CC, Rosenthal MS. Need and unmet need for care coordination among children with mental health conditions. Pediatrics 2014; 133(3): e530-7.

[25] Council on Children with Disabilities and Medical Home Implementation Project Advisory Committee. Patient- and family-centered care coordination: a framework for integrating care for children and youth across multiple systems. Pediatrics 2014; 133(5): e1451-60.

[26] Gopalan G, Goldstein L, Klingenstein K, Sicher C, Blake C, McKay MM. Engaging families into child mental health treatment: updates and special considerations. J Can Acad Child Adolesc Psychiatry J Académie Can Psychiatr Enfant Adolesc 2010; 19(3): 182-96.

[27]   Bartels SJ, Coakley EH, Zubritsky C, *et al.* Improving access to geriatric mental health services: a randomized trial comparing treatment engagement with integrated *versus* enhanced referral care for depression, anxiety, and at-risk alcohol use. Am J Psychiatry 2004; 161(8): 1455-62.

[28]   Briggs RD, Stettler EM, Silver EJ, *et al.* Social-emotional screening for infants and toddlers in primary care. Pediatrics 2012; 129(2): e377-84.

[29]   Lieberman A, Adalist-Estrin A, Erinle O, Sloan N. On-site mental health care: a route to improving access to mental health services in an inner-city, adolescent medicine clinic. Child Care Health Dev 2006; 32(4): 407-13.

[30]   Williams J, Shore SE, Foy JM. Co-location of mental health professionals in primary care settings: three North Carolina models. Clin Pediatr (Phila) 2006; 45(6): 537-43.

[31]   National Network of Child Psychiatry Access Programs, 2016. [cited 2016 Mar 11]. Available from: http://nncpap.org/

[32]   Straus JH, Sarvet B. Behavioral health care for children: the Massachusetts child psychiatry access project. Health Aff (Millwood) 2014; 33(12): 2153-61.

[33]   Ollendick TH, King NJ. Empirically supported treatments for children with phobic and anxiety disorders: current status. J Clin Child Psychol 1998; 27(2): 156-67.

[34]   Ollendick TH, King NJ, Chorpita BF. Empirically supported treatments for children and adolescents. In: Kendall PC, Ed. Child and adolescent therapy: Cognitive-behavioral procedures. 3rd ed. 2006; pp. 492-520.

[35]   Ollendick TH, Jarrett MA, Grills-Taquechel AE, Hovey LD, Wolff JC. Comorbidity as a predictor and moderator of treatment outcome in youth with anxiety, affective, attention deficit/hyperactivity disorder, and oppositional/conduct disorders. Clin Psychol Rev 2008; 28(8): 1447-71.

[36]   Brady EU, Kendall PC. Comorbidity of anxiety and depression in children and adolescents. Psychol Bull 1992; 111(2): 244-55.

[37]   Seligman LD, Ollendick TH. Comorbidity of anxiety and depression in children and adolescents: an integrative review. Clin Child Fam Psychol Rev 1998; 1(2): 125-44.

[38]   Russo MF, Beidel DC. Comorbidity of childhood anxiety and externalizing disorders. Prevalence, associated characteristics, and validation issues. Clin Psychol Rev 1994; 14(3): 199-221.

[39]   Seligman LD, Ollendick TH. Cognitive-behavioral therapy for anxiety disorders in youth. Child Adolesc Psychiatr Clin N Am 2011; 20(2): 217-38.

[40]   Chambless DL. Update, on empirically validated therapies. II Clinical Psychologist 1998; 51: 3-16.

[41]   Southam-Gerow MA, Prinstein M. Evidence Base Updates: The evolution of the evaluation of psychological treatments for children and adolescents. J Clin Child Adolesc Psychol 2013; 43(1): 1-6.

[42]   Dow SP, Sonies BC, Scheib D, Moss SE, Leonard HL. Practical guidelines for the assessment and treatment of selective mutism. J Am Acad Child Adolesc Psychiatry 1995; 34(7): 836-46.

[43]   Albano AM, Kendall PC. Cognitive behavioral therapy for children and adolescents with anxiety disorders: Clinical research advances. Int Rev Psychiatry 2002; 14: 129-34.

[44]   Kendall PC, Chu BC. Retrospective self-reports of therapist flexibility in a manual-based treatment for youths with anxiety disorders. J Clin Child Psychol 2000; 29(2): 209-20.

[45]   Kendall PC, Chu B, Gifford A, Hayes C, Nauta M. Breathing life into a manual. Cognit Behav Pract 1998; 5: 177-98.

[46]   Strawn JR, Sakolsky DJ, Rynn MA. Psychopharmacologic treatment of children and adolescents with anxiety disorders. Child Adolesc Psychiatr Clin N Am 2012; 21(3): 527-39.

[47]   Southammakosane C, Schmitz K. Pediatric psychopharmacology for treatment of ADHD, depression and anxiety. Pediatrics 2015; 136(2): 351-9.

[48]　Compton SN, Grant PJ, Chrisman AK, Gammon PJ, Brown VL, March JS. Sertraline in children and adolescents with social anxiety disorder: an open trial. J Am Acad Child Adolesc Psychiatry 2001; 40(5): 564-71.

[49]　Wagner KD, Berard R, Stein MB, *et al.* A multicenter, randomized, double-blind, placebo-controlled trial of paroxetine in children and adolescents with social anxiety disorder. Arch Gen Psychiatry 2004; 61(11): 1153-62.

[50]　Strawn JR, Keeshin BR, DelBello MP, Geracioti TD, Putnam FW. Psychopharmacologic treatment of posttraumatic stress disorder in children and adolescents: a review. J Clin Psychiatry 2010; 71(7): 932-41.

[51]　Robb AS, Cueva JE, Sporn J, Yang R, Vanderburg DG. Sertraline treatment of children and adolescents with posttraumatic stress disorder: a double-blind, placebo-controlled trial. J Child Adolesc Psychopharmacol 2010; 20(6): 463-71.

[52]　March J, Silva S, Petrycki S, *et al.* Fluoxetine, cognitive-behavioral therapy, and their combination for adolescents with depression: Treatment for Adolescents With Depression Study (TADS) randomized controlled trial. JAMA 2004; 292(7): 807-20.

[53]　Walkup JT, Albano AM, Piacentini J, *et al.* Cognitive behavioral therapy, sertraline, or a combination in childhood anxiety. N Engl J Med 2008; 359(26): 2753-66.

[54]　Piacentini J, Bennett S, Compton SN, *et al.* 24- and 36-week outcomes for the Child/Adolescent Anxiety Multimodal Study (CAMS). J Am Acad Child Adolesc Psychiatry 2014; 53(3): 297-310.

[55]　Ginsburg GS, Kendall PC, Sakolsky D, *et al.* Remission after acute treatment in children and adolescents with anxiety disorders: findings from the CAMS. J Consult Clin Psychol 2011; 79(6): 806-13.

[56]　Practice parameter for the assessment and treatment of children and adolescents with obsessive-compulsive disorder. J Am Acad Child Adolesc Psychiatry 2012; 51(1): 98-113.

[57]　Hammad TA, Laughren T, Racoosin J. Suicidality in pediatric patients treated with antidepressant drugs. Arch Gen Psychiatry 2006; 63(3): 332-9.

[58]　Cooper WO, Callahan ST, Shintani A, *et al.* Antidepressants and suicide attempts in children. Pediatrics 2014; 133(2): 204-10.

[59]　Bridge JA, Iyengar S, Salary CB, *et al.* Clinical response and risk for reported suicidal ideation and suicide attempts in pediatric antidepressant treatment: a meta-analysis of randomized controlled trials. JAMA 2007; 297(15): 1683-96.

[60]　Miller M, Swanson SA, Azrael D, Pate V, Stürmer T. Antidepressant dose, age, and the risk of deliberate self-harm. JAMA Intern Med 2014; 174(6): 899-909.

[61]　Schneeweiss S, Patrick AR, Solomon DH, *et al.* Comparative safety of antidepressant agents for children and adolescents regarding suicidal acts. Pediatrics 2010; 125(5): 876-88.

[62]　Jick H, Kaye JA, Jick SS. Antidepressants and the risk of suicidal behaviors. JAMA 2004; 292(3): 338-43.

[63]　March JS, Entusah AR, Rynn M, Albano AM, Tourian KA. A Randomized controlled trial of venlafaxine ER *versus* placebo in pediatric social anxiety disorder. Biol Psychiatry 2007; 62(10): 1149-54.

[64]　Rynn MA, Riddle MA, Yeung PP, Kunz NR. Efficacy and safety of extended-release venlafaxine in the treatment of generalized anxiety disorder in children and adolescents: two placebo-controlled trials. Am J Psychiatry 2007; 164(2): 290-300.

[65]　Simeon JG, Ferguson HB. Alprazolam effects in children with anxiety disorders. Can J Psychiatry Rev Can Psychiatr 1987; 32(7): 570-4.

[66]   Simeon JG, Ferguson HB, Knott V, *et al.* Clinical, cognitive, and neurophysiological effects of alprazolam in children and adolescents with overanxious and avoidant disorders. J Am Acad Child Adolesc Psychiatry 1992; 31(1): 29-33.

[67]   MD JRS. An evidence-based approach to treating pediatric anxiety disorders : Current Psychiatry , [cited 2016 Mar 26]; Available from: http://www.currentpsychiatry.com/home/article/ an-evidenc--based-approach-to-treating-pediatric-anxiety-disorders/c117f45012d5b42e4da46003090487a8.html

[68]   Graae F, Milner J, Rizzotto L, Klein RG. Clonazepam in childhood anxiety disorders. J Am Acad Child Adolesc Psychiatry 1994; 33(3): 372-6.

[69]   Mancuso CE, Tanzi MG, Gabay M. Paradoxical reactions to benzodiazepines: literature review and treatment options. Pharmacotherapy 2004; 24(9): 1177-85.

[70]   Renaud J, Birmaher B, Wassick SC, Bridge J. Use of selective serotonin reuptake inhibitors for the treatment of childhood panic disorder: a pilot study. J Child Adolesc Psychopharmacol 1999; 9(2): 73-83.

[71]   Marseglia L, Manti S, D'Angelo G, *et al.* Potential use of melatonin in procedural anxiety and pain in children undergoing blood withdrawal. J Biol Regul Homeost Agents 2015; 29(2): 509-14.

[72]   Isik B, Baygin O, Bodur H. Premedication with melatonin *vs* midazolam in anxious children. Paediatr Anaesth 2008; 18(7): 635-41.

[73]   Birmaher B, Brent DA, Chiappetta L, Bridge J, Monga S, Baugher M. Psychometric properties of the Screen for Child Anxiety Related Emotional Disorders (SCARED): a replication study. J Am Acad Child Adolesc Psychiatry 1999; 38(10): 1230-6.

[74]   Spence SH. A measure of anxiety symptoms among children. Behav Res Ther 1998; 36(5): 545-66.

[75]   Seligman LD, Ollendick TH, Langley AK, Baldacci HB. The utility of measures of child and adolescent anxiety: a meta-analytic review of the Revised Children's Manifest Anxiety Scale, the State-Trait Anxiety Inventory for Children, and the Child Behavior Checklist. J Clin Child Adolesc Psychol Off J Soc Clin Child Adolesc Psychol Am Psychol Assoc Div 53 2004; 33(3): 557-65.

[76]   van Gastel W, Ferdinand RF. Screening capacity of the multidimensional anxiety scale for children (MASC) for DSM-IV anxiety disorders. Depress Anxiety 2008; 25(12): 1046-52.

[77]   Higa-McMillan CK, Francis SE, Rith-Najarian L, Chorpita BF. Evidence base update: 50 years of research on treatment for child and adolescent anxiety. J Clin Child Adolesc Psychol Off J Soc Clin Child Adolesc Psychol Am Psychol Assoc Div 53 2016; 45(2): 91-113.

[78]   Freeman J, Garcia A, Frank H, Benito K, Conelea C, Walther M. Evidence base update for psychosocial treatments for pediatric obsessive-compulsive disorder. J Clin Child Adolesc Psychol Off J Soc Clin Child Adolesc Psychol Am Psychol Assoc Div 53 2014; 43(1): 7-26.

[79]   Abramowitz JS, Taylor S, McKay D. Obsessive-compulsive disorder. Lancet Lond Engl 2009; 374(9688): 491-9.

[80]   Silverman WK, Ortiz CD, Viswesvaran C, *et al.* Evidence-based psychosocial treatments for children and adolescents exposed to traumatic events. J Clin Child Adolesc Psychol Off J Soc Clin Child Adolesc Psychol Am Psychol Assoc Div 53 2008; 37(1): 156-83.

[81]   Woods DW, Houghton DC. Evidence-based psychological treatments for pediatric body-focused repetitive behavior disorders. J Clin Child Adolesc Psychol Off J Soc Clin Child Adolesc Psychol Am Psychol Assoc Div 2015; 53: 1-14.

[82]   Franklin ME, Zagrabbe K, Benavides KL. Trichotillomania and its treatment: a review and recommendations. Expert Rev Neurother 2011; 11(8): 1165-74.

# SUBJECT INDEX

## A

AAP guidelines 176, 177, 179, 180
Acanthosis nigricans 105, 106, 107, 121, 125, 126, 131
Acid suppression therapy 83, 84, 85, 219, 220, 222
Acute 1, 2, 3, 4, 5, 6, 7, 8, 9, 11, 13, 174, 175, 301, 307
  anxiety 301, 307
  otitis media (AOM) 1, 2, 3, 4, 5, 6, 7, 8, 9, 11, 13, 174, 175
Adenoidectomy 12, 26, 34, 46, 52, 56, 57, 58, 59, 60, 72, 73, 206, 207, 211
Adenoiditis 2, 12, 51
Adenoids 34, 36, 40, 46, 206, 207, 242
Adenotonsillectomy 34, 47, 203, 265
Adrenergic antagonists 152, 153, 155, 157
Airflow obstruction 65, 160, 161, 203, 205
Airway 66, 67, 73, 74, 161, 163, 164, 169
  evaluation 66, 67, 73, 74
  remodeling 161, 163, 164, 169
Albright hereditary osteodystrophy (AHO) 119, 120
Allergen 162, 166, 259, 260, 262, 264, 272, 275, 276, 278, 279, 280, 281
  indoor 260
  inhalant 260
  injected 276
  offending 276, 278, 280
Allergic 152, 166, 253, 258, 259, 260, 262, 263, 264, 265, 266, 272, 275, 278
  asthma 166, 262, 264
  conjunctivitis 258, 262, 263
  disease 258, 260, 263, 264, 265, 266
  emergencies 272
  reactions 152, 253, 266, 272, 275
  rhinitis and asthma 258, 259, 264
  rhinitis and rhinosinusitis 258, 263
  rhinitis patients 262
  symptoms 260, 278
Allergy, drug 272, 274
Alternative treatments for autism 286

American academy of pediatrics (AAP) 111, 132, 175, 176, 177, 178, 179, 182, 210, 224, 286, 288, 292
American association of clinical endocrinologist (AACE) 150, 152
American diabetes association (ADA) 105, 131
American thyroid association (ATA) 150, 152, 154
Anaphylaxis 274, 276, 277, 278, 279, 280
  biphasic 279, 280
  diagnosis of 274, 276, 278
  symptoms of 274, 277
Anaphylaxis cases 274
Anemia 107, 110, 111, 197, 231, 232, 233, 234, 251, 252
  sickle cell 107, 231, 232, 233, 234
Anomalies, craniofacial 11, 67, 69, 72
Antacids 217, 225
Antibiotics 1, 8, 10, 12, 26, 38, 39, 40, 41, 42, 46, 48, 49, 53, 54, 56, 60, 176, 179, 274
  topical 12
  use of 40, 41, 42, 46, 48
Antibiotic therapy 8, 55, 176
Antihistamines 55, 237, 261, 262, 264, 279
  oral 261, 262
Antiseptic creams 252, 253
Anxiety 152, 291, 299, 300, 301, 302, 303, 304, 305, 306, 307, 308
  child's 301, 302, 308
  generalized 301, 307
  social 301, 306
  total 301
Anxiety 42, 299, 300, 303, 304, 306, 307
  disorders 42, 299, 303, 306, 307
  symptoms 299, 300
  treatment 299, 304
AOM, episodes of 6, 7
Apnea 66, 67, 174, 188, 189, 190, 191, 193, 195, 196, 197, 209, 210, 242
  -hypopnea index (AHI) 189, 195, 209, 210
Apparent life-threatening events (ALTE) 66, 67, 190, 191, 192
Approach, endoscopic 254, 255

www.ingramcontent.com/pod-product-compliance
Lightning Source LLC
Chambersburg PA
CBHW041725210326
41598CB00008B/777